A Christian Guide to Body Stewardship, Diet and Exercise

Third Edition, 2nd Printing

Written by:

David Peterson, Ed.D

Jeremy Kimble, Ph.D

Trent Rogers, Ph.D

Cedarville University

School of Allied Health

Cedrus Press 2023

Use the following URL to access weblinks referenced throughout the text:

https://digitalcommons.cedarville.edu/cedrus_press_publications/25/

A Christian Guide to Body Stewardship, Diet and Exercise

3rd Edition, 2nd Printing

© David Peterson, Ed.D: Jeremy Kimble, Ph.D: Trent Rogers, Ph.D

Cedrus Press

251 N. Main Street, Cedarville, OH 45314

Cover Design by Cam Davis, M.F.A.

All rights reserved. This book, or any portion thereof, may not be reproduced or used in any manner whatsoever without the express written permission of the copyright owners except for the use of brief quotations in a book review or scholarly journal.

ISBN (print version): 978-0-9967250-8-8

ISBN (electronic version): 978-0-9967250-9-5

About Cedrus Press

Cedrus Press is the digital and print-on-demand publishing service of DigitalCommons@Cedarville, the institutional repository of Cedarville University. Though not an official university press, the work of Cedrus Press is authorized by Cedarville University and thus submissions for publication must be in harmony with the mission and doctrinal statements of the university. Publication by the Press does not represent the endorsement of the University unless specified otherwise. The opinions and sentiments expressed by the authors do not necessarily reflect the views of DigitalCommons@Cedarville, the Centennial Library, or Cedarville University. The authors are solely responsible for the content of this work.

About the Authors

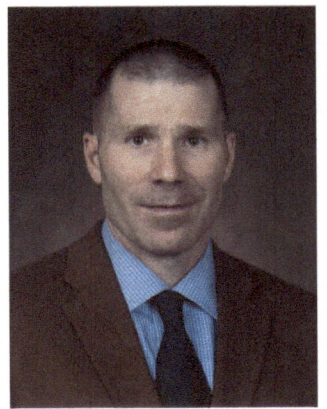

David "Pete" Peterson, Ed.D, CSCS*D. Program Coordinator, Multi-Age Physical Education; Assistant Professor of Kinesiology

Dr. David Peterson is a retired U. S. Navy Aerospace/Operational Physiologist with more than 20 years of active-duty service. He has earned multiple degrees in exercise science and is a former competitive powerlifter. Dr. Peterson has published numerous peer-reviewed journal articles, a textbook (in addition to this one), and presented at multiple state, national and international conferences on the topics of body composition and physical fitness testing. He is an active member of the National Strength and Conditioning Association.

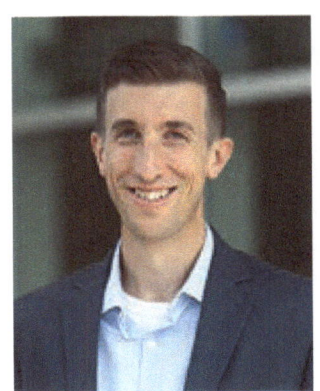

Jeremy Kimble, Ph.D. Director, Center for Biblical Integration; Associate Professor of Theology

Dr. Kimble is passionate about teaching college students the truth of God's Word. His hope is that through his courses, students will grow in their love for God and others, rightly understand the grand narrative of Scripture, and apply theological truths to everyday life. Dr. Kimble served in pastoral ministry for eight years and currently serves as a co-leader of an adult Sunday School class at Grace Baptist Church in Cedarville. Dr. Kimble's academic interests include biblical and systematic theology, ecclesiology, hermeneutics and homiletics, biblical worldview, and Jonathan Edwards.

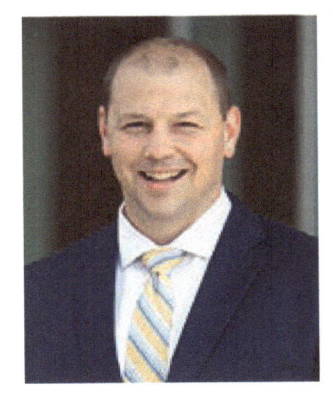

Trent Rogers, Ph.D. Dean of the School of Biblical and Theological Studies; Assistant Professor of New Testament and Greek

Dr. Trent Rogers teaches courses in New Testament and Greek. He is passionate about teaching the Bible and leading students to love and serve God, who has revealed Himself in the Bible. He has published in the areas of the Pauline Epistles, New Testament Greek, and Hellenistic Judaism. Prior to coming to Cedarville University, Trent served as Pastor for Adult Ministries at Grace Baptist Church in Cedarville, Ohio, where he is still an active member.

Acknowledgements

Editors:

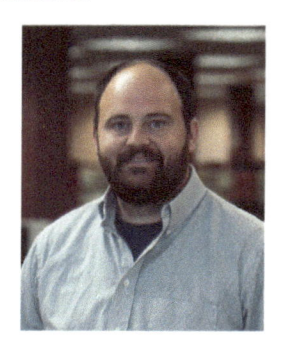

Nathanael Davis, M.E.S.
Assistant Professor of
Library Science

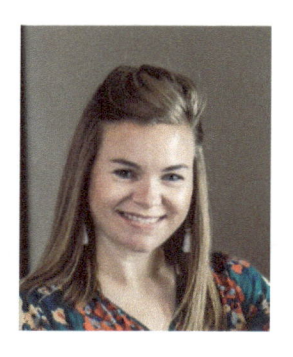

Christa Smith, MCN, RDN, LD
Adjunct Instructor
School of Allied Health

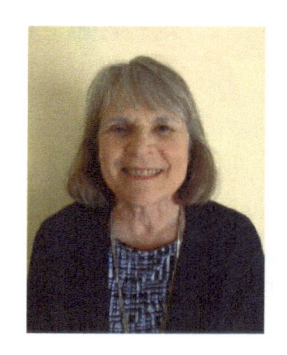

Sandra Shortt, Ed.D
Adjunct Faculty
School of Allied Health

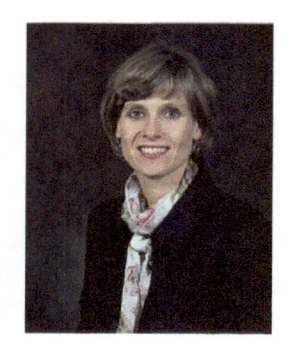

Elizabeth Sled, Ph.D
Associate Professor
School of Allied Health

Illustrators:

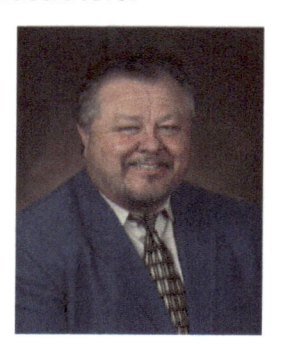

Cam Davis, M.F.A.
Assoc. Professor of
Visual Communication
Design

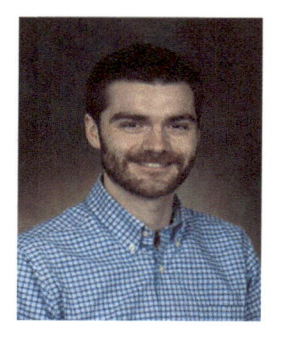

Jacob Lashuay
Instructional Media
Producer

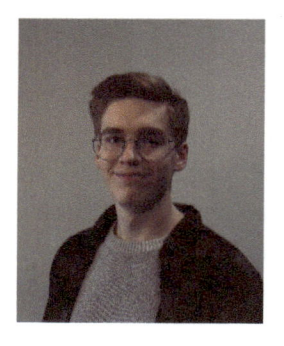

Max Lair
Student Illustrator

Table of Contents

Chapter 1
Biblical Foundations 1

Written by Jeremy Kimble, Ph.D and Trent Rogers, Ph.D

    Introduction 2
    Common Misconceptions about the Body and Physical Fitness 2
    Theology of the Human Body 5
    Biblical Theological Foundations of Physical Fitness and Body Care 8
    Summary 11
    25 Important Verses About the Body 11

Chapter 2
Basic Nutrition 15

Written by David Peterson, Ed.D, CSCS*D (with contributions from Christa Smith, MCN, RDN, LD)

    Introduction 16
    Determining Daily Caloric Intake 17
    Carbohydrates 18
    Glycemic Index vs. Glycemic Load 19
    Protein 20
    Fat 21
    Water 22
    Micronutrients 24
    Healthy Eating Patterns 25
    Eating Disorders / Disordered Eating 30
    Identifying Fad Diets 31
    Fad Diet Examples 32
    Other Diets 34
    Supplements 34
    Summary 36

Chapter 3
Weight Management 39

Written by David Peterson, Ed.D, CSCS*D (with contributions from Christa Smith, MCN, RDN, LD)

    Introduction 40
    Prevalence of Obesity in America 40

Table of Contents

Obesity Statistics 43
What Causes Weight Gain? 43
Other Factors Contributing to Weight Gain 44
Determining Daily Energy Requirements 45
Effective Weight Loss Strategies 46
Hierarchy of Fat Loss 47
Healthy Weight Gain 50
Body Composition and Percent Body Fat 52
Techniques for Assessing Body Composition 53
Meal Planning Made Easy 57
MPME Directions for Use 58
Summary 64

Chapter 4
Stress Management and Sleep 67

Written by David Peterson, Ed.D, CSCS*D (with contributions from Sandra Short, Ed.D)

Introduction 68
What is Stress? 68
Stress Theories 68
Stress Response 70
Male vs. Female Response to Stress 72
Stress and the College Student 73
Emotional Intelligence and Relational Wisdom 75
Effective Ways to Manage Stress 76
Anxiety, Depression, and Hope 77
What to Do if Someone is Suicidal 78
Sleep 79
Sleep Regulation 80
Sleep Architecture 81
Sleep Deprivation 81
How Much Sleep Is Recommended? 82
Factors That Affect Sleep 83
Tips for Getting a Good Night's Sleep 84
Summary 84

Chapter 5
Training for Endurance **89**

*Written by David Peterson, Ed.D, CSCS*D*

Introduction 90
Biological Energy Systems 91
Factors Related to Endurance Performance 93
Types of Endurance Training 98
Treadmill Tempo Run 100
Measuring Intensity for Endurance Training 102
Developing a Personalized Endurance Training Program 104
How to Choose a Running Shoe 106
Tips for Selecting the Right Running Shoe for You 109
When to Replace Your Running Shoes 110
Summary 110

Chapter 6
Training for Strength **113**

*Written by David Peterson, Ed.D, CSCS*D*

Introduction 115
Basic Strength Training Terms and Concepts 115
Impact of Strength Training on Body Composition and Bone Density 118
Major Muscle Groups and Fiber Types 121
Muscle Hypertrophy 122
Physiological Differences Between Males and Females 123
Load and Repetition Assignments Based on Training Goal 124
Periodization 125
Developing a Personalized Strength Training Program 127
Training Considerations for Advanced Lifters 132
Summary 133

Chapter 7
Training for Mobility **135**

*Written by David Peterson, Ed.D, CSCS*D*

Introduction 136
Common Mobility-Related Terms and Concepts 136
Factors Influencing Mobility and Flexibility 137
Warm-Up and Cool-Down Purpose and Recommendations 139

Table of Contents

    Stretching Types 139
    Prehab 142
    Stretching Recommendations and Precautions 143
    Low Back Pain Causes 144
    Techniques for Assessing Posture 145
    Low Back Pain Prevention and Treatment 146
    A Case Against Sit-Ups 148
    Exercises and Stretches for Low Back Pain 149
    Summary 152

Chapter 8
Exercise Programming 155
*Written by David Peterson, Ed.D, CSCS*D*

    Introduction 156
    Components of Physical Fitness 156
    Physical Activity Guidelines 156
    Fitness Testing 158
    Scheduling the Physical Activity Guidelines 160
    Intensity, Volume and Frequency 161
    Other Exercise Programming Variables 163
    Stimulus-Recovery Adaptation Curve 164
    Designing a Comprehensive Exercise Program 165
    3 Steps of Program Design 167
    Top 10 Takeaway Points 170
    Summary 171

Appendix A
Glycemic Index and Glycemic Load for Common Foods 175

Appendix B
Estimated Percent Body Fat Based on Waist Circumference 179

Appendix C
Meal Planning Made Easy 189

    Recommended Serving Size per Food Group 190
    Fruit Group Examples 191
    Vegetable Group Examples 191
    Grain Group Examples 192

A CHRISTIAN GUIDE TO BODY STEWARDSHIP, DIET AND EXERCISE

    Protein Group Examples 192
    Dairy Group Examples 193
    Sample Meal Plan 194
    Meal Planning Made Easy Template 195

Appendix D
Stress Assessment **197**

Appendix E
1 Repetition Max (RM) Testing Protocol **201**

Appendix F
Predicted 1RM Based on Reps to Fatigue **203**

Appendix G
Strength Standards **205**
    Bench Press 206
    Bent-Over Row 207
    Pendlay Row 208
    Shoulder Press 209
    Squat 210
    Conventional Deadlift 211
    Sumo Deadlift 212
    Hex Bar Deadlift 213

Appendix H
Adjustment Procedure for Nautilus Equipment **215**

Appendix I
Sample Strength Training Exercises for Weekly Exercise Log **217**

Appendix J
QR Codes for Instructional Content **219**

Glossary of Terms **221**

TABLE OF CONTENTS

Chapter 1
Biblical Foundations
Human Body, Fitness and Care

Key Terms:

Appearance	Creation	Incarnation	Stewardship
Beauty	Discipline	Resurrection	Suffering
Body	Embodiment	Sanctification	Temple
Character	Image of God	Self-control	Worship

Learning Objectives:

- Demonstrate an awareness of common misconceptions about physical fitness and appearance
- Articulate a Christian theology of the human body
- Explain biblical foundations for care of the body, expressed in part through physical fitness and healthful diet

CHAPTER 1: BIBLICAL FOUNDATIONS

Introduction

The primary concern of the Bible is not the same as the primary concern of this textbook. The Bible does not set out primarily to answer the role of physical well-being in the human life. Rather, God's salvation through Jesus Christ has implications for all of our lives, including issues about fitness, health, and **appearance**. And because God rightly rules everything, including our bodies, questions about how we use or operate anything must be grounded in the Bible. Unfortunately, many Christians derive their understandings about the human body, physical fitness, and **beauty** from cultural projections, and these projections often directly contradict the Bible.

We begin this chapter by stating and countering common cultural views of the human **body** and fitness. This section should begin the process of thinking critically about how we understand these issues and challenge us not to be conformed to ungodly views that we might even subconsciously adopt. While the list of misconceptions is nearly endless and constantly changing, the Christian understanding of the body has been fixed since **creation** and made explicit in Scripture. We begin with an understanding of the human body as foundational for understanding the use of the body, in things such as diet and fitness. Christian thoughts on topics like physical fitness are derived from a proper understanding of the body as the Bible as a whole describes it. With the foundation of a biblical view of the human body, we are in a position to discuss what are the Christian implications for topics like diet, exercise, and appearance.

Common Misconceptions about the Body and Physical Fitness

Turning on the TV or scrolling through social media instantly presents the Christian with an expression of how the body ought to be understood. The constant streaming of media also entails a constant reinforcement of viewpoints, many of which involve a view of the human body. The Christian must ask if these viewpoints are biblical, compatible with Christianity, or fundamentally opposed to it. The faithful Christian must be engaged in thinking critically about cultural projections and being shaped by the Bible rather than the culture. This brief list is a step in the right direction toward thinking critically about cultural viewpoints of the body and physical fitness. What are common cultural and personal misconceptions about physical fitness and exertion?

The body doesn't matter. The Creator God made all things and sustains all things. He has made all things for his glory (Ps. 19:1-2) and with a purpose to glorify his name, including us (Isa. 43:6-7). Thus, everything about us matters, including the bodies he has given to us. From the very beginning of creation God made his people, made in his image, as **embodied** creatures (Gen. 1:26-27; 2:7, 18-25). What he ordained that we do, he determined would be done as a people who would do so in a physical body. To strengthen this point, one need only look at the **incarnation** of Jesus Christ. The God-man took on flesh, demonstrating his full humanity, and dwelt among us (John 1:14; Phil. 2:5-11). In his resurrected state, Jesus appears to the disciples in his glorified embodied state (Luke 24:36-43), and someday when Christ returns we will see him and be like him as he is, namely, glorified and embodied (1 John 3:2). Thus, one can see that God made us with a body, our glorified state will be embodied, and, therefore, God deems that we exist with bodies, which gives purpose to this aspect of our created being.

What I do with my body is disconnected from my soul. This notion often comes up when people consider themselves in a dichotomous way, where all that really matters is the spiritual and not the physical. While we are made up of both material (body) and immaterial aspects (soul/spirit; these terms are often used interchangeably), we affirm that the Bible depicts us as essentially holistic beings. We should not depreciate the value of our physical bodies. They are neither evil nor unimportant as there is continual interaction between our body and spirit (Prov. 17:22). Christian growth includes all aspects of our lives, as we are called to love God with all our heart, soul, mind, and strength (Luke 10:27), cleanse ourselves from every defilement of body and spirit (2 Cor. 7:1), and be sanctified completely in both body and spirit (1 Thess. 5:23). Thus, while the body is distinct from the soul, one cannot minimize the importance of either nor relegate the essence of our humanity in some way that divides one aspect from the other in terms of their intertwined reality.

Exercise doesn't matter. If, as seen in answer to previous questions, God made us as embodied beings and the bodies we possess are able to be used in **worship** of God (Rom. 12:1-2), then the **stewardship** of our bodies matters. Our bodies are meant to be used for the Lord and his purposes (1 Cor. 6:13), and when we put them to work for his service, he delights in it. We are to love God with our mind (Luke 10:27), and studies have demonstrated that regular exercise improves alertness, attention, and motivation. In other words, exercise can encourage the peak use of our minds so our thoughts can be in the best form to love and glorify God. We are also to love the Lord with our strength. We should use our body's ability to glorify God, and this can be enhanced and improved through exercise to use that might for his name's sake. While not guaranteed, as we do not know the days God will give to us (Ps. 90:9-12), exercise can bring about a greater amount of time with greater effectiveness to minister to others and glorify God, as fitness does offer a better chance of longer life expectancy. **Discipline** in the area of physical exercise can also help one to be disciplined in other areas of life. As Paul beat his body into submission so as to preach the gospel with integrity (1 Cor. 9:24-27), so also, we must be disciplined in the physical realm as all areas of our lives are interconnected. Exercise can become an idol, like anything in life, and it is not more valuable than the pursuit of godliness (1 Tim. 4:7-8), but it is of value in bringing about overall discipline in our lives and enabling us to better love God with our heart, soul, mind, and strength.

Physical appearance and athletic accomplishments define me. Pursuing athletic accomplishments or a sculpted physique have the temptation of becoming idols that define what you do, how you spend money, what you wear, where you spend your time, and with whom you interact. The questions of time, activity, clothing, and friends can be determined primarily on account of one's union with Christ. When our identity is rightly centered on our union with Christ (John 1:12–13; Rom. 8:29–30; 2 Cor. 5:21; Gal. 3:26; Eph. 2:19–22; 1 Pet. 2:9–10), appearance and accomplishments might describe us, but they can never define us. Previous to his conversion, Paul pursued a religious and social identity by what he achieved, but he came to realize that his identity must be in Christ's work, not his own: "I count everything as loss because of the surpassing worth of knowing Christ Jesus my Lord" (Phil. 3:8). Similarly, people can seek to have their identity in outward appearance, or their identity can be fixed inwardly on Christ which affects how

CHAPTER 1: BIBLICAL FOUNDATIONS

they understand outward appearances. Having an outward appearance that others recognize as beautiful is not a bad thing (Gen. 29:17; 1 Sam. 25:3; Esth. 2:7), but it is also not an ultimate thing (1 Sam. 16:7; Prov. 31:30), and it can be a temptation to self-glory (2 Sam. 14:25). The Christian can pursue a fit body or wear make-up, but these must be secondary to the real beauty of a heart set on God (1 Tim. 2:9-10; 1 Pet. 3:3–6).

Care for outward appearance is the best way to attract and keep a godly spouse. When this way of thinking is made explicit, most Christians recognize it to be deeply flawed; nevertheless, this seems to be a common deception into which Christians fall. It seems self-evident to state that Christians desiring marriage to a godly spouse should look primarily for traits of godliness in a prospective spouse. The Bible's descriptions of wives (Eph. 5; Col. 3:18, 1 Tim. 5:9; Tit. 2:4–5; 1 Pet. 3:1) and husbands (Eph. 5; Col. 3:19; 1 Tim. 3:2, 12; Titus 1:6; 1 Pet. 3:7) focus on **character** and dispositions of the heart rather than on their appearances. Husbands should be characterized by leadership, love, provision, and protection. Wives should be characterized by honorable character, a disposition to honor leadership, and a nurturing heart. Physical beauty and physical attraction among spouses are good things, but there are repeated warnings that physical beauty is not an ultimate thing, nor can it provide the foundation for a godly marriage. (As a pastoral note, it might be helpful for younger Christians to know that attraction often heightens and intensifies over the course of a godly marriage, even as bodies deteriorate.) Peter prohibits ostentatious, self-seeking cultivation of external appearance to the neglect of godly character, "Do not let your adorning be external—the braiding of hair and the putting on of gold jewelry, or the clothing you wear— but let your adorning be the hidden person of the heart with the imperishable beauty of a gentle and quiet spirit, which in God's sight is very precious" (1 Pet. 3:3–4; see also 1 Tim. 2:9-10). Christian young men should pursue becoming godly men that godly young women would want to marry, and so with Christian young women.

Philippians 4:13 is about my bench press and 1 Corinthians 6:19 is about my diet. Christians appropriately cling to certain verses to help inform and motivate their daily lives. But when the verses are not interpreted properly, the results are disappointment and discouragement when Christians expect God to fulfill promises that he has never made. More than a few professional athletes confidently display Phil. 4:13 claiming God's guarantee of their athletic success, but this verse is really about enduring all things for the sake of the gospel. The whole context of the passage is that God has called Paul to both great hardships and times of relative ease. Paul confidently asserts that God will empower him to endure all the hardships of ministry to which God has called him. Paul is actually not pursuing anything other than faithfulness to God's call in ministry, and he trusts God to empower his ministry endurance. Similarly, 1 Cor. 6:19 is sometimes claimed as a justification for the most meticulous diet. Again, the context of the passage is not addressing a Christian's personal physical well-being but the Christian's engagement with sin, specifically sexual sin. There is a fundamental incompatibility of being united with Christ and thus indwelt by the Holy Spirit and engaging in bodily sin. This personal indwelling of the believer parallels the corporate indwelling of the church (1 Cor. 3:16). Improper interpretation, while temporarily inspirational, ultimately leads to disappointment and despair. It is incorrect to take two passages out of context, one about the hardships of ministry and the other about sexual holiness, and apply them to athletic pursuits. These passages do address how the Christian should understand their bodies, but they are informing the Christian that dedication to Christ involves hardship and holiness.

Theology of the Human Body

In light of those misconceptions about the human body, it is appropriate to ask how the Bible defines the human body. The body is the material aspect of our human nature, which is distinct from, but intimately linked with, the immaterial aspect (soul/spirit). God has ordained that the human body be an essential aspect of humanity during our earthly existence, as well as in the new creation where we will exist in a glorified, embodied state. Only between physical death and the return of Christ (i.e., the intermediate state) will human existence be a disembodied one. The soul/spirit will survive death and continue to exist, either with Christ in heaven (Phil. 1:20-24) or in Hades (Luke 16:19-31), but this is a temporary condition (2 Cor. 5:1-10). Embodiment is the state of human existence between conception and death, as well as after the **resurrection** of the body throughout eternity. The normal state of human existence, therefore, is an embodied existence.

Human beings are embodied beings because God purposed to create them in that fashion. He created Adam out of the dust of the ground (Gen. 2:7) and Eve out of the rib of man (Gen. 2:22), and every human being since has existed as an embodied being, whom God fashioned and formed (Ps. 139:13-16). By divine design we live and operate in human bodies, made up of both material and immaterial aspects. Embodiment, thus, is God's creation design for human beings, and thus we should be grateful for our bodily existence. As people made in the **image of God** (Gen. 1:26-28) we represent God on this earth as we subdue and have dominion over creation, and as we are fruitful and multiply. Even as God calls us to exercise certain functions as his image-bearers, one can see that such tasks are bodily in nature, and thus God created us with the capacities (body, mind, affections, will, soul/spirit) to accomplish the purposes he has set out for us.

Genesis 3 details the foolish rebellion of humanity against the decree of God, and because of this rebellion we are reaping the consequences. These consequences include guilt and shame (Gen. 3:7), distortions in relationships (Gen. 3:8-19), pain in childbirth (Gen. 3:14), cursing of the ground (likely work in general; Gen. 3:17), knowledge of good and evil (Gen. 3:22), original sin for Adam's descendants (Rom. 5:12-21), and death (Gen. 3:22-24; Gen. 5:1-32; Rom. 6:23; Rev. 2:11; 20:14-15). Within these ramifications for sin, one can observe how the human body has been affected by sin, particularly in the consequence of death, and, by implication, aging, disease, and decay. Accompanying these bodily realities, sin causes us to engage in self-deception (Ps. 36:2), dulls the conscience (1 Tim. 4:2), and hardens the heart (Heb. 3:12-13). Additionally, because of sin the body has become an instrument of wickedness (Rom. 6:12-13), the mind has become darkened (Eph. 4:17-19), the conscience is impure (Titus 1:15), the heart is deceitful (Jer. 17:9), emotions are at war (Jas. 4:1), and the will is enslaved to sin and Satan (John 8:34). The fall has had a tremendous and dire impact on all of creation (Rom. 8:19-23) and every facet of our being, including our bodies. We cannot restore ourselves; we are in need of someone to save us from

Chapter 1: Biblical Foundations

this plight, namely, eternal, bodily condemnation in hell (Rev. 20:14-15).

Praise God that in his love and mercy he has shown himself to be both just and justifier by sending his Son, Jesus Christ, to pay the price for our sins (Rom. 3:21-26). As human beings, we were made in the image of God (Gen. 1:26-28; Gen. 9:6), but that image was marred and distorted by our sin. Jesus, God in the flesh (John 1:14) came and dwelt among us. He is the perfect image of God, the exact representation of his nature and the radiance of the glory of God (2 Cor. 4:4; Col. 1:15; Heb. 1:3). Scripture demonstrates that while the image of God is marred within humanity due to their sin, because of Christ's work on our behalf we are called to be renewed in his image (Rom. 8:28-29; 1 Cor. 15:49; 2 Cor. 3:18; Eph. 4:22; Col. 3:10). The call to be renewed in the image of Christ involves ongoing transformation of our hearts and minds and the use of our entire being to do all in the name of the Lord Jesus (Col. 3:17). This includes the use of our body, as we use the capacities God has given us for intellect, emotions, will, words, and deeds to glorify him in all we do. Jesus came as the God-man, fully embodied, and he calls us toward growth in him in all that we are as embodied beings.

As new creations in Christ, humans have the capacity to worship God (2 Cor. 5:17–21). Humans cannot worship God as disembodied spiritual beings because God's good created order is for humans to worship as embodied souls. The choice for humans is not between embodied or disembodied worship, but rather between embodied worship or embodied idolatry. On the one hand, worship involves everything that a believer does (a total-life response to God), but worship also is recognized in particular acts and contexts. Old Testament practices of worship involved the very physical acts of sacrifices, ascending to the temple, singing, teaching, and prayer. Similarly, worship in the New Testament involves gathering as the church, singing, preaching, praying, and caring for the physical bodily needs of others (e.g., Acts 6:1–7; 1 Tim. 5:3–8; Jas. 2:14–17). The acts of worship that most closely express the physicality of Christian worship are ordinances of the church: baptism and the Lord's Supper. These ordinances are tangible, physical, embodied expressions of worship. The physical participation in the Lord's Supper is a spiritual participation with Christ himself (1 Cor. 10:14–22). Because Christ died bodily in our place, Christians no longer worship through offering animal sacrifices (Heb. 10:11–14); rather, their worship is to be expressed in a whole life of worship: "I appeal to you therefore, brothers, by the mercies of God, to present your bodies as a living sacrifice, holy and acceptable to God, which is your spiritual worship" (Rom. 12:1).

Worship of God involves obedience and growth in holiness. And **sanctification**, increasingly being conformed to the image of Christ in holiness (Rom. 8:29; 2 Cor. 3:18), necessarily is lived out in one's body (Gal. 2:20; 1 Thess. 5:23). While the term "sanctification" can refer to once-for-all cleansing that happens when a person receives Christ, it more commonly describes a Christian's growth in Christlikeness. In Romans 6, Paul explains how our union with Christ in his bodily life, death, and resurrection transforms us and impels us to pursue holiness. Through our union with Christ in his death, our "old self" was killed and abolished. And through our union with Christ in his resurrection life, we are given new life in holiness. Christian sanctification includes this understanding of our transformative union with Christ (Rom. 6:11; Col. 3:1) and the act of committing our bodies to God in holiness (Rom. 6:12–14; Rom. 12:1; Col. 3:5).

The empowering means of sanctification is God's Spirit working in the life of the one united to Christ (Rom. 8:1–17; 15:16; 2 Thess. 2:13), so that the Christian life is characterized as walking by the Spirit (Gal. 5:16, 22–26; in contrast to non-Christian rebellion Gal. 5:19–21). It is impossible to grow in Christlikeness if one is not growing in Christlikeness with the use of one's body. Thus, Christians should be characterized by **self-control** (Gal. 5:23; 1 Tim. 2:9; Tit. 2:2, 5, 6, 12; 1 Pet. 4:7; 2 Pet. 1:6), particularly with the way that they use their bodies: "For this is the will of God, your sanctification: that you abstain from sexual immorality; that each one of you know how to control his own body in holiness and honor, not in the passion of lust like the Gentiles who do not know God" (1 Thess. 4:3–5; see also 1 Cor. 6:14). While non-Christians are so driven by the simple impulses of bodily desires (Phil. 3:19), Christians dedicate their bodies to worship of God and service of others.

Although Christians use their bodies in a sanctified way for the worship of God, all human bodies still suffer the decay resulting from sin. The human body was not created for **suffering** and death, but they are tragic results of sin. Thus, even while bodily suffering and bodily death are experienced universally, they are unnatural in that they are not part of what God declared over his creation to be good. Following the fall of Adam and Eve into sin, they experience the suffering of broken relationship with God (Gen. 3:8–13), health issues (Gen. 3:16), relationship struggles (Gen. 3:16), struggles to provide (Gen. 3:17–19), and ultimately death (Gen. 3:22–24). Written on nearly every page of the Bible are stories of suffering, struggle, and death resulting from sin, sometimes one's personal sin, the sin of others, or just the effects of living in a sin-cursed world. Since the exit from Eden, bodies age, sickness ravages, and death reigns (Rom. 5:12; Heb. 9:27). The decay of the human body is one example of the larger category of natural evil, the terrible things that result from living in a world downstream from the fall in Eden. In Romans 8, Paul describes both the anguish of living in a sin-cursed world and the promise of God's deliverance: "For the creation was subjected to futility, not willingly, but because of him who subjected it, in hope that the creation itself will be set free from its bondage to corruption and obtain the freedom of the glory of the children of God" (Rom. 8:20–21).

All creation fell with humanity, suffers with humanity, and awaits the adoption of humanity. As we await the eternal realization of our adoption, our physical bodies are subject to decay. Physical activity and healthful food are common graces of God that make functioning in the sin-cursed world possible as we await the final undoing of the curse. Being united to Christ does not always entail immediate deliverance from bodily suffering (Jas. 5:13–15); rather, Christians suffer all the more because they risk their bodies for gospel-ministry (Acts 20:22–25; 2 Cor. 4:7–12) and experience persecution (e.g., Mark 8:34–35; 13:13; John 15:20; 2 Tim. 3:12). So, the human body is a frail yet resilient vessel through which to worship God and in which to carry the gospel message, "so that the life of Jesus may also be manifested in our bodies" (2 Cor. 4:10). This resiliency can and should be enhanced through careful stewardship.

Just as death was not the original intent for the human body, death is not the final end of the human body. God corrects the sin-caused distortion of his created goodness in the new creation through his Son. On account of Adam's sin, God subjected the whole world to the futility of suffering, decay, and death (Rom. 8:20). God did so with the plan of salvation and ultimately

Chapter 1: Biblical Foundations

glorification (Rom. 8:18–25). As Adam's sin plunged all creation, including the human body, into decay and death, so Christ as the Second Adam saves creation by his own death and defeats death in his resurrection (Rom. 5:12–20; 1 Cor. 15:20–23). Thus, Jesus Christ can declare, "I am the resurrection and the life. Whoever believes in me, though he die, yet shall he live, and everyone who lives and believes in me shall never die" (John 11:25–16). The promise of eternal resurrection life is for all those who believe and trust in the death and resurrection of Jesus for salvation. Even as Christians die physical deaths, they await physical resurrection. And just as Christ's resurrection body is a transformed physical body (John 20:19–29), so the Christian's resurrection body will be a transformed physical body (Rom. 8:11; 1 Cor. 15:35–53; Phil. 3:20–21). Christians' resurrection bodies will have both continuity and discontinuity with their earthly bodies, but the Bible does not give us much in the way of specific details.

Biblical Theological Foundations of Physical Fitness and Body Care

Though the Bible is not primarily about physical fitness and the care of the human body, that does not mean that the Bible does not address how Christians should think about these issues. How does this biblical theology of human embodiment described above affect the way that Christians should think about using their bodies? Even if it is not the main point of Paul's argument, we can also ask what is the value in physical discipline and exertion that Paul describes incidentally (1 Tim. 4:8)? What biblical categories or concepts should be primary when the Christian thinks about physical fitness and wellness?

Worship. Often people equate worship with singing, and this certainly is one form of worship (Rev. 5:9-10). However, the concept of worship is more encompassing than that. Paul tells us that we are to "present our bodies as a living sacrifice, holy and acceptable to God, and that this is our reasonable worship" (Rom. 12:1). As such, worship, which can be defined as ascribing worth and praise to God, is done as we offer our entire lives to him as a living sacrifice. This means all of life should be viewed in some measure as worship before God. This then includes something like exercise, which, the apostle Paul states, is of some value (1 Tim. 4:8). Your time in exercise can and should be done as an expression of worship to God. It is a chance to humble yourself and recognize that any level of fitness or athletic ability you possess is because God granted that to you (1 Cor. 4:7). Thus, worship can be accomplished in exercise by humbly thanking God for the gift of physical exertion. Also, stewarding all that God has given is an act of worship. Therefore, steward your body well, putting it through physical exertion as a means of worshipping God and for the sake of being able to use your body to worship him in a variety of ways for years to come, if he so wills.

Stewardship. The claim that a Christian should be a good steward of his body is an extension of the claim that everything belongs to God. The Parable of the Talents (Matt. 25:14–30) is a vivid description of God entrusting to people certain things and requiring that they make good use of them for his glory. Because God rightly owns everything, we will give an account for how we steward or faithfully use everything that is entrusted to us. This call for faithful stewardship includes how we use our bodies for his glory: for holiness not impurity, for worship not idolatry, and for gospel ministry not idleness or indifference.

Effectiveness in ministry. God created the human body to be active, and it is a modern convenience that many people do not need to be active to earn a living. In the New Testament, Paul's ministry is an example of the physical exertion of travel, manual labor, and tireless preaching in order to minister to others (1 Cor. 15:10; Col. 1:29). There are numerous practical benefits resulting from physical exercise that can enhance our ability to minister to others: sustained vigor, improved focus, emotional stability, and ability to travel to others. God has designed our bodies for physical activity, proper nutrition, and appropriate rest–all of these are his good gifts. While in the short term, a Christian might compromise any one of these, to sustain long-term ministry, the Christian must have each of them in balance. We glorify God by pursuing each of these habits in thankfulness to him and also by willingly sacrificing each of them at times for reasons of gospel risk (2 Cor. 11:23–31; 12:15). The believer might go without sleep for a night to minister to a friend in need or sacrifice bodily health taking the gospel to remote areas.

Character formation. Physical exercise can also benefit our growth in character. A person's character is the sum of his or her disposition, thoughts, intentions, desires, and actions. It is who we truly are, and we are called as Christians to develop Christ-like character (Rom. 8:28-29; 1 John 2:6). Everything in our lives is interconnected when it comes to the physical, mental, emotional, and spiritual disciplines. We are holistic beings with different facets to our being. Thus, overcoming laziness in exercise can help us overcome laziness in other areas of our lives. Enjoying the benefits of bodily activity can help us lean into, as opposed to draw away from, activity and God-centered ambition in life. Exercise can teach us to press through resistance in any difficulty and not simply give in and quit when it becomes hard. This is good training for life. We were promised tribulation in this life (John 16:33; Rom. 5:3-4; Jas. 1:2-4) and we are called to endure in the race set before us (1 Cor. 9:24-27; Heb. 12:1-3). Exercise can help to develop a mindset and promote habits of perseverance where we will actually gravitate toward dealing with the hard things of life in a healthy way. Physical exertion, thus, can be a means of growing in character and, by God's grace, following Jesus more effectively.

Pleasure. All people seek pleasure, and we were made by God to find our ultimate satisfaction in him (Ps. 16:11). This is sensible, since it is only in God, we can have infinite and eternal pleasure. We are to enjoy God above all things, lest we be guilty of idolatry (Ps. 115:1-8) and we are to enjoy God in all things (Ps. 43:4) since all of his good gifts ultimately point back to him, including exercise. A sedentary life is in actuality a more stressed life, physically, mentally, and emotionally. The remainder of this textbook will speak more to the scientific facts regarding physical fitness, but it cannot be denied that God designed our bodies to feel more pleasure as we use them in assertive ways. If you have not put physical fitness on your priority list, there is no doubt that pleasure may not be the first thing you feel as you get started. However, there truly is pleasure to be experienced, and it seems by divine design. God put chemicals into our bodies, like endorphins, serotonin, dopamine, and oxytocin, and these chemicals are brought up to raised levels in our bodies during intensive sessions of aerobic workouts. And these bodily chemicals produce feelings of pleasure that are undeniable. God made us to move, and made our movement to contribute to our health and happiness, and all of this is meant ultimately to draw our attention

CHAPTER 1: BIBLICAL FOUNDATIONS

and affections back to God himself.

Community. The Christian life is a life that is lived together, committing ourselves to other Christians, particularly in the context of the local church. We are called to exhort one another everyday so that we are not hardened by the deceitfulness of sin (Heb. 3:12-13) and to spur one another on to love and good works (Heb. 10:24-25). Certainly, this can and should be done on a Sunday morning as we gather for worship as a local church, but it needs to happen throughout the week if we are to grow and endure faithfully. There are many venues where this could happen, including exercising within that community of people. Exercise is an excellent opportunity to take some extended time to talk about the latest sermon you heard, review what you have been reading in Scripture, discuss theological questions and concepts, testify to God's hand of providence in your life, find accountability for issues of temptation, and provide ways you can pray for one another. This is a great way to redeem the time (Eph. 5:15-16) by exerting your body and encouraging one another in living as disciples of Jesus.

Evangelistic opportunity. Faithful Christians have a mindset of constantly sharing the good news about Jesus (1 Pet. 3:15), and the settings of physical activity provide unique opportunities for evangelism on account of the shared interest and pursuit. In 1 Corinthians 9, Paul describes the lengths that he is willing to go to share the gospel with people. He adapts personal practices "for the sake of the gospel, that I may share with them in its blessings" (1 Cor. 9:23). Christians and non-Christians alike recognize the benefits of physical exercise, even while Christians understand this as a common grace from God. In this way, a gym parallels a book club, in that both settings provide a context in which Christians can leverage their shared interest with a non-believer to share the gospel message. There is not something inherently effective about exercise-evangelism, but it provides a context for Christians to interact with non-Christians, form relationships, and share the gospel. Likewise, shared pursuits, such as team sports, can provide feelings of camaraderie that make a person more likely to listen to the gospel message. Every context is for evangelism, including those that involve bodily exercise.

Bodily Discipline. As described above, God created and then redeemed embodied souls to worship with their bodies. The implication is that I "belong—body and soul, in life and death—to my faithful Savior Jesus Christ" (Heidelberg Catechism Question 1; Rom. 14:7–9; 1 Cor. 6:19–20). Sanctification is lived out in the body through self-control, not asceticism. This means that Christians should enjoy physical joys while recognizing that any legitimate joy ought to point us to the ultimate joy experienced in relationship with God. The Bible assumes that bodily discipline is part of sanctification (e.g., 1 Cor. 9:27; the spiritual discipline of fasting; prohibitions on sexual immorality and drunkenness) and that bodily discipline produces a disposition to discipline that is transferable to other areas.

Summary

- God's Word, not cultural or self-perception, must ultimately determine how we understand and use our bodies.

- A proper theology of the body is dependent upon accurate biblical interpretation, including reading verses within their respective contexts.

- God created us as embodied image bearers. Though our bodies, like all creation, bear the effects of the Fall, redemption comes through God the Son embodied.

- We were made by God to glorify him through worship, which includes the use of our physical bodies. Therefore, sanctification necessarily incorporates what we do with our bodies (e.g., physical acts of worship, the ordinances of the church, self-control, service).

- The claim that a Christian should be a good steward of his body is an extension of the claim that everything belongs to God.

- Exercise can help to develop a mindset and promote habits of perseverance where we will actually gravitate toward dealing with the hard things of life in a healthy way.

- A properly stewarded body is more effective and typically more enduring in ministry, and venues of physical activity provide contexts for evangelism.

25 Important Verses About the Body

1. Genesis 1:27: So, God created man in his own image, in the image of God he created him; male and female he created them.

2. Genesis 1:31: And God saw everything that he had made, and behold, it was very good. And there was evening and there was morning, the sixth day.

3. Genesis 2:15: The LORD God took the man and put him in the garden of Eden to work it and keep it.

4. Deuteronomy 6:5: You shall love the LORD your God with all your heart and with all your soul and with all your might.

5. 1 Samuel 16:7: But the LORD said to Samuel, "Do not look on his appearance or on the height of his stature, because I have rejected him. For the LORD sees not as man sees: man looks on the outward appearance, but the LORD looks on the heart."

6. Proverbs 21:25: The desire of the sluggard kills him, for his hands refuse to labor.

7. Proverbs 31:30: Charm is deceitful, and beauty is vain, but a woman who fears the LORD is to be praised.

8. Song of Songs: A recognition of the goodness of the perceptions of beauty between spouses.

Chapter 1: Biblical Foundations

9. John 1:14: And the Word became flesh and dwelt among us, and we have seen his glory, glory as of the only Son from the Father, full of grace and truth.

10. John 20:27-28: Then he said to Thomas, "Put your finger here, and see my hands; and put out your hand, and place it in my side. Do not disbelieve, but believe." Thomas answered him, "My Lord and my God!"

11. Romans 6:11–13: So, you also must consider yourselves dead to sin and alive to God in Christ Jesus. Let not sin therefore reign in your mortal body, to make you obey its passions. Do not present your members to sin as instruments for unrighteousness, but present yourselves to God as those who have been brought from death to life, and your members to God as instruments for righteousness.

12. Romans 8:22–23: For we know that the whole creation has been groaning together in the pains of childbirth until now. And not only the creation, but we ourselves, who have the first fruits of the Spirit, groan inwardly as we wait eagerly for adoption as sons, the redemption of our bodies.

13. Romans 12:1: I appeal to you therefore, brothers, by the mercies of God, to present your bodies as a living sacrifice, holy and acceptable to God, which is your spiritual worship.

14. 1 Corinthians 6:19–20: Or do you not know that your body is a temple of the Holy Spirit within you, whom you have from God? You are not your own, for you were bought with a price. So, glorify God in your body.

15. 1 Corinthians 9:27: But I discipline my body and keep it under control, lest after preaching to others I myself should be disqualified.

16. 1 Corinthians 10:31: So, whether you eat or drink, or whatever you do, do all to the glory of God.

17. Ephesians 4:28: Let the thief no longer steal, but rather let him labor, doing honest work with his own hands, so that he may have something to share with anyone in need.

18. Ephesians 5:18–20: In the same way husbands should love their wives as their own bodies. He who loves his wife loves himself. For no one ever hated his own flesh, but nourishes and cherishes it, just as Christ does the church, because we are members of his body

19. Philippians 3:20-21: But our citizenship is in heaven, and from it we await a Savior, the Lord Jesus Christ, who will transform our lowly body to be like his glorious body, by the power that enables him even to subject all things to himself.

20. Colossians 3:17: And whatever you do, in word or deed, do everything in the name of the Lord Jesus, giving thanks to God the Father through him.

21. 1 Thessalonians 5:23: Now may the God of peace himself sanctify you completely, and may your whole spirit and soul and body be kept blameless at the coming of our Lord Jesus Christ.

22. 1 Timothy 2:8–10: I desire then that in every place the men should pray, lifting holy hands without anger or quarreling; likewise also that women should adorn themselves in respectable apparel, with modesty and self-control, not with braided hair and gold or pearls or costly attire, but with what is proper for women who profess godliness—with good works.

23. 1 Timothy 4:7–8: Have nothing to do with irreverent, silly myths. Rather train yourself for godliness; for while bodily training is of some value, godliness is of value in every way, as it holds promise for the present life and also for the life to come.

24. 1 Peter 3:3–4: Do not let your adorning be external—the braiding of hair and the putting on of gold jewelry, or the clothing you wear—but let your adorning be the hidden person of the heart with the imperishable beauty of a gentle and quiet spirit, which in God's sight is very precious.

25. I John 4:2–3: By this you know the Spirit of God: every spirit that confesses that Jesus Christ has come in the flesh is from God, and every spirit that does not confess Jesus is not from God. This is the spirit of the antichrist, which you heard was coming and now is in the world already.

Chapter 1: Biblical Foundations

A CHRISTIAN GUIDE TO BODY STEWARDSHIP, DIET AND EXERCISE

Chapter 2
Basic Nutrition

Key Terms:

Amino acids	Fad diet	Monounsaturated fat
Amenorrhea	Fat	Muscle dysmorphia
Anabolism	Fat-soluble vitamins	Non-celiac gluten sensitivity
Anorexia athletica	Fatty acids	Nonessential amino acids
Anorexia nervosa	Female athlete triad	Nutrient
Binge eating disorder	Fiber	Nutrition
Bulimia nervosa	Gluten	Phytochemicals
Carbohydrates	Glycemic index	Polysaccharides
Catabolism	Glycemic load	Polyunsaturated fat
Celiac disease	Incomplete protein	Protein
Cholesterol	Intermittent fasting	Saturated fat
Complete protein	Insoluble fiber	Soluble fiber
Conditional amino acid	Ketones	Trace mineral
Dietary reference intake	Ketoacidosis	Trans fat
Disaccharides	Micronutrients	Vegan
Disordered eating	Minerals	Vegetarian
Electrolytes	Monosaccharides	Vitamins
Essential amino acids	Macronutrients	Water-soluble vitamins

Learning Objectives:

- Identify and understand the function of the four macronutrients
- Distinguish the Glycemic Index and Glycemic Load
- Name at least 3 foods that are high in each macronutrient
- Identify and understand the function of micronutrients
- Name at least 3 vitamins and 3 minerals and their value in a healthy diet
- Know how to choose a healthy diet plan and recognize the features of a fad diet

CHAPTER 2: BASIC NUTRITION

Introduction

The simple fact that God gave food its flavor and human beings the ability to taste suggests that eating was meant, at least in part, to be enjoyable. Yet, God intended food to be more than just a source of enjoyment; it also serves an important and vital role in our overall health and well-being. For example, food provides the necessary nutrients the body needs to facilitate movement as well as the growth and repair of various bodily tissues. Therefore, when selecting foods to eat, it is important to consider which nutrients the body needs and not just how a particular food tastes.

Nutrition is an interdisciplinary science that studies the chemical and physiological processes involved in digesting and delivering the chemical components of food to cells all over the body as well as how those components impact our health (Pope & Nizielski, 2020). An important component of food are the **nutrients**, or the chemical substances that are required for growth and proper body functioning. Our bodies can make many of its own nutrients, but other essential nutrients must be supplied by the diet because the body cannot make them (or enough of them) on its own.

There are six major nutrients that the body needs and they are divided into two main categories: **macronutrients** and **micronutrients**. Although both need to be consumed daily for optimal health, the amount required of each differs significantly between the two categories. Macronutrients are required in large amounts because they provide energy (except for water), whereas micronutrients do not provide energy and are required in small amounts. All six classes of nutrients are important for normal body function and growth. **Table 2.1** lists the six major nutrients by category.

Table 2.1. 6 Major Nutrients

MACRONUTRIENTS	MICRONUTRIENTS
Carbohydrates	Vitamins
Protein	Minerals
Fat	-
Water	-

Phytochemicals are another important component of a heathy diet. Phytochemicals, or phytonutrients, are chemicals found in plants that provide certain health benefits. An example would be anthocyanins, or the chemical that give berries their blue and purple hues. Anthocyanins act as antioxidants to provide a protective effect to cells to fend off oxidative damage (Pope & Nizielski, 2020).

The best way to meet the intake recommendations for both macronutrients and micronutrients is to eat a variety of different nutrient-dense foods (foods that are high in nutrients as compared to calories) each day. Adequacy, variety, balance, and moderation are key components of a healthy eating pattern.

Now that we know about the six classes of nutrients, the next step is to determine what percentage of our daily calories should come by way of carbohydrates, protein and fats. The Institute of Medicine (2005) has provided **Acceptable Macronutrient Distribution Ranges (AMDR)** for each of the different macronutrients. Although these recommendations are suitable for the general public, they may not be ideal for all populations (e.g., athletes). As a result, sport-specific recommendations have also been developed. Current research also suggests that the IOM recommendations are likely better suited for males than they are for females as females tend to rely less on carbohydrates during exercise than men (Smith-Ryan & Antonio, 2013). **Table 2.2** below provides ranges for general population, sport- and female-specific macronutrient distribution ranges (IOM, 2005; Smith-Ryan & Antonio, 2013; Sheiko et al., 2018).

Table 2.2. General, Sport- and Female-Specific Macronutrient Distribution Ranges

	CARBOHYDRATES	**PROTEIN**	**FAT**
General Population	45-65%	10-35%	20-35%
Female	40-45%	20-25%	30-35%
Endurance Athlete	55-65%	15-25%	20-30%
Mixed Athlete	50-55%	20-25%	25-30%
Strength Athlete (whose goal is to lose weight)	40-50%	20-30%	25-30%
Strength Athlete (whose goal is to naintain weight)	45-50%	20-30%	20-30%
Strength Athlete (whose goal is to gain weight)	45-55%	15-20%	20-25%

In addition, the Health and Medicine division of the National Academies of Science, Engineering, and Medicine have developed **Dietary Reference Intake (DRI)** values for each nutrient. Although the DRIs cannot encompass all of the factors that impact nutrient needs, they do address the major factors for the general healthy population. They help to avoid deficiency, optimize health, and avoid toxicity by consuming too much. The DRIs are categorized into four values: the Recommended Dietary Allowances (RDA), Adequate Intakes (AI), the Estimated Average Requirements (EAR), and Upper Limits (UL).

The **Dietary Guidelines for Americans (DGA)** is another evidence-based resource that provides recommendations for dietary habits that promote health and reduce the risk for major chronic diseases. The DGAs are updated every five years by the U.S. Departments of Agriculture (USDA) and Health and Human Services (HHS) and reflect the goals of the nation in regards to nutrition and health.

Determining Daily Caloric Intake

Because water, **vitamins** and **minerals** do not contain calories, caloric intake is only determined by the consumption of **carbohydrates**, **protein**, and **fats**. Daily caloric needs are based on several factors (e.g., age, gender and physical activity level) and therefore differ from person to person,

CHAPTER 2: BASIC NUTRITION

and even day to day. **Table 2.3** provides specific recommendations for daily caloric intake as developed by the U.S. Department of Health and Human Services (2010).

To be clear, the calorie ranges are simple estimates and are not adjusted for specific individual needs. If information that includes specific numbers and quantities triggers a negative response, please disregard. Negative responses include obsessing over caloric ranges, disordered eating patterns such as restricting intake, and desiring a certain body type or a particular number on the scale. Calorie recommendations can be helpful as a baseline, but should not be adhered to above or below physical hunger and fullness cues.

Table 2.3. Daily Caloric Needs Based on Age, Gender and Activity Level

| MALES ||| AGE | FEMALES |||
SEDENTARY	MODERATELY ACTIVE	ACTIVE		SEDENTARY	MODERATELY ACTIVE	ACTIVE
1,000	1,000	1,000	2-3	1,000	1,000	1,000
1,200-1,400	1,400-1,600	1,600-2,000	4-8	1,200-1,400	1,400-1,600	1,400-1,800
1,600-2,000	1,800-2,200	2,000-2,600	9-13	1,400-1,600	1,600-2,000	1,800-2,200
2,000-2,400	2,400-2,800	2,800-3,200	14-18	1,800	2,000	2,400
2,400-2,600	2,600-2,800	3,000	19-30	1,800-2,000	2,000-2,200	2,400
2,200-2,400	2,400-2,600	2,800-3,000	31-50	1,800	2,000	2,200
2,000-2,200	2,200-2,400	2,400-2,800	51+	1,600	1,800	2,000-2,200

After we have determined how many calories we should be consuming per day, the next step is to determine what percentage of our daily calories should come by way of carbohydrates, protein and fats.

Carbohydrates

Carbohydrates are primarily a source of readily available energy. They also provide sweetness and flavor to foods, are a source of necessary fiber, and help to spare the use of protein as an energy source. **The AMDR for carbohydrates is 45-65%**, which means carbohydrates should make up 45-65% of total calories per day (for the general population). A helpful visual to consider when choosing foods is to aim for half your plate to be fruits and vegetables and about a quarter to be starchy vegetables or grains.

The primary function of carbohydrates is to provide energy for muscle contractions. Although the body can use proteins and fats for energy, it is not preferred and comes at a cost (e.g., decreased mental/athletic performance and muscle **catabolism** (breaking down of muscle tissue)). Carbohydrates come in simple forms such as sugars and complex forms such as starches and fiber. They can be broken down into three categories: **monosaccharides** (one sugar molecule), **disaccharides** (two sugar molecules), and **polysaccharides** (long chains of sugar molecules).

Monosaccharides and disaccharides are classified as simple carbohydrates as they are easily and quickly digested, whereas polysaccharides are classified as complex carbohydrates as they take longer for the body to digest. This is an important consideration for individuals with diseases like diabetes and glucose insensitivity as polysaccharides, due to their slower rates of digestion and absorption, help to prevent spikes in blood sugar. **Table 2.4** lists the different classifications of carbohydrates as well as sample foods in which they can be found.

Table 2.4. Classification of Carbohydrates

SIMPLE CARBOHYDRATES				COMPLEX CARBOHYDRATES	
MONOSACCHARIDES		DISACCHARIDES		POLYSACCHARIDES	
Glucose	Form of sugar circulating in the blood after foods are broken down	Maltose	Glucose + glucose; form of sugar found in bread and cereals	Glycogen	Chains of glucose stored in the muscles and liver
Fructose	Form of sugar found in fruits	Sucrose	Glucose + fructose (aka table sugar)	Starch	Chains of glucose found in grains, legumes, and starchy vegetables
Galactose	Form of sugar found in milk	Lactose	Galactose + glucose; form of sugar found in dairy products	Fiber	Chains of monosaccharides that cannot be separated by the body therefore less is absorbed

Carbohydrates can be found in a variety of foods such as grains (e.g., bread, rice, pasta, cereals, oatmeal), fruits, starchy vegetables and dairy products. **Fiber** is also a type of carbohydrate found in plants and cannot be broken down by the body. Fiber has several health benefits to include aiding in digestion and helping to prevent constipation. Additionally, fiber helps you feel full faster and stay full longer, which can be helpful in terms of weight management. Fiber also plays a crucial role in maintaining a healthy environment within our digestive tract (thereby decreasing the risk of disease), reducing the rise in blood sugar following a carbohydrate-containing meal, and helping maintain healthy lipid levels. There are two types of fiber: soluble and insoluble. **Soluble fiber** dissolves in water and is found in foods such as oat bran, barley, nuts, seeds, beans, lentils, peas and some fruits and vegetables. Eating foods high in soluble fiber may help to regulate blood cholesterol and sugar levels thereby reducing the risk for heart disease and diabetes. **Insoluble fiber** does not dissolve in water and is found in foods such as wheat bran, vegetables and whole grains. Insoluble fiber helps to promote bowel health and improve regularity by making the stool softer and easier to pass.

Glycemic Index vs. Glycemic Load

Blood glucose levels will naturally rise after ingestion of food containing carbohydrates. The rate at which blood glucose levels rise is determined by how quickly the carbohydrate is digested and absorbed. The **Glycemic Index** (GI) classifies food by how high and for how long it raises blood glucose levels. The faster the carbohydrate is digested and absorbed, the higher the GI ranking.

CHAPTER 2: BASIC NUTRITION

Research shows that regular consumption of high GI foods can increase an individual's risk for certain metabolic diseases such as cardiovascular disease, stroke, type 2 diabetes, metabolic syndrome, chronic kidney disease, gall stones and various types of cancer (Peterson & Rittenhouse, 2019).

While regular consumption of high GI foods is not recommended for improving general health, if timed correctly, they can be used strategically, such as immediately post-workout to help replace and replenish used carbohydrates during exercise. For example, waiting to eat your favorite sugary cereal until after your workout.

The Glycemic Index can be a useful tool, but has its limitations. The Glycemic Index rates food solely by the impact it has on blood glucose levels, and not by the quality or quantity of the carbohydrate being consumed. For example, watermelon has a GI rating of 80, which categorizes it as a high GI food and thus should be avoided. However, watermelon has few digestible calories in a typical serving. Conversely, a 2 oz. candy bar has a GI rating of 62, which categorizes it as medium GI food.

Because of these limitations, **Glycemic Load** (GL) was developed to provide a more accurate assessment of carbohydrate food choices. Glycemic Load evaluates both the quality and quantity of the carbohydrate in food and is calculated by multiplying the GI rating of a food by the grams of carbohydrate per serving, then dividing the sum by 100.

Watermelon, for instance, has 6 grams of sugar per serving, whereas a candy bar has 40 grams. This means that watermelon has a GL rating of 5 (i.e., GI rating of 80 x 6 g of sugar per serving / 100), which categorizes it as a low GL food. Conversely, a candy bar has a GL rating of 25 (GI rating of 62 x 40 g of sugar per serving / 100), which categorizes it as a high GL food. As you can see from this example, GL is likely the better and more accurate means for assessing and choosing foods containing carbohydrate. **Table 2.5** provides the various GI and GL classifications. **Appendix A** provides the GI and GL ratings for several common foods (Foster-Powell et al., 2002).

Table 2.5. Classifications for Glycemic Index and Glycemic Load

	HIGH	MEDIUM	LOW
Glycemic Index	70-100	55-69	0-55
Glycemic Load	≥ 20	11-19	≤ 10

Protein

Similar to carbohydrates, protein also plays an important role within the body. For example, protein is used to build and repair various bodily tissues, support numerous metabolic reactions as well as maintain proper pH and fluid balance. **The AMDR for protein is 10-35% of total calories.** Protein can be found in a variety of foods with the largest quantities being found in animal products (e.g., meat, poultry and dairy). Whole grains, beans, legumes, nuts and seeds are also good sources of protein.

Proteins are made up of smaller compounds called **amino acids**. There are 20 different amino acids: 9 essential, 7 conditional and 4 nonessential. **Essential amino acids**, also known as indispensable amino acids, cannot be produced by the body and therefore must be supplied through the diet. **Conditional amino acids** are usually not essential except during times of illness or stress. **Nonessential amino acids** can be made by the body and thus do not need to be provided in the diet. **Table 2.6** provides a comprehensive listing of the different essential, conditional and nonessential amino acids.

Table 2.6. Essential, Conditional and Nonessential Amino Acids

Essential Amino Acids		Conditional Amino Acids		Nonessential Amino Acids	
Histidine	Phenylalanine	Lysine	Arginine	Proline	Alanine
Isoleucine	Threonine	-	Asparagine	Serine	Aspartic Acid (Aspartate)
Leucine	Tryptophan	-	Glutamine	Tyrosine	Cysteine
Methionine	Valine	-	Glycine	-	Glutamic Acid (Glutamate)

Animal proteins are **complete proteins** because they contain all of the different essential amino acids, whereas most plant proteins are **incomplete proteins** because they are missing or are low in one or more of the essential amino acids. However, not all plant proteins are incomplete as both soybeans and quinoa are complete proteins. Moreover, it is possible to make a complete protein by combining two or more incomplete proteins (e.g., peanut butter on wheat bread) or by combining incomplete plant proteins with small amounts of animal protein (e.g., macaroni and cheese). It is not necessary to combine incomplete proteins at every meal, but rather assess the entire day as a whole to determine if adequate essential amino acids have been provided. Research suggests that protein sources should be spread out throughout the day. This can be achieved by aiming for about a quarter of the plate to be protein at meals (or about the size of your palm) and including a protein source with snacks (Fink & Mikesky, 2021). Frequent consumption of protein is recommended due to the body's inability to store excess protein as well as the high turnover rate of protein within the body.

Fat

Similar to carbohydrates and protein, fat also provides several vital functions. In fact, fat is essential for the transport and absorption of the fat-soluble vitamins (i.e., A, D, E and K), the conduction of nerve impulses, the maintenance of cell membranes, and the production of specific hormones. **The AMDR for dietary fat is 20-35% of total calories.** Fat also provides flavor to foods and contributes to satiety by delaying the time it takes for food to pass through the digestive tract. When fats are added to meals, foods are digested and absorbed more slowly. This is helpful in controlling blood sugar when high-carbohydrate foods are consumed.

Fat is the most energy dense of the macronutrients providing 9 calories per gram (as compared to carbohydrates and protein that provide only 4 calories per gram). Due to fat's high palatability in taste appeal combined with caloric density, eating patterns high in fat (specifically saturated and trans-fat) increase the risk for obesity and other chronic diseases (e.g., hypertension, diabetes, gallbladder disease, breast cancer). Healthy sources of fat can be obtained through a variety of foods such as nuts, nut butters, seeds, avocados, and oily fish (e.g., mackerel, salmon).

There are three primary types of fat: **monounsaturated fat, polyunsaturated fat,** and **saturated fat**. Both monounsaturated fats and polyunsaturated fats are thought to help lower low-density lipoprotein cholesterol levels (sometimes referred to as "bad cholesterol") and reduce the risk of heart disease. Sources of monounsaturated fat include nuts, seeds, avocados, olives, olive oil, and canola oil. Polyunsaturated fats, in their natural form, are liquid at room temperature. There are two types of polyunsaturated fats: omega-3 and omega-6 fatty acids. Sources of omega-3 fatty acids include fish, fish oil, flaxseed, and soybean oil. Sources of omega-6 fatty acids include poultry, eggs, nuts, cereals, whole grain breads, pumpkin seeds, and most vegetable oils (e.g., corn, safflower, soybean, sunflower, linseed).

Saturated fats are solid at room temperature. Sources of saturated fat include fatty cuts of meat, dark poultry meat, high-fat dairy, tropical oils (e.g., coconut oil, palm, cocoa butter) and lard. There is currently some debate regarding the health risks associated with diets high in saturated fats. For years there has been a long-standing bias that diets high in saturated fats are associated with an increased risk of heart disease. However, current research now seems to suggest there is no clear or direct correlation between saturated fat intake and heart disease (Hooper et al., 2020).

Trans fat is another type of fat that is created when converting liquid fats into solid fats. Examples of trans fat include shortening and some margarines. Unlike saturated fats, trans fats are believed to raise low-density lipoprotein cholesterol levels and lower high-density lipoprotein cholesterol levels. Similar to saturated fats, diets high in trans fats may increase blood cholesterol levels and risk of heart disease.

Table 2.7 provides recommendations for how much of your daily fat intake should come from the various types of fat (Israetel et al., 2019).

Table 2.7. Fat Intake Recommendations

Fat Type	% of Daily Fat Intake
Monounsaturated	45-60%
Polyunsaturated	35-50%
Saturated	5-20%
Trans fats	< 1%

Water

Although water does not contain any energy (calories), it is an important macronutrient and daily consumption is vital for life. In fact, up to 60% of the human body is comprised of water. The body uses water to absorb and transport nutrients, remove waste, regulate body temperature, and maintain other bodily functions. As a result, even a small amount of dehydration can have a large impact on mental and physical performance. Research shows that exercise performance can be impacted with as little as a 2% loss in body water. Water loss in excess of 5% can decrease work capacity by almost 30% and cause extreme fatigue and dizziness, while a 15-25% loss can result in death (Jeukendrup & Gleeson, 2010).

Water can be lost in several ways, including perspiration, sweating, urination, and defecation. Water balance (water intake equals water loss) is an important part of a healthy lifestyle. Those who exercise regularly in dry or cold climates or at high altitudes will need to pay extra attention to water balance. An individual's hydration status can easily be assessed by their urine color and frequency. For example, **Table 2.8** provides estimated hydration status based on urine color (Urine Colors, n.d.). In terms of frequency, optimal hydration is generally associated with urination of about every 1-2 hours while awake.

Table 2.8. Hydration Status Based on Urine Color.

WELL-HYDRATED	HYDRATED	PARTIALLY HYDRATED	PARTIALLY DEHYDRATED	DEHYDRATED
Drink water as normal	Drink a small glass of water now	Drink a ½ bottle (¼ liter) of water within the hour	Drink a ½ bottle (¼ liter) now	Drink 2 bottles (1 liter) of water now

The AI for water, published by the Institute of Medicine (2005), for men and women over the age of 19 is 3.7 liters (or about 15.5 cups) and 2.7 liters (or about 11.4 cups) per day, respectively. This includes water from both foods and beverages. The recommendation for beverages alone is 3 liters (or about 13 cups) and 2.2 liters (about 9 cups), respectively (Fink & Mikesky, 2021). Eating a well-balanced diet that includes fruits and vegetables can also help contribute to daily fluid intake. **Table 2.9** provides additional recommendations for daily water intake (Quinn, 2020).

Table 2.9. Water Intake Recommendations in Fluid Ounces per Day

	LOW END	HIGH END
General health (not including exercise)	Bodyweight (lbs.) x 0.5	Bodyweight (lbs.) x 1.0
2 hours before exercise	16 oz.	24 oz.
20-30 minutes before exercise	8 oz.	-
During normal exercise (≤ 60 min.)	8 oz. every 15 min.	-
During high-intensity exercise (≥ 90 min.) *	8 oz. every 15-30 min.	10 oz. every 15-30 min.
After exercise	16 oz. for every lb. lost	24 oz. for every lb. lost

* Carbohydrate/electrolyte replenishing sports drink with 60-100 kcal per 8 oz. serving

Chapter 2: Basic Nutrition

Micronutrients

Unlike macronutrients (excluding water), micronutrients do not provide energy (calories). Additionally, although vital for normal growth and development, micronutrients are only required in trace amounts. Micronutrients can be divided into four categories: water-soluble vitamins, fat-soluble vitamins, major minerals and trace minerals.

Vitamins are any group of organic compounds, either acquired from food or produced by the body, that are necessary for the regulation of certain metabolic processes. For example, vitamins help to support bone health, heal wounds, and bolster your immune system. There are two types of vitamins: water-soluble and fat-soluble. **Water-soluble vitamins** include vitamin C and the B vitamins. **Fat- soluble vitamins** include vitamins A, D, E and K. Any excess of water-soluble vitamins will be excreted in the urine; whereas excess of fat-soluble vitamins will be stored in the liver or fat tissue. **Table 2.10** provides a complete listing of the different water-soluble and fat-soluble vitamins. **Table 2.12** provides the recommended daily intake, sources, functions and signs of deficiency for the various vitamins (University of Michigan Health, 2019a).

Table 2.10. Water-Soluble and Fat-Soluble Vitamins

WATER-SOLUBLE			FAT-SOLUBLE	
Thiamine (Vitamin B1)	Pantothenic Acid	Folic Acid	Vitamin A	Vitamin K
Riboflavin (Vitamin B2)	Biotin	Cobalamin (Vitamin B12)	Vitamin D	-
Niacin (Vitamin B3)	Pyridoxine (Vitamin B6)	Ascorbic Acid (Vitamin C)	Vitamin E	-

Minerals are solid inorganic substances acquired from food that are essential to certain metabolic functions. The body uses minerals to perform many different functions ranging from building strong bones, transmitting nerve impulses, manufacturing hormones to maintaining a normal heart rhythm. **Major minerals** are required in amounts greater than 100 mg per day; whereas **trace minerals** are required in amounts less than 100 mg per day. **Electrolytes** are minerals dissolved in the body fluids that help to regulate nerve and muscle function, rehydrate, balance blood acidity and pressure, and rebuild damaged tissue. Some of the major electrolytes include sodium, potassium, calcium, magnesium and phosphate. **Table 2.11** provides a complete listing of the different major minerals and trace minerals. **Table 2.13** provides the recommended daily intake, sources, functions and signs of deficiency for the various minerals (University of Michigan Health, 2019b).

Table 2.11 Major Minerals and Trace Minerals

MAJOR MINERALS			TRACE MINERALS		
Sodium	Calcium	Sulfur	Iron	Copper	Selenium
Potassium	Phosphorus	-	Zinc	Manganese	Chromium
Chloride	Magnesium	-	Iodine	Fluoride	Molybdenum

Healthy Eating Patterns

A healthy eating pattern is one that includes a variety of foods in order to provide the necessary energy and essential nutrients we need. As a general rule of thumb, strive to have all three macronutrients (i.e., carbohydrates, protein, fat) represented at each meal.

A healthy eating pattern is also one that can be maintained over the course of a lifetime. Our bodies are very different and all have different calorie needs (even differing from day to day). God made us all unique and therefore calorie needs cannot be represented by a generalized number. Additionally, one pattern of eating may be sustainable for some individuals, but not others. For some individuals, it may be necessary to refrain from using calorie counters / calculator and diet trackers in order to maintain a healthy relationship with food and their body.

It is also important to remember that food holds no moral value (i.e., food is neither good or bad).

Food is consumed for a variety of reasons (e.g., preference, cultural / social norms, accessibility, mood) and all of them are valid. With that in mind, it is important not to demonize or avoid certain foods. While we should be mindful of nourishing our bodies well, we should also be careful not to place boundaries on what we eat. For example, it would be ultimately counterproductive and unrealistic to only consume "healthy" foods in the pursuit of health.

A healthy eating pattern should not be difficult to implement and follow. God has equipped each of us with an innate ability to assess our hunger and fullness. As a result, we should listen to and honor these hunger and fullness cues. However, unhealthy eating patterns can disrupt this ability thereby allowing this God-given ability to fade over time.

Chapter 2: Basic Nutrition

Table 2.12. Recommended Daily Intake, Sources, Functions and Signs of Deficiency for Vitamins

VITAMIN	REC. DAILY INTAKE	SOURCES	FUNCTIONS	SIGNS OF DEFICIENCY
Thiamine (Vitamin B1)	1.2 mg (Males) 1.1 mg (Females)	Found in all nutritious foods in moderate amounts: pork, whole-grain or enriched breads and cereals, legumes, nuts and seeds	Part of an enzyme needed for energy metabolism; important to nerve function	Edema or muscle wasting, mental confusion, anorexia, enlarged heart, abnormal heart rhythm, muscle degeneration and weakness, nerve changes
Riboflavin (Vitamin B2)	1.3 mg (Males) 1.1 mg (Females)	Milk and milk products; leafy green vegetables; whole-grain, enriched breads and cereals	Part of an enzyme needed for energy metabolism; important for normal vision and skin health	Cracks at corners of mouth, sore throat, skin rash, hypersensitivity to light, purple tongue
Niacin (Vitamin B3)	16 mg (Males) 14 mg (Females)	Meat, poultry, fish, whole-grain or enriched breads and cereals, vegetables (especially mushrooms, asparagus, and leafy green vegetables), peanut butter	Part of an enzyme needed for energy metabolism; important for nervous system, digestive system, and skin health	Weakness, diarrhea, dermatitis, inflammation of mucous membranes, mental illness
Pantothenic Acid	5 mg	Widespread in foods	Part of an enzyme needed for energy metabolism	Vomiting, insomnia, fatigue
Biotin	300 mcg	Widespread in foods; also produced in intestinal tract by bacteria	Part of an enzyme needed for energy metabolism	Abnormal heart action, muscle pain, fatigue, weakness
Pyridoxine (Vitamin B6)	1.3 mg	Meat, fish, poultry, vegetables, fruits	Part of an enzyme needed for protein metabolism; helps make red blood cells	Anemia, convulsions, cracks at corners of mouth, dermatitis, nausea, confusion
Folic Acid	400 mcg	Leafy green vegetables and legumes, seeds, orange juice, and liver; now added to most refined grains	Part of an enzyme needed for making DNA and new cells, especially red blood cells	Anemia, gastrointestinal disturbances, decreased resistance to infection, depression
Cobalamin (Vitamin B12)	2.4 mcg	Meat, poultry, fish, seafood, eggs, milk and milk products; not found in plant foods	Part of an enzyme needed for making new cells; important to nerve function	Anemia, fatigue, nervous system damage, sore tongue
Ascorbic Acid (Vitamin C)	90 mg (Males) 75 mg (Females)	Found only in fruits and vegetables, especially citrus fruits, vegetables in the cabbage family, cantaloupe, strawberries, peppers, tomatoes, potatoes, lettuce, papayas, mangoes, kiwifruit	Antioxidant; part of an enzyme needed for protein metabolism; important for immune system health; aids in iron absorption	Scurvy, anemia, reduced resistance to infection, bleeding gyms, weakness, loosened teeth, rough skin, joint pain, poor wound healing, hair loss, poor iron absorption

Vitamin A	900 mcg (Males) 700 mcg (Females)	Fortified milk, cheese, cream, butter, fortified margarine, eggs, liver Leafy, dark green vegetables; dark orange fruits (apricots, cantaloupe) and vegetables (carrots, winter squash, sweet potatoes, pumpkin)	Antioxidant, needed for vision, healthy skin and mucous membranes, bone and tooth growth, immune system health	Night blindness, dry skin, increased susceptibility to infection, loss of appetite, anemia, kidney stones
Vitamin D	15 mcg	Egg yolks, liver, fatty fish, fortified milk, fortified margarine. When exposed to sunlight, the skin can make vitamin D.	Needed for proper absorption of calcium; stored in bones	Rickets (children), bone softening, loss and factures (adults)
Vitamin E	15 mg	Polyunsaturated plant oils (soybean, corn, cottonseed, safflower); leafy green vegetables; wheat germ; whole-grain products; liver; egg yolks; nuts and seeds	Antioxidant; protects cell walls	Red blood cell breakage and anemia, weakness, neurological problems, muscle cramps
Vitamin K	120 mcg (Males) 90 mcg (Females)	Leafy green vegetables such as kale, collard greens, and spinach; green vegetables such as broccoli, brussels sprouts, and asparagus; also produced in intestinal tract by bacteria	Needed for proper blood clotting	Hemorrhage

Chapter 2: Basic Nutrition

Table 2.13. Recommended Daily Intake, Sources, Functions and Signs of Deficiency for Minerals

Mineral	Rec. Daily Intake	Sources	Functions	Signs of Deficiency
Sodium	1,500 mg	Table salt, soy sauce; large amounts in processed foods; small amounts in milk, breads, vegetables, and unprocessed meats	**Needed for proper fluid balance, nerve transmission, and muscle contraction**	Muscle weakness, loss of appetite, nausea, vomiting
Chloride	2,300 mg	Table salt, soy sauce; large amounts in processed foods; small amounts in milk, meats, breads, and vegetables	Needed for proper fluid balance, stomach acid	Muscle cramps, apathy, poor appetite
Potassium	3,500-4,700 mg	Meats, milk, fresh fruits and vegetables, whole grains, legumes	Needed for proper fluid balance, nerve transmission, and muscle contraction	Muscular weakness, nausea, drowsiness, paralysis, confusion, disruption of cardiac rhythm
Calcium	1,000 mg	Milk and milk products; canned fish with bones (salmon, sardines); fortified tofu and fortified soy milk; greens (broccoli, mustard greens); legumes	Important for healthy bones and teeth; helps muscles relax and contract; important in nerve functioning, blood clotting, blood pressure regulation, immune system health	Stunted growth (children), bone mineral loss (adults)
Phosphorus	700 mg	Meat, fish, poultry, eggs, milk, processed foods (including soda pop)	Important for healthy bones and teeth; found in every cell; part of the system that maintains acid-base balance	Nausea, weakness, confusion, loss of bone calcium
Magnesium	400-420 mg (Males) 310-320 mg (Females)	Nuts and seeds; legumes; leafy, green vegetables; seafood; chocolate; artichokes; "hard" drinking water	Found in bones; needed for making protein, muscle contraction, nerve transmission, immune system health	Neurological disturbances, impaired immune function, kidney disorders, nausea, weight loss, growth failure (children)
Sulfur	Not determined	Occurs in foods as part of protein: meats, poultry, fish, eggs, milk, legumes, nuts	Found in protein molecules	Reduced protein synthesis, joint pain or disease
Iron	8 mg (Males) 18 mg (Females)	Organ meats; red meats; fish; poultry; shellfish (especially clams); egg yolks; legumes; dried fruits; dark, leafy greens; iron-enriched breads and cereals; and fortified cereals	Part of a molecule (hemoglobin) found in red blood cells that carries oxygen in the body; needed for energy metabolism	Anemia, weakness, impaired immune function, cold hands and feet, gastrointestinal distress, pale appearance

A Christian Guide to Body Stewardship, Diet and Exercise

Zinc	11 mg (Males) 8 mg (Females)	Meats, fish, poultry, leavened whole grains, vegetables	Antioxidant, part of many enzymes; needed for making protein and genetic material; has a function in taste perception, wound healing, normal fetal development, production of sperm, normal growth and sexual maturation, immune system health	Growth failure, reproductive failure, loss of appetite, impaired taste acuity, skin rash, impaired immune function, poor wound healing, night blindness
Iodine	150 mcg	Seafood, foods grown in iodine-rich soil, iodized salt, bread, dairy products	Found in thyroid hormone, which helps regulate growth, development, and metabolism	Goiter, mental retardation, hearing loss, growth failure (newborns)
Selenium	55 mcg	Meats, seafood, grains	Antioxidant	Muscle pain and tenderness, heart failure, Keshan disease
Copper	900 mcg	Legumes, nuts and seeds, whole grains, organ meats, drinking water	Part of many enzymes; needed for iron metabolism	Seizures, anemia, growth retardation
Manganese	2.3 mg (Males) 1.8 mg (Females)	Widespread in foods, especially plant foods	Antioxidant, Part of many enzymes	Impairs energy metabolism, produces bone abnormalities
Fluoride	4 mg (Males) 3 mg (Females)	Drinking water (either fluoridated or naturally containing fluoride), fish, and most teas	Involved in formation of bones and teeth; helps prevent tooth decay	Tooth decay
Chromium	50-200 mcg	Unrefined foods, especially liver, brewer's yeast, whole grains, nuts, cheeses	Works closely with insulin to regulate blood sugar (glucose) levels	Weight loss, poor glucose control
Molybdenum	45 mcg	Legumes; breads and grains; leafy greens; leafy, green vegetables; milk; liver	Part of some enzymes	Rapid heartbeat, nausea, vomiting, coma

Eating Disorders / Disordered Eating

While nurturing our bodies through sound nutrition and exercise is wise practice, we must recognize there is a fine line between a healthy relationship with food and exercise and a disordered one. Unfortunately, it is not uncommon for some individuals to innocently embark upon a weight loss journey and end up with an eating disorder. Disordered eating can lead to serious health complications like malnourishment and altered levels of various bodily hormones. A listing of various types of eating and psychological disorders is provided in **Table 2.14** (Fink & Mikesky, 2021).

Table 2.14. Various Types of Eating and Psychological Disorders Associated with Body Image

Eating Disorder	Description
Anorexia Nervosa	A clinical condition characterized by extreme fear of becoming obese, a distorted body image, and avoidance of food.
Bulimia Nervosa	A clinical condition characterized by repeated and uncontrolled food binging in which a large number of calories are consumed followed by an immediate purge (e.g., vomiting or use of laxatives / diuretics).
Binge Eating Disorder	A clinical condition characterized by the inability to control what or how much food is being consumed.
Muscle Dysmorphia	A psychological disorder characterized by a negative body image and obsessive desire to have a muscular physique.
Anorexia Athletica	A subclinical condition characterized by inappropriate eating behaviors and weight control methods to prevent weight and/or fat gain. Although the condition does not meet the clinical criteria for an eating disorder, the associated behaviors can lead to a clinically recognized eating disorder.
Female Athlete Triad	A condition characterized by the combination of disordered eating, **amenorrhea** (absence or abnormal cessation of menstruation), and osteoporosis.

Some of the key warning signs of disordered eating include:

- Obsessing over calories
- Constantly tracking food and/or exercise
- Withdrawing from social situations involving food
- Feeling out of control about food
- Believing food must be earned through exercise
- Only eating "clean"
- Disordered view of body image
- Extreme desire to be thin

Weight is not the only clinical risk factor for developing an eating disorder. For example, certain personality types, sports, and professions can be more likely to develop eating disorders than others (e.g., individuals diagnosed with obsessive compulsive disorder (OCD), gymnasts and other aesthetic sport athletes). It is also worth mentioning that some individuals may not meet the criteria for an eating disorder but follow a pattern of disordered eating.

Unfortunately, the consequences of disordered eating often go unnoticed, even by seasoned medical professionals. As a result, individuals with an eating disorder may not recognize the gravity of the situation until after serious health complications arise. Therefore, early detection, prevention, and treatment are essential. Additionally, it is important to seek help from qualified medical professionals as soon as some of the early warning signs of disordered eating have been detected.

Education on how to identify, eliminate, and reduce contributing factors for disordered eating is an effective prevention strategy. Other strategies include limiting negative social media intake, avoiding fad diets, and developing a healthy relationship with exercise and sports (e.g., focus on developing various skills rather than on weight or body composition).

Identifying Fad Diets

Fad diets are weight-loss programs that promise fast results with minimal effort. Unfortunately, many of these programs involve the severe restriction or elimination of certain foods or food groups which can lead to nutritional deficiencies (e.g., dietary **fiber**, select vitamins and minerals). Examples include fat-free, low-carbohydrate, and high protein diets. Most of the weight loss associated with these diets is a result of reduced water retention caused by decreased carbohydrate intake.

Dehydration and reduced glycogen stores then result in reduced athletic performance as well as early onset of fatigue (Peterson & Rittenhouse, 2019). Research shows that the majority of weight lost on these diets come from body water and lean muscle mass, not body fat (Williams, 2007). Some of the long-term risks associated with fad diets include dehydration, weakness/fatigue, nausea, headaches, constipation, and vitamin/mineral deficiencies. Provided below are some of the characteristics of a fad diet:

- Recommendations to limit or eliminate certain foods or food groups
- Claims of weight loss greater than 1-2 pounds per week
- Need to purchase proprietary products in order to be successful
- Use of non-peer reviewed studies to substantiate claims
- Formulate simple conclusions from complex studies
- Recommendations taken from studies ignore differences among individuals or groups

CHAPTER 2: BASIC NUTRITION

Fad Diet Examples

Low-carbohydrate diet (e.g., Adkins / Keto / Carnivore). As the name suggests, these diets promote either severely restricting or eliminating carbohydrate intake. As previously mentioned, although seemingly effective, the weight loss associated with these diets is primarily a result of a temporary decrease in water weight due to reduced carbohydrate intake. When carbohydrate intake is significantly reduced, glycogen stores in the muscle are depleted, which results in weight loss due to reduced water retention. However, once carbohydrates are reintroduced, the muscles begin to store water again resulting in weight gain. Additionally, since most foods contain at least some carbohydrates, some of the weight loss associated with these diets is a result of an overall reduction in the number of calories consumed per day.

It is important to note that carbohydrates are the body's preferred source of energy. When inadequate amounts of carbohydrates are consumed, the body produces **ketones** (chemical produced by the body when fats are broken down for energy) as an alternative energy source. However, burning of ketones instead of carbohydrates, leads to decreased mental and physical performance. **Figure 2.1** shows the impact that various diets (i.e., high-carbohydrate intake, normal carbohydrate intake, and low-carbohydrate/high-fat intake) can have on muscle glycogen levels and exercise duration (Balsom et al., 1999). Some of the common side effects reported with a keto diet include: excessive thirst, frequent urination, fatigue, hunger, confusion, anxiety, irritability, tachycardia, lightheadedness, sweating and chills. Additionally, prolonged use of a keto diet can also lead to a condition called **ketoacidosis**, which can be fatal.

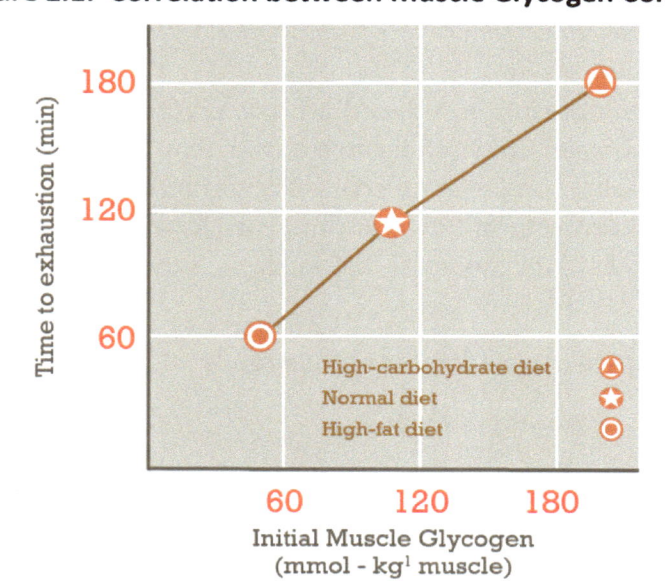

Figure 2.1. Correlation between Muscle Glycogen Content and Exercise Duration

Time to exhaustion (min) vs. Initial Muscle Glycogen (mmol - kg^1 muscle)

- High-carbohydrate diet ▲
- Normal diet ☆
- High-fat diet ●

Intermittent fasting. Intermittent fasting is not as much a diet as it is a particular pattern of eating. Some of the more common types of intermittent fasting include: 16:8 (i.e., 16-hour fast with 8-hour eating window); 20:4 (i.e., 20-hour fast with 4-hour eating window); 5:2 (i.e., 5 days no restrictive with 2-days of fasting); 24-hour fast; 36-hour fast; alternate day fasting; and spontaneous fasting / skipping meals. The theory behind intermittent fasting is that the body burns more fat in a fasted state than when food is consumed on a more regular basis.

Some research suggests that intermittent fasting may be an effective weight loss strategy for obese individuals; however, there is only limited data to suggest similar benefits for healthy, normal-weight individuals (Anton et al., 2017). In terms of performance, research has shown that eating before exercise, as compared to exercising on an empty stomach, helps to improve athletic performance (Aird et al., 2018). In terms of aesthetics, current research shows that fasting can be used when performing low-intensity endurance training to improve body composition. However, it is not recommended to perform fasted exercise for bouts lasting more than 60 minutes or when performing high-intensity exercise (Guillermo & Barakat, 2020). This is because being in a fasted state while performing long duration or high-intensity exercise can result in a catabolic state where the body is forced to break down muscle tissue in order to produce and provide available energy.

Although intermittent fasting may work for some individuals, it isn't for everyone. For example, intermittent fasting is not recommended for individuals who require a more frequent feeding schedule due to current or previous medical conditions (e.g., pregnancy, breast feeding, diabetes, history of disordered eating, taking medication that requires food with consumption).

Due to the potential impact on daily protein intake, intermittent fasting may be less suitable for athletes - especially strength athletes. As depicted in **Table 2.4**, consuming 1.0 gram of protein per pound of bodyweight is appropriate for most individuals (to include athletes). However, consuming that much protein is extremely different for individuals who are only eating three or less times per day. For example, a 150 lb. individual would have to consume 50 grams of protein per setting if on a three-meal per day schedule or 75 grams of protein per setting if on a two-meal per day schedule. A much easier and effective strategy would be to consume 30 grams of protein over a five-meal per day schedule.

Gluten-free diet. This diet excludes the consumption of **gluten**, a complex combination of proteins found in wheat, rye and barley that are not easily digestible. One of the problems associated with this diet is that not all gastrointestinal issues (e.g., constipation, gas, bloating) are related to the consumption of gluten. As a result, individuals can be unnecessarily restricting nutrient-dense foods from their diet that are high in whole grains, fiber and B vitamins. Therefore, it is recommended that individuals with gastrointestinal issues work with their physician, or possibly a registered dietitian, to identify the underlying cause of their symptoms as well as foods to include and/or avoid in order to help manage those symptoms.

Only individuals with **Celiac disease** need to completely avoid gluten in their diet. Celiac disease is an autoimmune disorder where the body enacts an immune response when gluten is consumed, that causes damage to the small intestine. This damage causes symptoms like diarrhea, bloating, gas and possibly other non-gastrointestinal issues (e.g., headaches, fatigue). **Non-celiac gluten sensitivity** (NCGS, sometimes called gluten intolerance or gluten sensitivity), on the other hand, is when there are gastrointestinal issues related to gluten consumption but without the autoimmune response and damage. Most people with NCGS have a threshold for gluten and only after that threshold is exceeded do they experience symptoms. Instead of avoiding whole grain foods altogether, a better strategy for individuals with NCGS may be to determine, through systematic trial and error, the amount of whole grain foods they can tolerate per day without experiencing symptoms.

Another problem with the gluten-free diet is that it was never intended to be a strategy for weight loss, although many people use it as one. Gluten-free foods are not necessarily low-calorie foods and therefore, just as with foods containing gluten, weight gain is possible with overconsumption.

Other Diets

Paleolithic (paleo) diet. The paleo diet can be a healthy eating strategy, if done correctly, due to its incorporation of high quality, nutrient-dense foods such as nuts, seeds, eggs, fruits, vegetables and grass-fed beef. However, limiting oneself to just these foods can be expensive. Another concern is that most of the recommended foods are very low in carbohydrates, which may hinder athletic performance. Additionally, some users of this diet unnecessarily restrict or eliminate certain nutrient- dense foods such as sweet potatoes, dairy, beans and legumes. Again, the paleo diet can be a healthy dietary strategy if an individual does not avoid or restrict certain food groups from their diet (e.g., starches, whole grains, dairy).

Vegetarian diet. Similar to intermittent fasting, there are several different types of vegetarian diets: **vegan** (i.e., diet consists of plant products only); lacto-vegetarian (i.e., diet consists of plant and milk products); ovo-vegetarian (i.e., diet consists of plant and egg products); and lacto-ovo-vegetarian (i.e., diets consists of plant, milk and egg products). Similar to the paleo diet, the vegetarian diet can be a healthy dietary strategy if done correctly. Since most plant products are incomplete proteins, careful attention must be made to ensure all essential (indispensible) amino acids and other key nutrients are included in the diet. For example, vegetarians sometimes have a hard time getting enough of the following nutrients in their diet: vitamin D, vitamin B_{12}, iron, zinc and calcium. As a result, it may be necessary to take a daily dietary supplement and/or follow-up with a healthcare provider to ensure they do not develop any nutritional deficiencies.

Supplements

Although there are numerous dietary supplements on the market, research has shown that very few actually do what they claim to do. The few supplements that seem to live up to the hype include: protein shakes, chocolate milk, creatine and caffeine. Supplements not listed do not have credible support for their use in the literature and therefore are not included in the discussion.

Protein shakes. There are several different types of protein: whey (comprises 20% of milk protein), casein (comprises 80% of milk protein) soy, egg, and pea. Whey protein is digested and absorbed very quickly (i.e., within 20 minutes), whereas, casein and soy proteins are digested and absorbed more slowly (i.e., 2-4 hours). As a result, whey protein consumption is recommended immediately after a workout due to its fast absorption; whereas casein protein consumption is recommended before bed due its slower rate of absorption (Dunford & Doyle, 2015; Rosenbloom & Coleman, 2012). Research suggests consuming 20-30 grams of protein 5-6 times per day is the best way to promote muscle **anabolism** (building up of muscle tissue) and prevent muscle catabolism (Prevost, 2015). Pea protein may be a good source of protein for those individuals looking for non-meat or dairy alternatives to whey and casein. However, plant proteins have a lower absorption rates than animal proteins and therefore slightly more than the normal 20-30 grams per serving may be required.

Chocolate Milk. Flavored milk (e.g., chocolate milk) is one of the most cost-effective post-workout beverages on the market. Additionally, research has shown time and again that flavored milk is an effective and nutritionally sound dietary supplement. In fact, numerous studies have reported flavored milk, due to its high carbohydrate (i.e., 3 grams per ounce) and moderate protein (i.e., 1 gram per ounce) intake, to be an ideal post-workout recovery beverage and superior to most other high-carbohydrate recovery beverages with the same number of calories (Dunford & Doyle, 2015; Rosenbloom & Coleman, 2012). Consumption of flavored milk post-workout has also shown to aid in rehydration as well as provide a variety of essential nutrients needed for recovery after strenuous physical activity. In terms of quantity, if the goal is to consume at least 20-30 grams of protein post-workout, one would need to drink at least three 8-ounce glasses of flavored milk.

Creatine. Similar to flavored milk, creatine is one of the most researched supplements on the market. Creatine is produced in the liver, kidneys and pancreas and stored in the muscle. Adequate consumption increases creatine levels in the muscle thereby allowing adenosine triphosphate (ATP) to regenerate more rapidly. Creatine can be taken as a supplement or acquired naturally in the diet by consuming adequate amounts of meat and fish. The average individual needs about 2 grams of creatine per day in order to maintain normal creatine levels (Peterson & Rittenhouse, 2019). Creatine supplementation has been shown to:

- Increase muscle size (hypertrophy)
- Increase muscle endurance
- Increase intra-set recovery
- Increase maximal force / strength

Caffeine. Caffeine is a potent stimulant that affects the body's central nervous system and metabolism. Caffeine has been shown to increase neural activity and alertness as well as decrease perceived level of effort, which makes its use well suited for endurance athletes. The rate at which caffeine enters the bloodstream is dependent upon the product being consumed. For example, caffeine from caffeinated gum enters the bloodstream in about 10 minutes, whereas caffeine from caffeinated beverages (e.g., coffee, tea, soft drinks) enters the bloodstream in about 45 minutes (Peterson & Rittenhouse, 2019). This is an important consideration when taking a caffeinated product in conjunction with an endurance event. The benefits of caffeine supplementation occur at rather low dosages. In fact, research shows that dosages greater than 5 mg per kilogram do not offer any additional benefit (U.S. Department of Health and Human Services, 2015). Up to 400 mg per day of caffeine is thought to be safe for most individuals; however, overconsumption can lead to dizziness or gastrointestinal distress, especially if taken on an empty

CHAPTER 2: BASIC NUTRITION

stomach. Caffeine supplementation has been shown to:

- Increase motivation for training
- Increase pain tolerance during training
- Increase ability to sustain high-volume training

Summary

- The four macronutrients are carbohydrate, fat, protein and water
- Micronutrients are vitamins and minerals essential for healthy bodily function
- Vitamins are classified as either water-soluble or fat-soluble and perform hundreds of roles in the body
- Healthy eating patterns are sustainable and include consuming all food groups as well as honoring hunger and fullness cues
- There are no "good" or "bad" foods as food doesn't have a moral value
- Fad diets are weight-loss programs or supplements that promise to deliver fast results with minimal effort and pose potential harm to the body
- Supplements like creatine, whey and chocolate milk are healthy options for post-exercise recovery and building muscle

References

1. Aird, T., Davies, R., & Carson, B. (2018). *Effects of Fasted vs. Fed-State on Performance and Post-Exercise Metabolism: A Systematic Review and Meta-Analysis.* Scand J Med Sci Sports, 28(5):1476-1493.

2. Anton, S., Moehl, K., Donahoo, W., Marosi, K., Lee, S., Mainous, A., Leeuwenburgh, C. & Mattson, M. (2017). *Flipping the Metabolic Switch: Understanding and Applying the Health Benefits of Fasting.* Obesity, 26(2):254-268.

3. Balsom, P., Gaitanos, G., Soderlund, K., Ekblom, B. (1999). *High-Intensity Exercise and Muscle Glycogen Availability in Humans.* Acta Physiol Scand, 65(4):337-45.

4. Dietary Guidelines for Americans. (2020-2025). *Executive Summary.* Retrieved from https://www.dietaryguidelines.gov/sites/default/files/2020-12/DGA_2020-2025_ExecutiveSummary_English.pdf.

5. Dunford, M., & Doyle, A. (2015). *Nutrition for Sport and Exercise.* (3rd Ed). Boston, MA: Cengage.

6. Fink, H, & Mikesky, A. (2021). *Practical Applications in Sports Nutrition (6th ed)*. Burlington, MA: Jones & Bartlett Learning.

7. Foster-Powell, K., Holt, S., Brand-Miller, J. (2002). *International Tables of Glycemic Index and Glycemic Load Values*. American Journal of Clinical Nutrition, 62:5-56.

8. Guillermo, E., & Barakat, C. (2020). *Fasted Versus Nonfasted Aerobic Exercise on Body Composition: Considerations for Physique Athletes*. Strength and Conditioning Journal.

9. Hooper, L., Martin, N., Jimoh, O., Kirk, C., Foster, E., & Abdelhamid, A. (2020). *Reduction in Saturated Fat Intake for Cardiovascular Disease*. Cochrane Database of Systemic Reviews.

10. Institute of Medicine. (2005). *Dietary Reference Intakes for Energy, Carbohydrate, Fiber, Fat, Fatty Acid, Cholesterol, Protein and Amino Acids*. Retrieved from http://www.nap.edu/read/10490/chapter/1.

11. Israetel, M., Davis, M., Case, J., & Hoffman, J. (2019). *The Renaissance Diet 2.0: Your Scientific Guide to Fat Loss, Muscle Gain and Performance* [eBook]. Renaissance Periodization.

12. Jeukendrup, A., & Gleeson, M. (2010). *Sport Nutrition: An Introduction to Energy Production and Performance*. (2nd Ed.). Champaign, IL: Human Kinetics.

13. Pope, J., & Nizielski S. (2020). *Scientific American Nutrition for a Changing World (2nd ed)*. Macmillan Learning.

14. Prevost, M. (2015). *Built to Endure* [eBook]. Retrieved from http://built-to-endure.blogspot.com/.

15. Quinn, E. (16 March 2020). *Recommended Water Intake for Athletes during Exercise: Calculating Your Need and Hydration Schedule*. Retrieved from https://www.verywellfit.com/how-much-water-should-you-drink-3120428.

16. Rosenbloom, C., & Coleman, E. (2012). *Sports Nutrition A Practice Manual for Professionals*. (5th Ed). Chicago, IL: Academy of Nutrition and Dietetics.

17. Sheiko, B., Israetel, M., & Wilcox, D. (2018). *Powerlifting Foundations and Methods*. Renaissance Periodization.

18. Smith-Ryan, A., & Antonio, J. (2013). *Sports Nutrition & Performance Enhancing Supplements*. Ronkonkoma, NY: Linus Learning.

19. University of Michigan Health. (21 August 2019a). *Vitamins: Their Functions and Sources*. Retrieved from https://www.uofmhealth.org/health-library/ta3868.

20. University of Michigan Health. (21 August 2019b). Minerals: Their Functions and Sources. Retrieved from https://www.uofmhealth.org/health-library/ta3912.

21. Urine Colors (n.d.). *Urine Colors: Everything You Need to Know*. Retrieved from www.urine-colors.com.

22. U.S. Department of Health and Human Services and U.S. Department of Agriculture. (2010). *Dietary Guidelines for Americans.* (7th Ed). Retrieved from http://www.health.gov/dietaryguidelines/ 2010.asp.

23. U.S. Department of Health and Human Services and U.S. Department of Agriculture. (2015). *2015 – 2020 Dietary Guidelines for Americans.* (8th Ed.). Retrieved from http://health.gov/dietaryguidelines/ 2015/guidelines/.

24. Williams, M. (2007). *Nutrition for Health, Fitness, & Sport.* New York, NY: Mc-Graw Hill.

Chapter 3
Weight Management

Key Terms:

Android	Gynoid	Physical activity level factors
Basal metabolic rate	Hierarchy of fat loss	Positive energy balance
Body composition	High-intensity interval training	Positive nitrogen balance
Body mass index	Hyperthyroidism	Set point theory
Caloric balance	Hypertrophy	Subcutaneous fat
Caloric expenditure	Low-intensity steady state	Thermal effect of food
Circuit training	Meal planning made easy	Traditional resistance training
Circumference measurements	Metabolic resistance training	Visceral fat
Exercise activity thermogenesis	MyPlate	Waist circumference
Fat cell theory	Non-exercise activity thermogenesis	Waist-to-hip ratio
Food composition	Nutrient timing	Weight cycling
Food deserts	Obesity	Weight management
Glandular disorder theory	Percent body fat	

Learning Objectives:

- Understand the prevalence of obesity in America and the associated health problems
- Identify the current theories which describe and the factors which lead to weight gain
- Determine how to calculate individual daily caloric intake
- Outline strategies to lose weight effectively and maintain an overall healthy weight
- Describe various ways to assess body composition
- Learn to set realistic fat-loss goals through making permanent lifestyle changes
- Learn how to establish a healthy meal plan habit based on appropriate weight goals

CHAPTER 3: WEIGHT MANAGEMENT

Introduction

According to a 2010 online poll, 64% of Americans said the first thing they noticed about someone was how attractive they were. Another online poll reported that the majority of U.S. men admitted looks were more important than personality when determining a mate. Similarly, a 2017 study, found that men must be at least "moderately attractive" in order for a woman to consider his personality. And finally, a 2018 study found that 76% of Americans favor appearance over reliability when selecting their next car. These collective results are neither unexpected or surprising. American culture, as evidenced by the majority of reality television shows, clearly suggests that one's appearance is more important than their character.

But what about Christians? Is it wrong for Christians to consider looks when choosing a mate? And, how much time (if any) should Christians put into bettering their appearance? The Bible makes it clear that appearance is overrated and, at best, a temporary attribute (Prov. 11:22; 31:30). Additionally, the Bible shows that God is more concerned with a person's heart than he is the outward appearance (1 Sam. 16:7). This means that although our culture may value appearance over character; as Christians, our identity should not be found in how we look but rather in whom we serve (Eph. 1).

Prevalence of Obesity in America

Due to numerous advances in both nutrition and training, today's athletes are becoming bigger, stronger and faster than ever before. In fact, most of the current world records have been set in the last 5 - 10 years. **Table 3.1** lists some of the current world records in various endurance and strength sports.

Table 3.1. Current World Records in Various Endurance and Strength Sports

ENDURANCE SPORTS			STRENGTH SPORTS		
Event	Year Set	Record Holder	Event	Year Set	Record Holder
100-m	2009	Usain Bolt	Squat	2018	Vlad Alhazov
400-m	2016	Wayde van Niekerk	Bench Press	2019	Julius Maddox
1-Mile	1999	Hicham El Guerrouj	Deadlift	2020	Hafthor Bjornsson
Marathon	2018	Eliud Kipchoge	Snatch	2016	Lasha Talakhadze

How is it that athletes are becoming faster and stronger, yet the average U.S. adult is becoming more overweight and unfit? These physiological differences illustrate the disparity between technological advances and socioeconomic factors. **Figure 3.1.** illustrates the prevalence of **obesity** in U.S. adults by state and territory as reported by the Centers for Disease Control and Prevention (2020). The results depict the following:

- No state had an obesity trend < 20%
- Only the District of Columbia had an obesity trend between 20% and < 25%

- 8 states had an obesity trend between 25% and < 30%
- 22 states had an obesity trend between 30% and < 35%
- 17 states had an obesity trend between 35% and < 40%
- 2 states had an obesity trend ≥ 40%
- Southern states had the highest prevalence of obesity (36.3%), followed by the Midwest (35.4%), the Northeast (29.9%), and the West (28.7%)

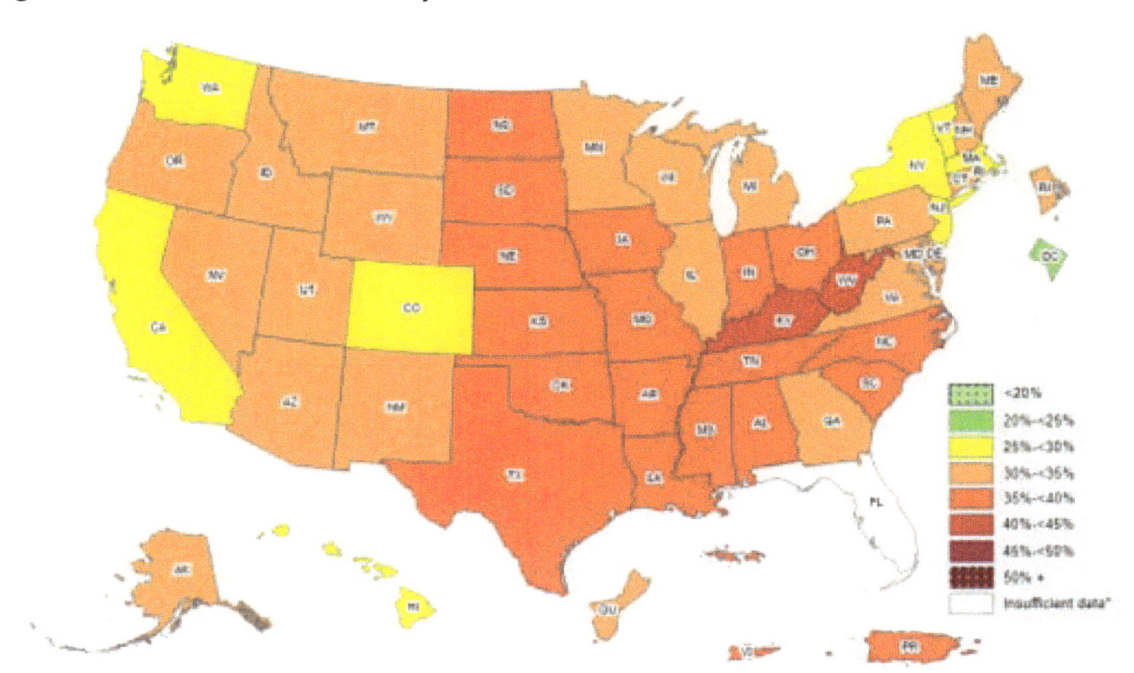

Figure 3.1. Prevalence of Obesity in U.S. Adults in 2021

According to the Centers for Disease Control and Prevention (2020), only Colorado and the District of Columbia reported obesity trends below 25%. According to their findings, the lower obesity trend, at least for Colorado, is likely due in part to a culture of outdoor recreation (e.g., hiking, skiing). In fact, 82.3% of the individuals surveyed admitted to being physically active within the past month (compared to a 76.2% median for the other states). However, the obesity trend for Colorado has doubled in just a little over a decade and is currently ranked higher for childhood obesity as compared to the other states. Due to relatively low number of participants and the transient nature of those interviewed, the Centers for Disease Control and Prevention estimates the actual obesity trend for the District of Columbia is much higher than that currently reported. The takeaway message is that the obesity trend for all Americans, regardless of state or territory, is on the rise.

Obesity rates also tend to be higher in areas of the country that are considered to be **food deserts** (i.e., areas that do not have easy access to a grocery store or transportation and are low-income households). Research shows that those living in food deserts also experience higher incidence of diabetes and lower access to healthcare (Pope, 2020; Lantz, 2010). **Figure 3.2** illustrates low access to grocery stores and low-income households.

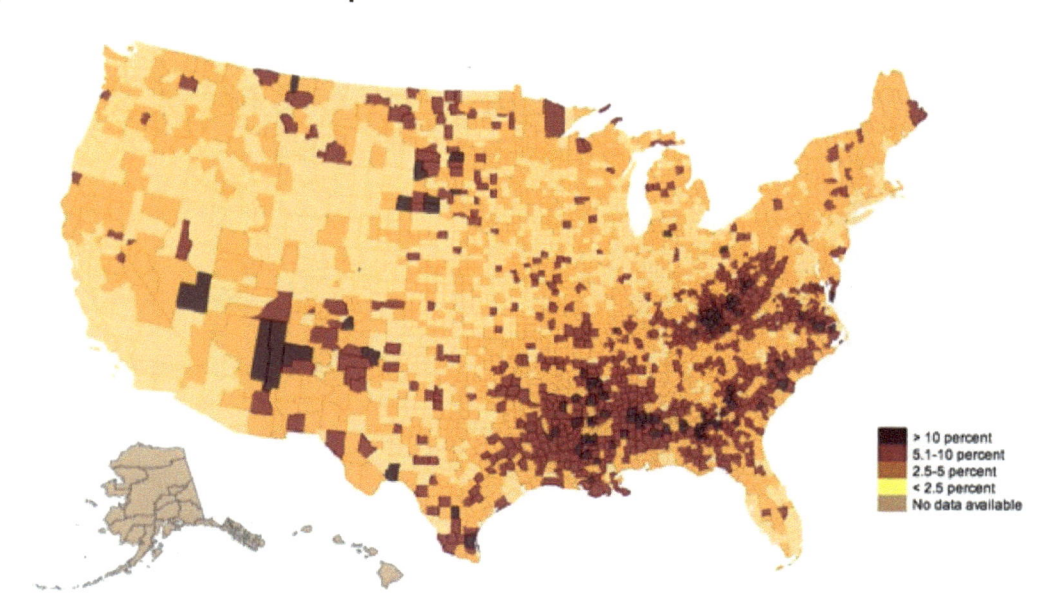

Figure 3.2. No Car and No Supermarket within a Mile

Obesity is a common, serious, and costly disease. Individuals with obesity are at greater risk for multiple diseases or conditions including:

- Heart disease
- Type 2 diabetes
- Gallbladder disease
- Certain types of cancer (e.g., endometrial, colon, gallbladder, prostate, kidney, breast)
- Sleep apnea
- Asthma
- Arthritis
- Incontinence (loss of bladder control)
- Depression

It is important to note that these conditions are correlated or related to obesity, not caused by obesity. There are numerous factors that contribute to the onset of various medical conditions to include family history, smoking, and lifestyle factors (e.g., diet, exercise, sleep, stress). The notion that an individual's eating habits is the only factor related to and contributing to obesity is simply unfair and biased. Similarly, **weight cycling** (aka yo-yo dieting or the process of repeated dieting resulting in the same few pounds being lost and then regained) is also associated with numerous negative health outcomes such as systemic inflammation, hypertension, insulin resistance, and hyperlipidemia (Montani et al., 2015; Strohacker & McFarlin, 2010).

Obesity Statistics

The Centers for Disease Control and Prevention (2022) provides the following statistics regarding the prevalence of obesity in the United States:

- In 2019, the estimated annual medical cost of obesity was $173 billion.

- From 1999 to 2020, the prevalence of obesity increased from 30.5% to 41.9%.

- From 1999 to 2020, the prevalence of severe obesity increased from 4.7% to 9.2%.

- In terms of ethnicity, non-Hispanic black adults had the highest prevalence of obesity (49.9%), followed by Hispanic adults (45.6%), non-Hispanic White adults (41.4%), and non-Hispanic Asian adults (16.1%).

- In terms of age, adults aged 40-59 years had the highest prevalence of obesity (44.3%), followed by adults aged 60 and older (41.5%), and adults aged 20-39 years (39.8%).

- In terms of socioeconomic status, adults without a high school degree or equivalent had the highest prevalence of obesity (37.8%), followed by adults with some college (35.6%) or high school graduates (35.5%), and then by college graduates (26.3%). Additionally, prevalence of obesity was lower in the lowest and highest income groups as compared with the middle-income group.

If current trends continue, it is estimated that 50% of American adults will be classified as obese (i.e., body mass index (BMI) values ≥30) by the year 2030 (Wang et al., 2011). The remedy seems to be in ensuring access to nutritious food and preventative healthcare, increasing physical activity, smoking cessation, stress and sleep management, and eating in a flexible manner that honors hunger, satiety, and appetite (Bacon et al., 2002; Bacon et al., 2005).

What Causes Weight Gain?

There are several theories as to what actually causes or leads to weight gain (Thygerson & Thygerson, 2016).

- **Fat cell theory.** This theory says that obese individuals have too many fat cells. People with an above-average number of fat cells may have been born with them or developed them over time as a result of overeating. It is believed that, through proper diet and exercise, individuals can decrease the size of fat cells but not the number.

- **Set point theory.** This theory says that obese individuals are genetically predisposed to carry a certain amount of weight. This predisposition is set and determined by the hypothalamus. This theory also states that losing weight, and keeping it off, is often times hard to do because the body strives to get back to its predisposed set point. In order to lose weight, and keep it off, the individual must somehow change their set point.

- **Glandular disorder theory.** This theory says that **hypothyroidism**, a condition in which the body does not produce enough thyroid hormone, is responsible for excessive weight gain and obesity. However, research has shown that overt hypothyroidism only causes modest weight gain (Sanyal & Raychaudhuri, 2016). Additionally, thyroid hormone treatment generally does not lead to significant weight loss.

- **Positive energy balance theory.** This theory says that weight gain occurs when caloric intake exceeds energy expenditure. In essence, the relationship between calories consumed and calories burned can result in one of the following three scenarios:
    - *Weight gain* = calories consumed > calories burned
    - *Weight loss* = calories consumed < calories burned
    - *Maintain weight* = calories consumed = calories burned

Other Factors Contributing to Weight Gain

There are several additional factors believed to contribute to weight gain and obesity to include (Thygerson & Thygerson, 2016):

- **Genetics.** More than 400 different genes are implicated in the development of obesity. Genes can contribute to obesity in several ways such as affecting appetite, satiety, metabolism, food cravings, fat distribution, and stress eating.

- **Diseases.** Certain illnesses affect the endocrine glands which can in turn cause weight gain. Some of these illnesses include hypothyroidism, polycystic ovarian syndrome and tumors on the pituitary gland, adrenal glands and/or pancreas.

- **Drugs.** Several drugs can increase appetite and/or slow metabolism thereby causing weight gain as a side effect. Some of these drugs include: corticosteroids, estrogen and progesterone, specific anti-cancer medications, antidepressants and certain psychiatric drugs.

- **Socioeconomic status.** Individuals who are below-average income, less-educated and/or unemployed have a higher incidence of obesity.

- **Age.** Fat mass tends to increase with age through adulthood and eventually decline when elderly.

- **Gender.** Obesity is more prevalent in women than in men.

- **Ethnicity.** Obesity is more prevalent in African-American, Hispanic, Native American and Pacific Islander populations. Although the exact causes for these disparities are not fully understood, it is believed to be due, at least in part, to differences in social and economic advantage related to ethnicity (Krueger & Reither, 2015).

- **Psychological factors.** Some individuals have used food as a means of coping with stress. Binge eating, and other unhealthy eating habits, can develop when eating becomes the primary means of dealing with stress (Fahey et al., 2011).

- **Dieting.** When an individual embarks on a diet, the body enacts self-protective measures in response to a perceived famine or starvation. When eating patterns are normalized, the body returns to a weight it prefers to be at for optimal function and health (Tomiyama et al., 2012).

Determining Daily Energy Requirements

Figure 3.3 depicts the percentages of caloric expenditure associated with the four major bodily processes: **basal metabolic rate** (i.e., rate at which the body uses energy at rest), **non-exercise activity thermogenesis** (i.e., amount of energy expended performing daily tasks), **thermal effect of food** (i.e., amount of energy expended processing food for use and storage), and **exercise activity thermogenesis** (i.e., amount of energy expended while exercising). As you can see from the pie chart, basal metabolic rate requires the most caloric expenditure and exercise requires the least, which may be a surprise to some. However, the percentage associated with exercise can increase significantly (e.g., up to 20-25%) for those individuals training at extremely high levels of intensity and/or volume (e.g., > 6 hours of training per day).

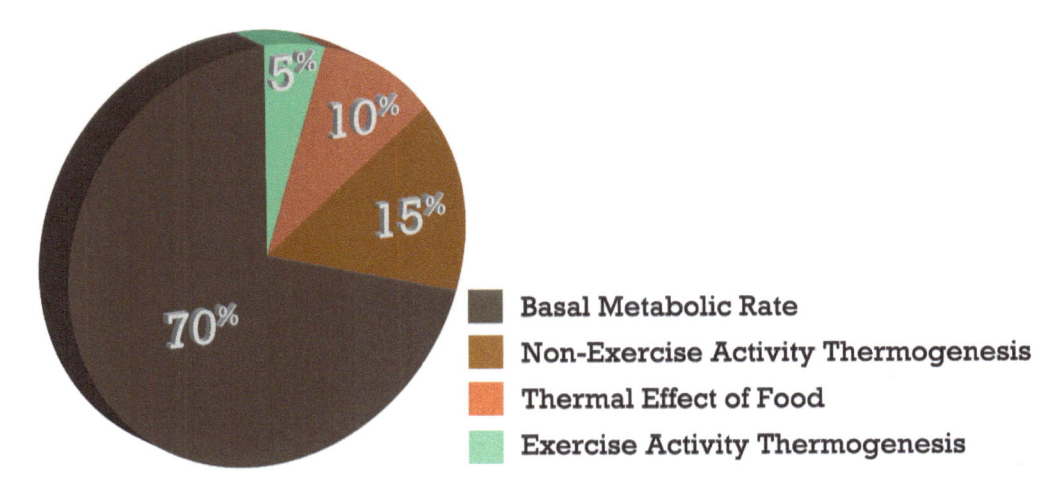

Figure 3.3. Components of and Their Contribution to Caloric Expenditure

An individual can determine the recommended number of calories by multiplying their target bodyweight (in lbs.) by the appropriate physical activity level (PAL) factor. **Table 3.2** assigns the associated factor with each of the different physical activity levels.

CHAPTER 3: WEIGHT MANAGEMENT

Table 3.2. Physical Activity Level (PAL) Factors

FACTOR	PHYSICAL ACTIVITY LEVEL
10-12	Sedentary
12-14	Lightly active (e.g., 30-60 min. of physical activity per day; 3-4 times a week)
14-16	Moderately active (e.g., 30-60 min. of physical activity per day; 4-6 times a week)
16-18	Very active (e.g., 1-2 hours of physical activity per day; 4-5 times a week)
19-23	Super active (e.g., 2-4 hours of physical activity per day; 5-6 times a week)

Using this information, for example, we can determine what the desired daily caloric intake should be for a 165-pound female who is lightly active and has a target (goal) weight of 135 pounds. This equates to a recommended daily intake of between 1,620 - 1,890 calories (i.e., 135 x 12 = 1,620; 135 x 14 = 1,890).

It is worth mentioning, that even if your goal is to lose weight, daily caloric intake should never go below 1,800 calories per day for males or 1,200 calories per day for females (Johnson & Morris, 2012). Additionally, Gilbert (2019) recommends that caloric intake should never go below 30 calories per kilogram, or 13.6 calories per pound, of lean body mass - regardless of gender. Going below these recommendations could result in failing to meet the minimum number of calories required by the basal metabolic rate. This will lower basal metabolic rate resulting in a cascade of negative responses including slowed metabolism and altered gastrointestinal (GI) processes. Failing to meet basic energy needs impacts bone health, sex hormones, the cardiovascular system, mood, and virtually every other vital body process.

Using our prior example, let's assume the female subject had an estimated percent body fat of 34% body, which equates to a lean body mass of 109 pounds (i.e., 165 x 0.34 = 56; 165 -56 = 109). So, the calculation for a daily caloric intake of somewhere between 1,620 - 1,890 calories per day is credible as it complies with both of the above recommendations: greater than 1,200 calories per day for females and greater than 13.6 calories per pound of lean body mass (i.e., 109 x 13.6 = 1,482).

Effective Weight Loss Strategies

In an attempt to lose weight and/or keep it off, many Americans have resorted to using various **weight management** strategies that have proven to be either unsafe or ineffective (e.g., severe calorie restriction, excessive exercise, weight loss pills and products). Fortunately, there are several weight management strategies that have proven to be both safe and effective (Fahey et al., 2011; Polivy & Herman, 2005; Thygerson & Thygerson, 2016). Some of these strategies include:

- Set reasonable and achievable goals (e.g., body weight, caloric intake, exercise requirements)
- Maintain a negative energy balance (e.g., 250 calorie deficit + 250 calorie increase in physical activity)
- Increase the amount of daily physical activity

- Make small, but permanent, changes in your diet:
    - Drink more water
    - Eat more lean protein
    - Eat more fruits and vegetables
    - Eat more high-fiber foods (e.g., whole grains, beans, legumes)
    - Eat small amounts of healthy fats
- Make small, but permanent, changes in your eating habits:
    - Eat less added sugar
    - Be conscious of portion sizes
    - Establish regular eating patterns (e.g., not going too long between meals and snacks)
    - Honor hunger and fullness cues (as restriction can lead to binging)

Hierarchy of Fat Loss

As mentioned previously, regular exercise is considered an effective weight management strategy. However, not all types of exercise will produce the same results. Research suggests that low-intensity steady-state exercise is relatively ineffective at promoting fat loss (Miller et al., 1997; Thorogood et al., 2011) and, despite decades of research, the physiological mechanisms by which exercise is used to regulate fat mass is still not clearly understood (Cosgrove, 2019; Melanson et al., 2009). Despite this uncertainty, current research suggests there may be a hierarchy of factors to consider in terms of losing body fat and keeping it off (Gilbert, 2019). **Figure 3.4** depicts this **hierarchy of fat loss**.

Figure 3.4. Hierarchy of Factors for Fat Loss

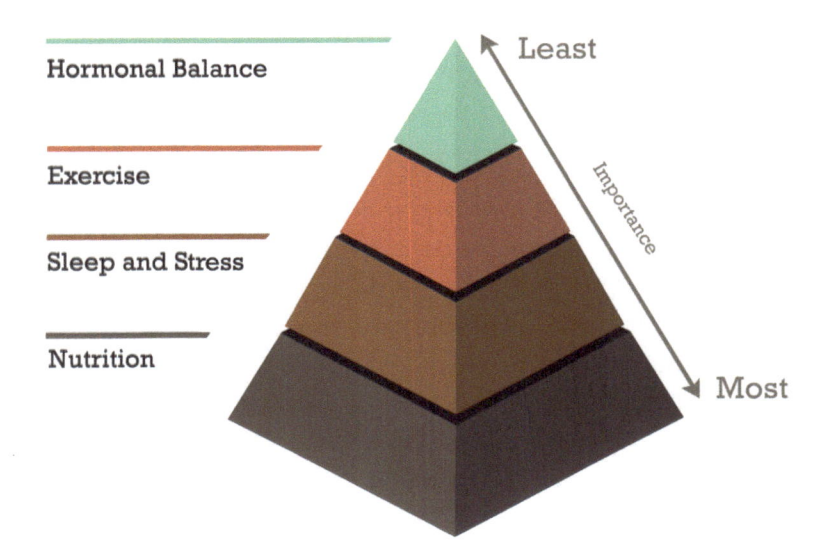

Chapter 3: Weight Management

Notice in **Figure 3.4**, nutrition is the most important factor and is fundamental in order to achieve fat loss. Israetel et al. (2019) proposes there is also a hierarchy in terms of nutritional priorities (**Figure 3.5**). Specifically, **caloric balance** (i.e., calories consumed vs. calories burned), macronutrient amounts (i.e., grams of carbohydrate, protein, and fat consumed per day), **nutrient timing** (i.e., when and how macronutrients are spread out across daily meals), **food composition** (i.e., sources of macronutrients consumed), and supplement use.

Figure 3.5. Hierarchy of Factors for Nutrition

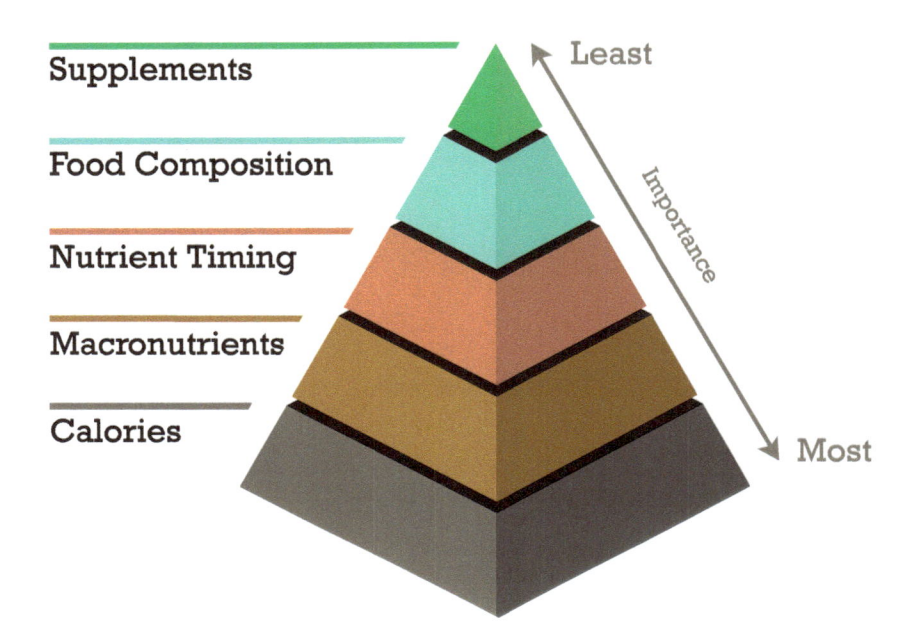

Just above nutrition, proper sleep and stress management plays the next most important role in effective weight management. We will be talking more about sleep and stress in **Chapter 4**. At the top of the list is hormonal balance. Although this topic will not be discussed in detail, hormones play a critical role in weight management. In addition to controlling blood sugar levels and insulin balance, hormones regulate our metabolism and therefore are intricately connected to the amount of fat gained or lost.

After sleep and stress management, exercise is the next most important factor in effective weight management. Just as with nutrition, there also seems to be a hierarchy in terms of the effectiveness of exercise in promoting fat loss (Cosgrove, 2019). As depicted in **Figure 3.6**, strength training (ST) and endurance training (ET) performed in combination is likely the best approach to losing body fat and keeping it off. However, current research would suggest that ST performed in isolation may be more effective than ET performed in isolation in terms of promoting fat loss. Additionally, some forms of ST seem to be more effective than others. According to Cosgrove (2019), **metabolic resistance training (MRT)** and **circuit training** (aka high-intensity resistance training) seem to be more effective in terms of promoting fat loss than **traditional resistance**

training. Both MRT and circuit training involve performing multiple sets of the compound lifts. For MRT, the last set is comprised of at least three micro-sets with short intra-set rest periods interspersed (e.g., 20 seconds). The unique programming and execution of MRT is believed to result in a higher post-exercise caloric expenditure, up to four times higher, than traditional low-intensity steady state exercise (Cosgrove, 2019). Similarly, some forms of ET may be more effective than others. According to Swain & Franklin (2006), vigorous-intensity endurance training (e.g., high-intensity interval training (HIIT)) seems to promote more favorable results than low- to moderate-intensity endurance training (e.g., low-intensity steady state exercise (LISS)).

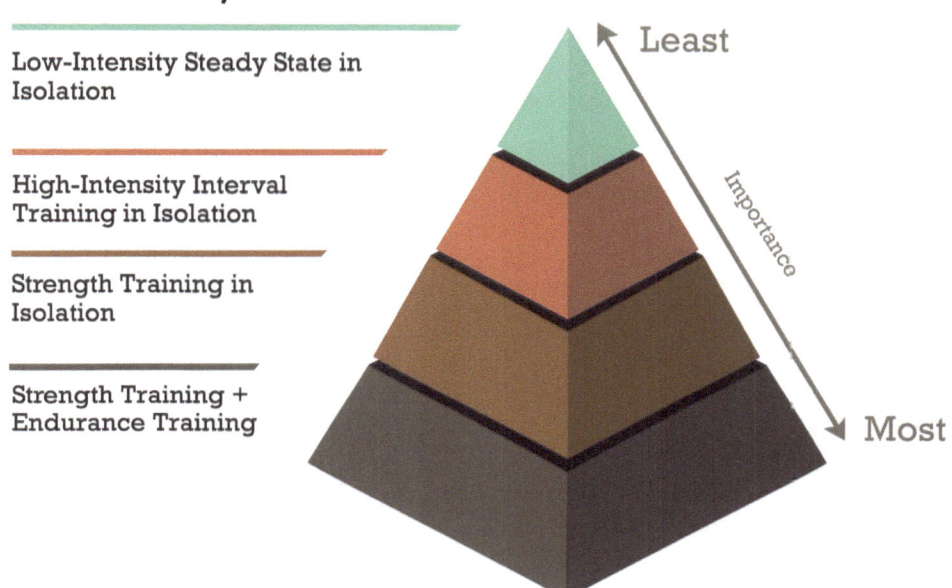

Figure 3.6. Hierarchy of Exercise for Fat Loss

Pyramid from top (Least Importance) to bottom (Most Importance):
- Low-Intensity Steady State in Isolation
- High-Intensity Interval Training in Isolation
- Strength Training in Isolation
- Strength Training + Endurance Training

As a result, Cosgrove (2019) assigns recommendations (**Table 3.3**) as to when and how to prioritize the different types of training based on the available amount of time to exercise each week. For example, if you only have 3 hours or less to exercise each week, and your primary fitness goal is to lose weight, then you should only perform ST, preferably MRT and/or circuit training. However, if you have between 3-6 hours or more to exercise each week, then you could engage in both ST and HIIT. If you have more than 6 hours to exercise each week you could engage in ST, HIIT, as well as LISS. Sample ST workouts for fat loss are provided in **Table 3.4**. Sample ET workouts for fat loss are provided in **Table 3.5**.

Table 3.3. Prioritizing Training for Fat Loss

Available Time	Recommended Exercise Type
≤ 3 hours per week	ST
3-6 hours per week	ST & HIIT
> 6 hours per week	ST, HIIT & LISS

Chapter 3: Weight Management

Table 3.4. Sample Strength Training Workouts for Fat Loss

METABOLIC RESISTANCE TRAINING (MRT)	CIRCUIT TRAINING	TRADITIONAL ST
4 sets of 8-10 reps: • Bench super-setted w/ Bent-Over Row 4 sets of 8-10 reps: • Squat super-setted w/ Overhead Press Deadlift Finisher: • Set 1: 70% of 5RM x 5 • Set 2: 75% of 5RM x 5 • Set 3: 80% of 5RM x 5 • Set 4: 65% of 5RM: • 20 reps then 20 sec rest • 10 reps then 20 sec rest • 5 reps 4 sets of 8-10 reps Hip Thrusters	3-5 rounds of 12-15 reps: • Chest Press • Lat Pulldowns • Overhead Press • Leg Press • Leg Curls • Back Extension No rest between exercises 2-3 min. rest between sets	• 3 x 6 Bench Press • 3 x 6 Bent Over Row • 3 x 6 Shoulder Press • 3 x 6 Back Squat • 3 x 6 Hex Bar Deadlift

Table 3.5. Sample Endurance Training Workouts for Fat Loss

SAMPLE HIIT	SAMPLE LISS
10 sets of: • 1-min at 90% of maximum intensity • 1-min at 50% of maximum intensity (Protocol can be performed using a variety of aerobic activities to include running, stationary bike, elliptical trainer, rower)	60 minutes of walking

Healthy Weight Gain

While the primary weight management goal for many is to lose weight (i.e., fat), for others the goal is to gain weight and increase muscle mass. Implementing an appropriate weight gain strategy will help individuals to safely gain weight by increasing the amount of muscle mass with little to no increase in fat mass. **Figure 3.7** depicts the three primary factors necessary for healthy weight gain.

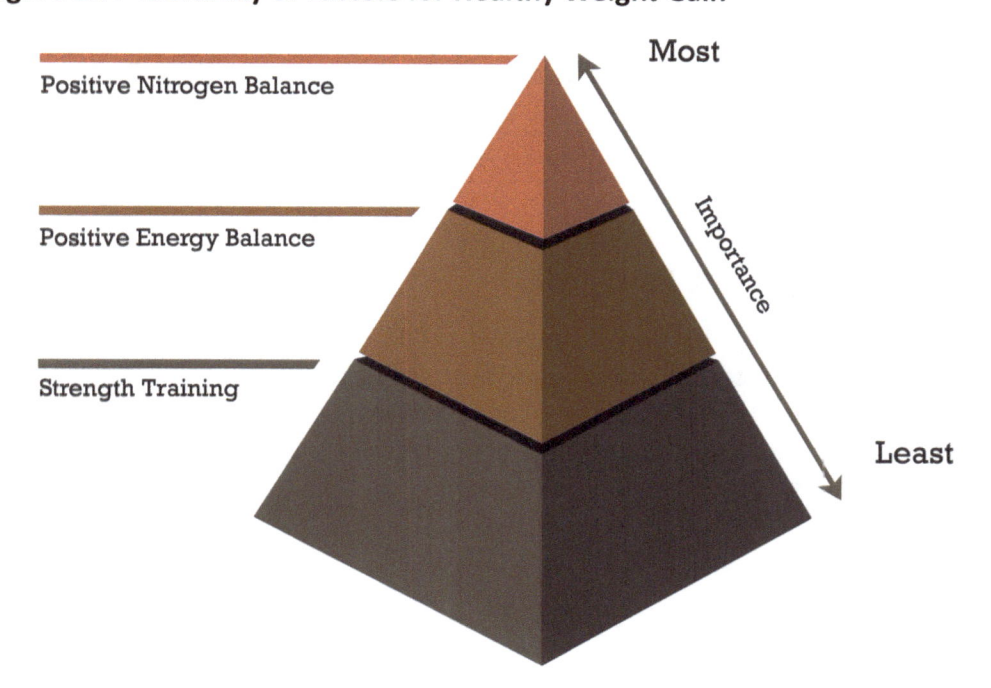

Figure 3.7. Hierarchy of Factors for Healthy Weight Gain

- Positive Nitrogen Balance
- Positive Energy Balance
- Strength Training

(Importance: Most → Least)

As depicted in **Figure 3.7**, the first factor necessary for healthy weight gain is regular participation in ST. Although we will go into more detail in **Chapter 6**, some basic recommendations regarding ST for healthy weight gain include performing multiple sets of 6-12 reps as well as participation in each of the compound lifts (i.e., bench, row, press, squat, deadlift) at least once per week.

The second factor necessary for healthy weight gain is maintaining a **positive energy balance**. In other words, regularly consuming more calories in the diet than is expended via exercise. A realistic goal for healthy weight gain is to increase body weight by 0.5 to 1.0 pound per week. For most individuals, this is best achieved by consuming an additional 300-500 calories per day. The composition of calories should also be considered. Specifically, it is recommended that 55-60% of the calories consumed per day should come from carbohydrates as this helps to prevent muscle protein breakdown and encourage protein synthesis.

The third factor necessary for healthy weight gain is maintaining a **positive nitrogen balance** (i.e., protein intake exceeds protein loss). Although carbohydrates are necessary in order to prevent muscle protein breakdown and encourage protein synthesis, it is important to note that protein intake also plays an important role in this process. If the primary goal is to gain weight, then protein should be elevated to about twice the recommended dietary allowance (RDA) for general health. This can be achieved by prioritizing lean protein sources at each meal (to include snacks). It is also recommended that the additional protein come from whole food sources instead of from sport foods and/or supplements as often as possible. **Table 3.6** provides specific macronutrient intake recommendations for those individuals interested in general health as well as those interested in gaining muscle mass (Israetel et al., 2019).

CHAPTER 3: WEIGHT MANAGEMENT

Table 3.6. Macronutrient Intake Recommendations

	CARBOHYDRATES	PROTEIN	FAT
General Health	0.3 - 5.0 g / lb. / day	0.3 - 2.0 g / lb. / day	0.3 g / lb. / day
Hypertrophy (Size)	1.0 - 2.5 g / lb. / day	0.7 - 2.0 g / lb. / day	0.3 g / lb. / day

Body Composition and Percent Body Fat

Now that we know how to safely and effectively lose weight (fat), let's learn how much fat body fat is needed for good health. Body composition is any method of measure (e.g., skinfolds, hydrostatic weighing, air displacement plethysmography) used to determine the percentages of fat, muscle, bone, and water within the body. **Table 3.7** provides the ideal body fat percentages for adult males and females (Bryant & Green, 2010).

Table 3.7. Ideal Body Fat Percentages

DESCRIPTION	MALES	FEMALES
Essential Fat	2 - 5%	10 - 13%
Athlete	6 - 13%	14 - 20%
Fitness	14 - 17%	21 - 24%
Average	18 - 24%	25 - 31%
Obese	25% +	32% +

There are two basic types of fat: subcutaneous and visceral. **Subcutaneous fat** is stored immediately below the dermis layer of the skin and is not necessarily hazardous to your health. However, **visceral fat**, which is the unseen fat stored around your internal organs, is considered to be hazardous to your health. In fact, visceral fat is linked to several metabolic disorders and diseases such as: insulin resistance, impaired glucose tolerance, type 2 diabetes, dyslipidemia (abnormal amount of lipids (e.g., triglycerides, cholesterol) in the blood), and cancer. **Figure 3.8** depicts the different types and location of fat.

Figure 3.8. Visceral vs. Subcutaneous Fat

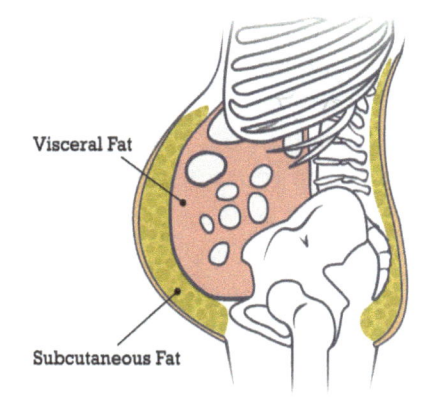

A CHRISTIAN GUIDE TO BODY STEWARDSHIP, DIET AND EXERCISE

The location of body fat also seems to play an important role in health and disease risk. Individuals who carry more fat around their waist are at a greater health and disease risk than individuals who carry it elsewhere in the body. Generally speaking, males accumulate more fat around their waist thus giving them an apple-shaped (aka **android**) appearance. Conversely, females generally accumulate more fat around their hips and buttocks thus giving them a pear-shaped (aka **gynoid**) appearance. **Figure 3.9** depicts the two primary body fat distribution patterns.

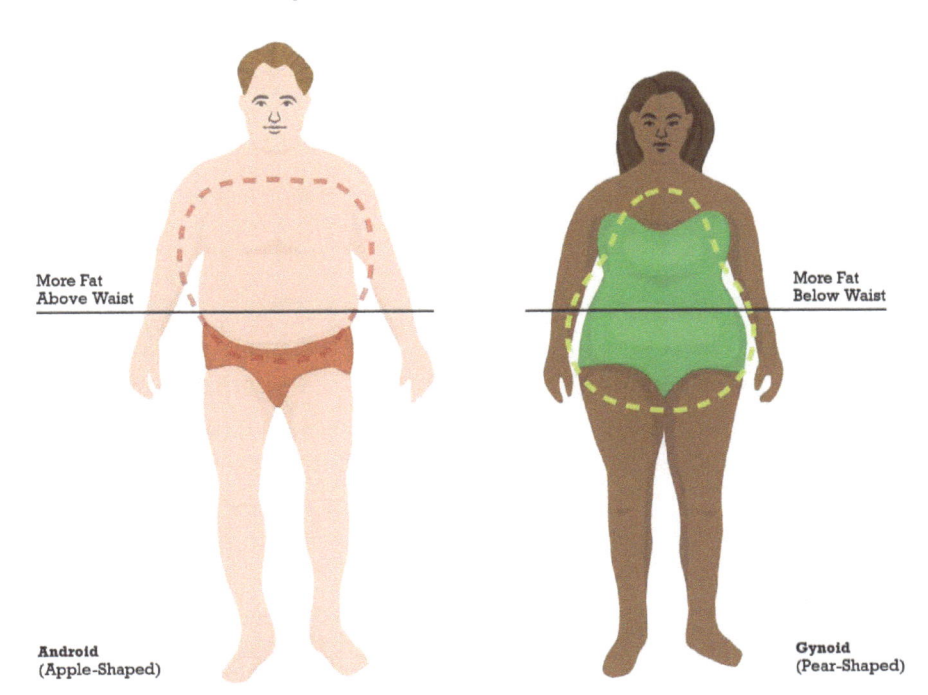

Figure 3.9. Android and Gynoid Fat Distribution Patterns

Techniques for Assessing Body Composition

Circumference Measurements (aka Girth Measurements). Circumference measurements are measurements taken at specific anatomical sites that can be used to assess body size. Although circumference measurements by themselves, tell us very little about actual body composition, this can be an effective means of assessing progress toward meeting body composition goals. For example, increases in upper arm girth can be testament of muscle **hypertrophy** as a result of regular ST. Similarly, a decrease in waist girth can be testament of fat loss as a result of regular exercise and healthy dietary practices. **Figure 3.10** depicts some of the positive changes that can occur in body composition as a result of regular exercise. For this reason, regular circumference measurement should be performed in addition to weekly weigh-ins. Weigh-ins alone cannot determine if fluctuations in weight following exercise and/or dieting are a result of fat loss, muscle gain or both. Estimated percent body fat percentages based on waist circumference are provided in **Appendix B** (Latour et al., 2019).

Figure 3.10. Changes in Body Composition as a Result of Regular Exercise

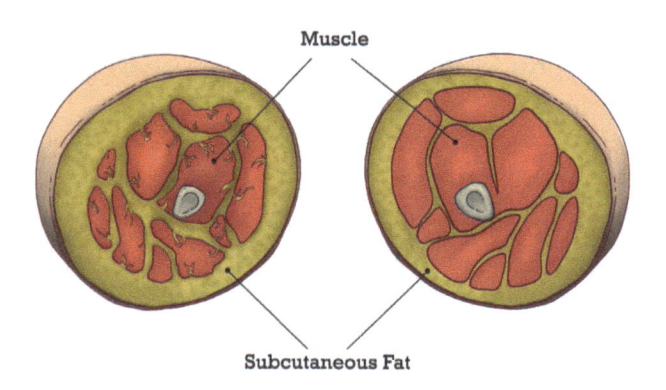

Waist circumference (WC). Waist circumference is a measurement taken around the abdomen at the level of the umbilicus and used to assess health risk. As mentioned previously, there is a strong correlation between excessive abdominal fat and a number of metabolic disorders and diseases. In fact, research has shown an increase in health risk with every one-inch increase in waist circumference (Peterson & Rittenhouse, 2019). The relative risk categories for WC are provided in **Table 3.8**.

Table 3.8. Relative Health Risk Categories for Waist Circumference

HEALTH RISK CATEGORY	MALES	FEMALES
Very Low	< 31.5 in.	< 27.5 in.
Low	31.5 - 39.0 in.	27.5 - 35.0 in.
High	39.5 - 47.0 in.	35.5 - 43.0 in.
Very High	> 47.0 in.	> 43.5 in.

Waist-to-hip ratio (WHR). Waist-to-hip ratio is the ratio of the circumference of the waist to that of the hips. WHR is calculated by dividing the waist measurement (taken at the level of the umbilicus) by the hip measurement [waist (in.) / hips (in.)]. WC and WHR may be even better predictors of health risk than percent body fat since both methods take into consideration the location of fat and not just the amount. Relative risk ratings for WHR are provided in **Table 3.9**.

Table 3.9. Relative Health Risk Ratings for Waist to Hip Ratio

GENDER	EXCELLENT	GOOD	AVERAGE	AT RISK
Males	< 0.85	0.85 - 0.89	0.90 - 0.95	≥ 0.95
Females	< 0.75	0.75 - 0.79	0.80 - 0.86	≥ 0.86

Body mass index (BMI). BMI provides a descriptive ratio between body weight and height. Although BMI may be a relatively accurate predictor of health risk for most individuals, it has been shown to over predict health risk for individuals who are extremely muscular or have large frames. Additionally, BMI has been shown to under predict health risk for older individuals with decreased muscle mass and excess body fat. BMI is calculated by dividing one's weight in kilograms (kg) by the square of one's height in meters (m) [BMI = wt (kg) / ht^2 (m)]. **Table 3.10.** provides the different BMI classifications. **Table 3.11** is a quick reference chart to determine BMI classification.

Table 3.10. BMI Classifications.

Weight Categories	BMI (kg / m²)
Underweight	18.5
Healthy Weight	18.5 - 24.9
Overweight	25 - 29.9
Obese	30 - 34.9
Severely Obese	35 - 39.9
Morbidly Obese	≥ 40

Chapter 3: Weight Management

Table 3.11. Body Mass Index

BMI	19	20	21	22	23	24	25	26	27	28	29	30	31	32	33	34	35	36	37	38	39	40	41	42	43	44	45	46	47	48	49	50	51	52	53	54
	Normal						Overweight					Obese										Extremely Obese														
58	91	96	100	105	110	115	119	124	129	134	138	143	148	153	158	162	167	172	177	181	186	191	196	201	205	210	215	220	224	229	234	239	244	248	253	258
59	94	99	104	109	114	119	124	128	133	138	143	148	153	158	163	168	173	178	183	188	193	198	203	208	212	217	222	227	232	237	242	247	252	257	262	267
60	97	102	107	112	118	123	128	133	138	143	148	153	158	163	168	174	179	184	189	194	199	204	209	215	220	225	230	235	240	245	250	255	261	266	271	276
61	100	106	111	116	122	127	132	137	143	148	153	158	164	169	174	180	185	190	195	201	206	211	217	222	227	232	238	243	248	254	259	264	269	275	280	285
62	104	109	115	120	126	131	136	142	147	153	158	164	169	175	180	186	191	196	202	207	213	218	224	229	235	240	246	251	256	262	267	273	278	284	289	295
63	107	113	118	124	130	135	141	146	152	158	163	169	175	180	186	191	197	203	208	214	220	225	231	237	242	248	254	259	265	270	278	282	287	293	299	304
64	110	116	122	128	134	140	145	151	157	163	169	174	180	186	192	197	204	209	215	221	227	232	238	244	250	256	262	267	273	279	285	291	296	302	308	314
65	114	120	126	132	138	144	150	156	162	168	174	180	186	192	198	204	210	216	222	228	234	240	246	252	258	264	270	276	282	288	294	300	306	312	318	324
66	118	124	130	136	142	148	155	161	167	173	179	186	192	198	204	210	216	223	229	235	241	247	253	260	266	272	278	284	291	297	303	309	315	322	328	334
67	121	127	134	140	146	153	159	166	172	178	185	191	198	204	211	217	223	230	236	242	249	255	261	268	274	280	287	293	299	306	312	319	325	331	338	344
68	125	131	138	144	151	158	164	171	177	184	190	197	203	210	216	223	230	236	243	249	256	262	269	276	282	289	295	302	308	315	322	328	335	341	348	354
69	128	135	142	149	155	162	169	176	182	189	196	203	209	216	223	230	236	243	250	257	263	270	277	284	291	297	304	311	318	324	331	338	345	351	358	365
70	132	139	146	153	160	167	174	181	188	195	202	209	216	222	229	236	243	250	257	264	271	278	285	292	299	306	313	320	327	334	341	348	355	362	369	376
71	136	143	150	157	165	172	179	186	193	200	208	215	222	229	236	243	250	257	265	272	279	286	293	301	308	315	322	329	338	343	351	358	365	372	379	386
72	140	147	154	162	169	177	184	191	199	206	213	221	228	235	242	250	258	265	272	279	287	294	302	309	316	324	331	338	346	353	361	368	375	383	390	397
73	144	151	159	166	174	182	189	197	204	212	219	227	235	242	250	257	265	272	280	288	295	302	310	318	325	333	340	348	355	363	371	378	386	393	401	408
74	148	155	163	171	179	186	194	202	210	218	225	233	241	249	256	264	272	280	287	295	303	311	319	326	334	342	350	358	365	373	381	389	396	404	412	420
75	152	160	168	176	184	192	200	208	216	224	232	240	248	256	264	272	279	287	295	303	311	319	327	335	343	351	359	367	375	383	391	399	407	415	423	431
76	156	164	172	180	189	197	205	213	221	230	238	246	254	263	271	279	287	295	304	312	320	328	336	344	353	361	369	377	385	394	402	410	418	426	435	443
Ht. (in.)																						Weight (lbs.)															

Meal Planning Made Easy

As mentioned previously, proper nutrition is likely the most important factor in effective weight management. As a result, implementing a safe eating strategy that can be maintained is imperative for both long-term health and keeping the weight off. To help develop healthy dietary habits, the U.S. Department of Agriculture (n.d.) developed the **MyPlate** initiative which provides dietary guidelines regarding daily caloric intake and consumption of the five major food groups: fruits, vegetables, grains, protein and dairy. Likewise, **Meal Planning Made Easy (MPME)** was developed using these MyPlate guidelines. Additional information regarding the recommended timing, serving size, and specific examples for the different food groups is provided in **Appendix C**.

Meal Planning Made Easy is not a diet plan, but rather a proposed eating strategy. In essence, MPME helps users to meet their goal number of calories, based on their physical activity classification and desired weight management goal (i.e., lose weight, gain weight, maintain weight), as well as maintain the recommended number of servings for each food group per day.

As with any eating strategy, there are potential benefits and limitations associated with this program. Provided below are some potential pros and cons associated with MPME.

Pros:
- No counting calories
- Helps to prevent / limit nutritional deficiencies
- Allows for a vast array of food choices
- Can be tailored to vegan, vegetarian and dairy-free diet plans

Cons:
- Proposed timing of certain food subgroups may not work for everyone
- Serving sizes within some food groups vary considerably
- Does not account for food combinations (e.g., casseroles, soups, stews)

Figure 3.11 provides some healthy plate options for breakfast, lunch and dinner. These options are designed to help MPME users meet the daily caloric intake and consumption recommendations proposed by MyPlate for the five major food groups (i.e., fruits, vegetables, grains, protein and dairy).

Figure 3.11. Healthy Plate Options for Specific Meals

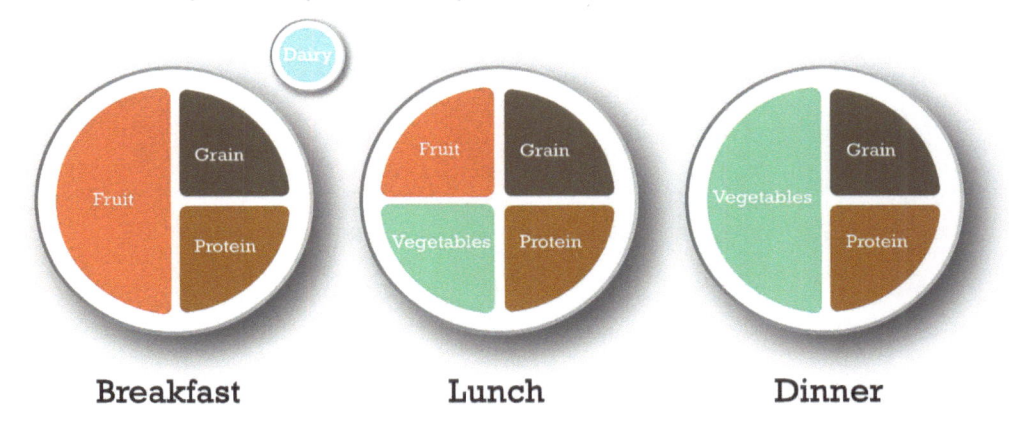

Breakfast   Lunch   Dinner

MPME Directions for Use

1. Use Chart A (**Table 3.12**) to determine which meal plan to use based on your bodyweight and activity level (using **Table 3.13**).

2. Use Chart B (**Table 3.14**) to determine how many servings of each food group you should consume at each meal.

3. If lactose intolerant, substitute dairy requirements with items from the protein food group.

4. If vegan / vegetarian, select only non-animal items from the protein food group.

5. Click on the link at the bottom for additional choices from each food group.

    NOTE: If alternative food items are selected, additional research will be required in order to determine the appropriate serving size to meet the goal number of kcal from each food group (e.g., 75 kcal for fruit, etc.).

6. If your goal is to **lose weight**, consider using a meal plan one letter down the chart (e.g., C → B).

7. If your goal is to **gain weight**, consider using a meal plan one letter up the chart (e.g., C → D).

8. Evaluate progress by weighing yourself **once** a week. For consistency purposes, weigh in on the same day and same time each week.

    For weight loss: Strive to lose 1-2 lbs. per week

    For weight gain: Strive to gain 0.5-1 lb. per week

9. Adjustments may be required to your meal plan in order to achieve weight management goals.

    Not losing weight? Consider using a meal plan two letters down the chart (e.g., C → A).

    Not gaining weight? Consider using a meal plan two letters up the chart (e.g., C → E).

Table 3.12. Chart A: Meal Plan Assignment

Bodyweight (lbs.)	Sedentary	Lightly Active	Moderately Active	Very Active
100	A	A	B	C
105	A	A	B	D
110	A	A	C	D
115	A	B	D	E
120	A	B	D	F
125	A	C	E	F
130	B	C	E	G
135	B	D	F	H
140	B	D	F	H
145	C	E	F	I
150	C	E	G	I
155	D	E	H	J
160	D	F	H	J
165	D	F	I	K
170	E	G	I	K
175	E	H	J	L
180	F	H	J	L
185	F	I	K	L
190	F	I	K	M
195	G	I	K	N
200	G	J	L	N
205	H	J	L	O
210	H	J	M	O
215	H	K	M	P
220	I	K	N	P
225	I	L	N	Q

*Continued on next page

CHAPTER 3: WEIGHT MANAGEMENT

BODYWEIGHT (LBS.)	SEDENTARY	LIGHTLY ACTIVE	MODERATELY ACTIVE	VERY ACTIVE
230	J	L	O	R
235	J	L	O	S
240	J	L	P	S
245	J	M	P	T
250	K	N	Q	T
255	K	N	Q	U
260	K	N	R	U
265	L	O	S	U
270	L	O	S	V
275	L	P	T	V
280	M	P	T	W
285	M	P	T	W
290	M	Q	U	X
295	N	Q	U	X
300	N	R	V	X

TABLE 3.13. PHYSICAL ACTIVITY CLASSIFICATIONS

	DESCRIPTION
Sedentary	Little to no planned physical activity per week
Lightly Active	30-60 min. of physical activity per day 3-4 times per week
Moderately Active	30-60 min. of physical activity per day 4-6 times per week
Very Active	1-2 hours of physical activity per day 4-6 times per week

A Christian Guide to Body Stewardship, Diet and Exercise

Table 3.14. Chart B: Proposed Meal Plan

Meal Plan		A		B		C		D		E		F		G		H	
Breakfast		Fruit	1	Fruit	2	Fruit	2	Fruit	2	Fruit	2	Fruit	2	Fruit	2	Fruit	2
		Grain	1	Grain	1	Grain	1	Grain	1	Grain	1	Grain	1	Grain	1	Grain	1
		Protein	1	Protein	1	Protein	1	Protein	1	Protein	1	Protein	1	Protein	1	Protein	1
		Dairy	1	Dairy	1	Dairy	1	Dairy	1	Dairy	1	Dairy	1	Dairy	1	Dairy	1
Snack		Fruit	-	Fruit	-	Fruit	-	Fruit	-	Fruit	2	Fruit	2	Fruit	2	Fruit	1
		Dairy	-	Dairy	-	Dairy	-	Dairy	1	Dairy	1	Dairy	1	Dairy	1	Dairy	1
Lunch		Fruit	1	Fruit	1	Fruit	2	Fruit	2	Fruit	2	Fruit	2	Fruit	2	Fruit	2
		Vegetable	1	Vegetable	2	Vegetable	2	Vegetable	2	Vegetable	2	Vegetable	2	Vegetable	2	Vegetable	2
		Grain	1	Grain	1	Grain	1	Grain	1	Grain	1	Grain	1	Grain	1	Grain	1
		Protein	1	Protein	1	Protein	1	Protein	1	Protein	1	Protein	1	Protein	1	Protein	2
Snack		Grain	-	Grain	-	Grain	-	Grain	-	Grain	-	Grain	-	Grain	1	Grain	1
		Dairy	-	Dairy	-	Dairy	-	Dairy	-	Dairy	-	Dairy	1	Dairy	1	Dairy	1
Dinner		Vegetable	1	Vegetable	1	Vegetable	2	Vegetable	2	Vegetable	2	Vegetable	2	Vegetable	2	Vegetable	2
		Grain	1	Grain	1	Grain	1	Grain	1	Grain	1	Grain	1	Grain	1	Grain	1
		Protein	1	Protein	1	Protein	1	Protein	1	Protein	1	Protein	1	Protein	1	Protein	1

61

Chapter 3: Weight Management

Meal Plan		I		J		K		L		M		N		O		P	
Breakfast		Fruit	2	Fruit	2	Fruit	2	Fruit	2	Fruit	2	Fruit	2	Fruit	2	Fruit	2
		Grain	1	Grain	1	Grain	1	Grain	2	Grain	2	Grain	2	Grain	2	Grain	2
		Protein	1	Protein	2	Protein	2	Protein	2	Protein	2	Protein	2	Protein	2	Protein	2
		Dairy	1	Dairy	1	Dairy	1	Dairy	1	Dairy	1	Dairy	2	Dairy	2	Dairy	2
Snack		Fruit	1	Fruit	1	Fruit	1	Fruit	1	Fruit	1	Fruit	1	Fruit	1	Fruit	1
		Dairy	1	Dairy	1	Dairy	1	Dairy	1	Dairy	1	Dairy	1	Dairy	2	Dairy	2
Lunch		Fruit	2	Fruit	2	Fruit	2	Fruit	2	Fruit	2	Fruit	2	Fruit	2	Fruit	2
		Vegetable	2	Vegetable	2	Vegetable	2	Vegetable	2	Vegetable	2	Vegetable	2	Vegetable	2	Vegetable	2
		Grain	1	Grain	1	Grain	2	Grain	2	Grain	2	Grain	2	Grain	2	Grain	2
		Protein	2	Protein	2	Protein	2	Protein	2	Protein	2	Protein	2	Protein	2	Protein	2
Snack		Grain	1	Grain	1	Grain	1	Grain	1	Grain	1	Grain	1	Grain	1	Grain	1
		Dairy	1	Dairy	1	Dairy	1	Dairy	1	Dairy	1	Dairy	1	Dairy	1	Dairy	2
Dinner		Vegetable	2	Vegetable	2	Vegetable	2	Vegetable	2	Vegetable	2	Vegetable	2	Vegetable	2	Vegetable	2
		Grain	1	Grain	1	Grain	1	Grain	2	Grain	2	Grain	2	Grain	2	Grain	2
		Protein	2	Protein	2	Protein	2	Protein	2	Protein	2	Protein	2	Protein	2	Protein	2

A Christian Guide to Body Stewardship, Diet and Exercise

Meal Plan		Q		R		S		T		U		V		W		X	
Breakfast		Fruit	2	Fruit	3	Fruit	3	Fruit	3	Fruit	3	Fruit	3	Fruit	3	Fruit	3
		Grain	2	Grain	2	Grain	2	Grain	2	Grain	2	Grain	2	Grain	3	Grain	3
		Protein	2	Protein	2	Protein	2	Protein	2	Protein	2	Protein	2	Protein	2	Protein	2
		Dairy	2	Dairy	2	Dairy	2	Dairy	2	Dairy	2	Dairy	2	Dairy	2	Dairy	2
Snack		Fruit	1	Fruit	2	Fruit	2	Fruit	3	Fruit	3	Fruit	3	Fruit	3	Fruit	3
		Dairy	2	Dairy	2	Dairy	2	Dairy	2	Dairy	2	Dairy	2	Dairy	2	Dairy	2
Lunch		Fruit	2	Fruit	2	Fruit	2	Fruit	3	Fruit	3	Fruit	3	Fruit	3	Fruit	3
		Vegetable	2	Vegetable	2	Vegetable	3	Vegetable	3	Vegetable	3	Vegetable	3	Vegetable	3	Vegetable	3
		Grain	2	Grain	2	Grain	2	Grain	2	Grain	3	Grain	3	Grain	3	Grain	3
		Protein	2	Protein	2	Protein	2	Protein	2	Protein	2	Protein	2	Protein	2	Protein	2
Snack		Grain	2	Grain	2	Grain	2	Grain	2	Grain	2	Grain	2	Grain	2	Grain	2
		Dairy	2	Dairy	2	Dairy	2	Dairy	2	Dairy	2	Dairy	2	Dairy	2	Dairy	2
Dinner		Vegetable	2	Vegetable	2	Vegetable	3	Vegetable	3	Vegetable	3	Vegetable	3	Vegetable	3	Vegetable	3
		Grain	2	Grain	2	Grain	2	Grain	2	Grain	2	Grain	3	Grain	3	Grain	3
		Protein	2	Protein	2	Protein	2	Protein	2	Protein	2	Protein	2	Protein	2	Protein	3

CHAPTER 3: WEIGHT MANAGEMENT

Summary

- Obesity is a common, serious, and costly disease where individuals with obesity are at greater risk for multiple diseases and unhealthy bodily conditions.

- There are several factors related to the cause of weight gain including an individual's genetics, age, socioeconomic status, gender, current diseases, drug interactions, ethnicity and psychological state.

- Total daily calorie expenditure can be calculated by evaluating resting metabolic rate, exercise expenditure and the thermic effect of food.

- Effective strategies for weight loss require reasonable weight loss goals, a positive energy balance, an increase in physical activity, and small, but permanent changes in diet and eating habits.

- There is a hierarchy of factors to consider in terms of losing body fat and keeping it off starting with balanced nutrition, adequate sleep and stress management, regular resistance training and normal hormone levels.

- Understanding the location of body fat plays an important role in managing health and disease risk and requires appropriate techniques for assessing body composition

- Implementing a safe and sustainable eating strategy is imperative for both long-term health and keeping weight off.

References

1. Bacon, L., Keim, N., Van Loan, M., Derricote, M., Gale, B., Kazaks, A., Stern, J. (2002). *Evaluating a 'Non-Diet' Wellness Intervention for Improvement of Metabolic Fitness, Psychological Well-Being and Eating and Activity Behaviors.* International Journal of Obesity & Related Metabolic Disorders, 26(6), 854-865.

2. Bacon, L., Stern, J., Van Loan, M., & Keim, N. (2005). *Size Acceptance and Intuitive Eating Improve Health for Obese, Female Chronic Dieters.* Journal of the American Dietetic Association, pp.929-936.

3. Bryant, C. X., & Green, D. J. (Eds.). (2010). *ACE Personal Trainer Manual: The Ultimate Resource for Fitness Professionals.* (4th ed.). San Diego, CA: American Council on Exercise.

4. Centers for Disease Control and Prevention (2022, September). *Adult Obesity Prevalence Maps.* Retrieved from https://www.cdc.gov/obesity/data/prevalence-maps.html.

5. Cosgrove, A. (2019, August). *Unlocking Fat Loss.* Seminar presented at Perform Better Functional Training Summit, Providence, RI.

6. Fahey, T., Insel, P., & Roth, W. (2011). *Fit & Well: Core Concepts and Labs in Physical Fitness and Wellness.* (9th Ed.). New York, NY: McGraw Hill.

7. Gilbert, A. (2019, August). *But I'm Doing Everything Right*. Seminar presented at Perform Better Functional Training Summit, Providence, RI.

8. Israetel, M., Davis, M., Case, J., & Hoffman, J. (2019). *The Renaissance Diet 2.0: Your Scientific Guide to Fat Loss, Muscle Gain and Performance* [eBook]. Renaissance Periodization.

9. Johnson, P., & Morris, D. *Physical Fitness and the Christian.* (5th Ed.). Dubuque, IA: Kendall Hunt.

10. Krueger, P., & Reither, E. (2015). *Mind the Gap: Race/Ethnic and Socioeconomic Disparities in Obesity*. Curr Diab Rep, 15(11):95.

11. Lantz PM, Golberstein E, House JS, Morenoff J. (2010). Socioeconomic and behavioral risk factors for mortality in a national 19-year prospective study of U.S. adults. *Social Science & Medicine*, 70, 1558-1566.

12. Latour, A., Peterson, D., & Riner, D. (2019). *Comparing Alternate Percent Body Fat Estimation Techniques for United States Navy Body Composition Assessment.* International Journal of Kinesiology in Hight Education, 3(4):1-13.

13. Melanson, E.L., Maclean, P.S., & Hill, J.O. 2009. *Exercise Improves Fat Metabolism in Muscle but does not Increase 24-hour Fat Oxidation.* Exer Sport Sci, 37(2):93-101.

14. Miller, W.C., Koceja, D.M., & Hamilton, E.J. 1997. *A Meta-Analysis of the Past 25 Years of Weight Loss Research using Diet, Exercise or Diet plus Exercise Intervention.* Int J Obes Relat Metab Disord, 21(10):941-947.

15. Montani, J., Schutz, Y, & Dulloo, A. (2015), Weight Cycling and Cardiometabolic Risks. Obes Rev, 16: 7-18.

16. Polivy, J., Herman, P. (2005). *The Effect of Deprivation on Food Cravings and Eating Behavior in Restrained and Unrestrained Eaters.* Int J Eat Disord., 38:301–309.

17. Pope, J., & Nizielski, S. (2020). *Scientific American Nutrition for a Changing World (2nd ed).* Macmillan Learning: Boston, MA.

18. Sanyal, D., & Raychaudhuri, M. (2016). Hypothyroidism and Obesity: An Intriguing Link. Indian J Endocrinol Metab, 20(4):554-557.

19. Strohacker, K., McFarlin, B. (2010). *Influence of Obesity, Physical Inactivity, and Weight Cycling on Chronic Inflammation.* Laboratory of Integrated Physiology, 2:98-104.

20. Swain, D., & Franklin, B. (2006). *Comparison of Cardioprotective Benefits of Vigorous Versus Moderate Intensity Aerobic Exercise.* Am J Cardiol, 97(1):141-7.

21. Thorogood, A., et al. 2011. *Isolated Aerobic Exercise and Weight Loss: A Systematic Review and Meta-Analysis of Randomized Controlled Trials.* Am J Med, 124(8):747-755.

22. Thygerson, A., & Thygerson, S. (2016). *Fit to be Well: Essential Concepts.* (4th Ed.). Burlington, MA: Jones & Bartlett Learning.

23. Tomiyama, A., Ahlstrom, B., & Mann, T. (2013). *Long-term Effects of Dieting: Is Weight Loss Related to Health?* Social and Personality Psychology Compass, 7:861-877.

24. U.S. Department of Agriculture. (n.d.). *ChooseMyPlate*. Retrieved from https://www.choosemyplate.gov/.

A CHRISTIAN GUIDE TO BODY STEWARDSHIP, DIET AND EXERCISE

Chapter 4
Stress Management and Sleep

Key Terms:

Alarm stage	Exhaustion stage	Self-induced stressors
Anxiety	Fight-or-flight response	Sleep deprivation
Chronic sleep deprivation	Insomnia	Sleep hygiene
Circadian biological clock	Inverted-U theory	Sleep-wake homeostasis
Cortisol	IZOF theory	Stress
Depression	Jet lag	Stress management
Distress	Melatonin	Stress response
Drive theory	Norepinephrine	Stressor
Emotional intelligence	Oxytocin	Sympathetic nervous system
Epinephrine	Relational wisdom	Tend-and-befriend response
Eustress	Resistance stage	

Learning Objectives:

- Explore what the Bible says about trials, anxiety, tribulation and sleep
- Understand what stress is, its causes and the difference between stress and stressors
- Explain the basic physiology of the stress response
- List signs and symptoms of prolonged stress and identify ways in which one can minimize self-caused stressors
- Understand the causes and treatment of depression and suicide
- Understand the scope, causes and effects of sleep deprivation
- Understand how much sleep one needs and identify ways to improve one's quality of sleep

CHAPTER 4: STRESS MANAGEMENT AND SLEEP

Introduction

Some people would like to believe that if they become a Christian everything will be okay; that God will somehow protect them from the different trials and tribulations of life. Unfortunately, Scripture does not support this theology. In fact, John 16:33 warns us that life in this world won't be easy and that we should expect "trouble." Fortunately, the passage goes on to say that because Christ has overcome the world, we can find peace in him. While the bad news is the stress we encounter in life is inevitable, the good news is that God is aware of our stress and desires to be our source of strength and refuge during stressful times (Psalm 46:1; Matthew 11:28-30). Additionally, God uses the stresses of life to produce godly character (James 1:2-4).

Research shows that, if left unchecked, chronic stress can lead to an array of serious health problems including physical illness, anxiety, and depression. So, effective stress management is important for long-term physical and mental health. Unfortunately, many people turn to unhealthy behaviors to deal and cope with stress (e.g., food, alcohol, drugs) instead of turning to God for help.

What is Stress?

Stress is the combination of mental, emotional, psychological, and physiological responses made by the body in response to a perceived harmful event or threat (Walters & Byl, 2021). These collective responses help the body to overcome or flee from physical threats. This phenomenon is sometimes called the **fight or flight response**. The events or situations that bring about stress are called **stressors**.

It is important to note that not all stress is bad stress. For example, **eustress** is considered to be good or beneficial stress. An example of eustress would be a class assignment that is perceived as neither too difficult nor too easy or a strenuous strength training workout. **Distress**, on the other hand, is considered to be bad or harmful stress. An example of distress would be having a crippling fear of public speaking yet being required to give an in-class presentation or coping with the death of loved one. In general, eustress helps to enhance performance, whether physical or mental, and distress tends to impair performance. There seems to be a fine line between eustress and distress. Any challenging event or situation will result in a **stress response**. Whether the event or situation is considered eustress or distress depends on how we perceive the stressor and whether it is transient or prolonged (Johnson & Morris, 2012).

Stress Theories

Research has shown a strong correlation between stress, performance and health (Selye, 1974). How the stress is perceived and the body's response can either positively or negatively impact performance. There are several theories that attempt to describe or define the relationship between stress and performance.

Drive Theory. The drive theory was one of the first theories to be developed and suggested a linear relationship between **arousal** (stress) and performance. It theorized that any stress, whether eustress or distress, would have a positive impact on performance. In essence, the greater the stress, the greater the performance (Hill, 1957). The drive theory is illustrated in **Figure 4.1**.

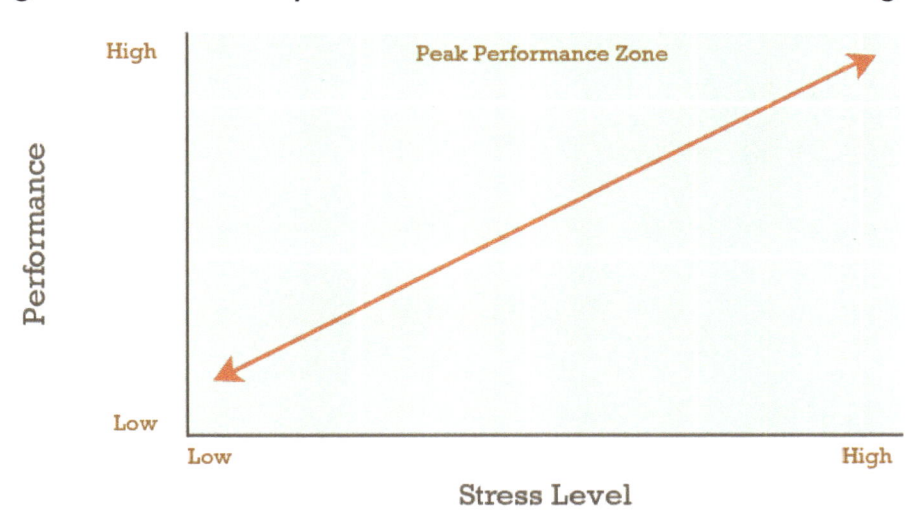

Figure 4.1. Relationship Between Stress and Performance According to the Drive Theory

Inverted-U Theory. Contrary to the drive theory, other studies suggest that the relationship between stress and performance is not always linear (Yerkes & Dodson, 1908). Additionally, although stress does enhance performance, it does so only to a certain level. In essence, there is a point where continual increases in stress start to decrease performance rather than increase it. Researchers referred to this phenomenon as the inverted- U theory of stress. As demonstrated in **Figure 4.2**, low to moderate levels of stress enhance performance, whereas, extremely high levels decrease it.

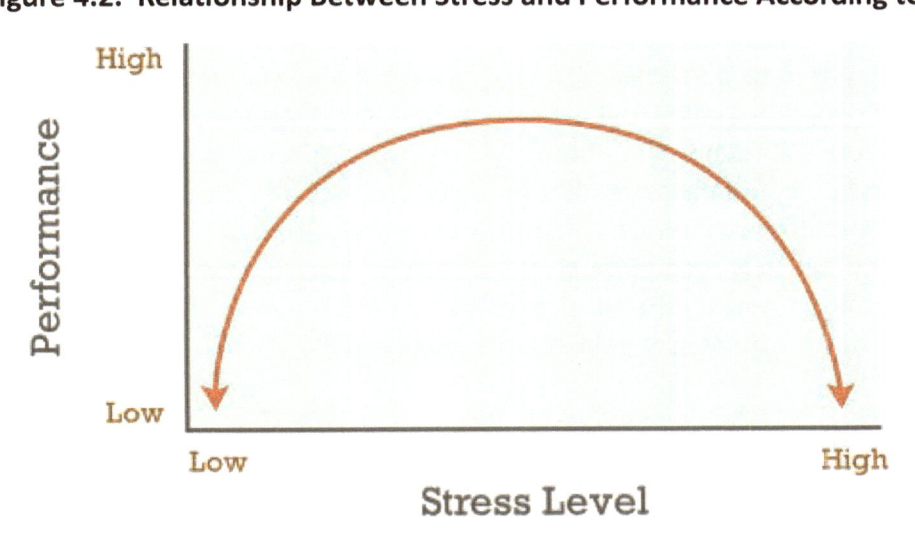

Figure 4.2. Relationship Between Stress and Performance According to the Inverted-U Theory

CHAPTER 4: STRESS MANAGEMENT AND SLEEP

Individual Zones of Optimal Functioning (IZOF). The individualized zones of optimal functioning (IZOF) is yet another theory, currently growing in popularity. This theory tries to describe the relationship between stress and performance and suggests that each person has a unique zone of optimal stress, rather than a specific point as suggested in the inverted-U model (Hanin et al., 1986). Additionally, this optimal zone of stress doesn't always occur at the midpoint of the stress continuum but rather varies from person to person. The IZOF theory is illustrated in **Figure 4.3**.

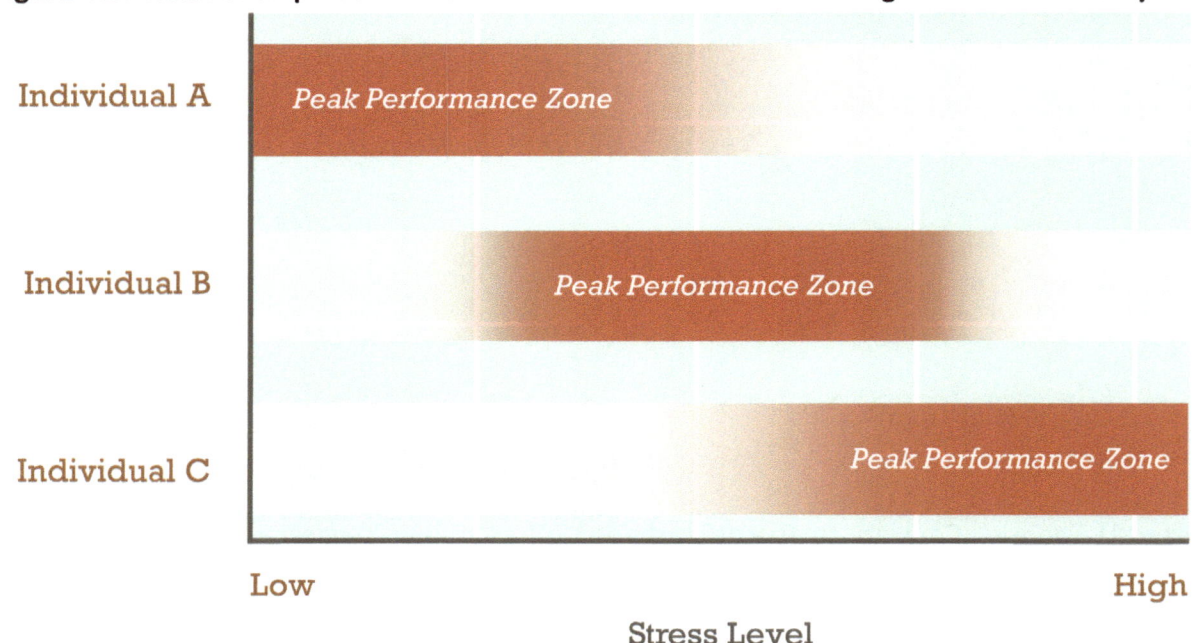

Figure 4.3. Relationship Between Stress and Performance According to the IZOF Theory

Stress Response

There are three stages to the stress response: alarm, resistance, and exhaustion (Selye, 1974). The first stage of the stress response is called the **alarm stage** or the fight-or-flight stage. In the alarm stage, the hypothalamus stimulates both the pituitary gland and **sympathetic nervous system** (part of the nervous system responsible for providing a rapid and involuntary response to dangerous or stressful situations). The pituitary gland responds by releasing adrenocorticotrophic hormone (ACTH), which in turn stimulates the adrenal glands. The adrenal glands respond by releasing the hormones cortisol, epinephrine, and norepinephrine into the blood. Collectively, these hormones and the sympathetic nervous system produce a heightened state of physical awareness. Some of the physiological responses to stress include increases in blood pressure, heart rate, respiratory rate, blood flow to the muscle as well as activation of the sweat glands (Johnson & Morris, 2012). These responses are depicted in **Figure 4.4**.

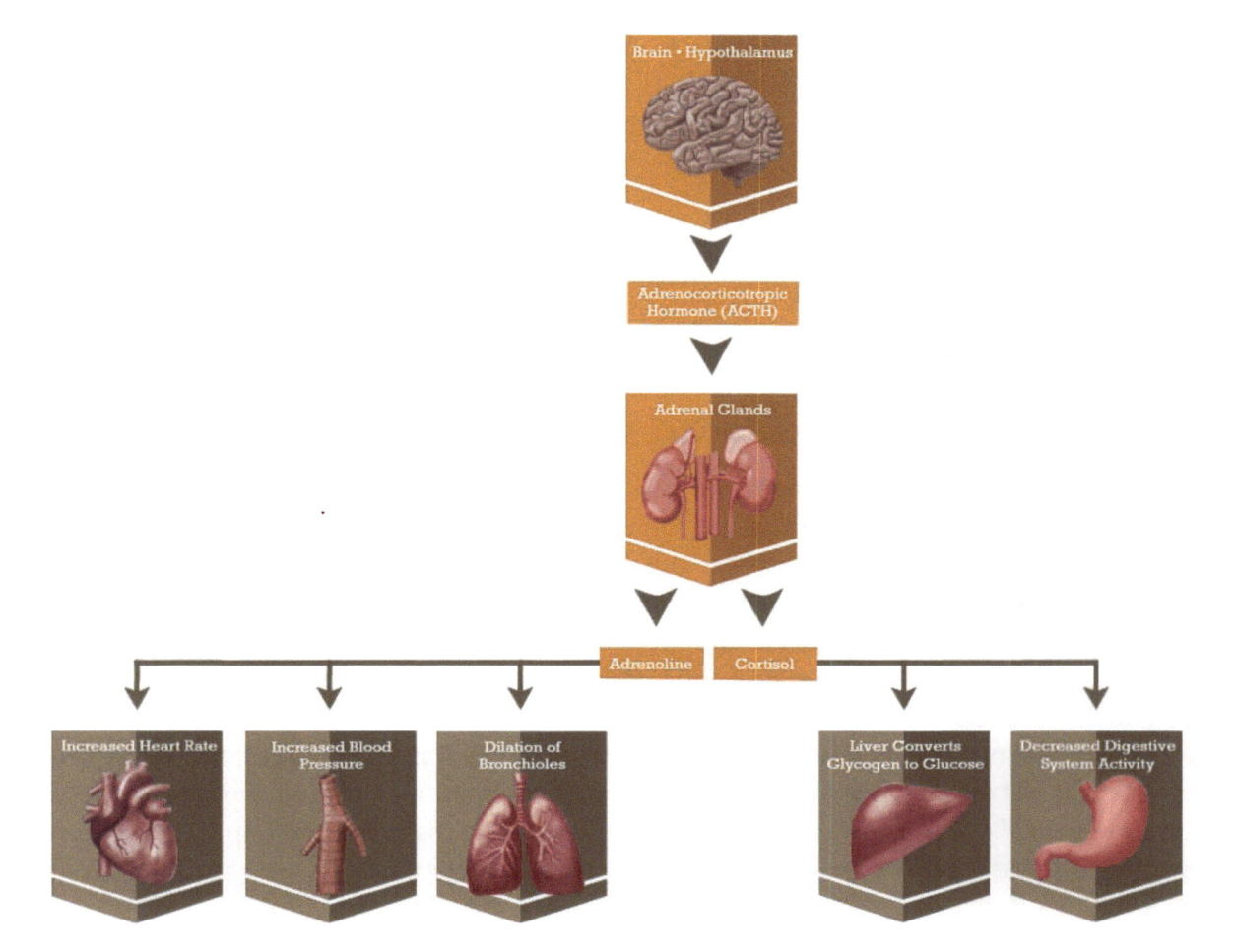

A Christian Guide to Body Stewardship, Diet and Exercise

Figure 4.4. The Physiological Response to Acute Stress

The second level of the stress response, called the **resistance stage**, occurs when stress is prolonged. If a stressful event or situation is prolonged, heart rate, blood pressure and other physiological responses associated with the alarm stage begin to decline, yet still remain above normal, resting levels. These levels remain elevated due to the higher than normal amount of cortisol in the blood, which can increase the risk for heart disease.

Unless the stressful situation or event is eliminated, or the person is able to change their perception of the situation or event (i.e., eustress versus distress), then the third stage, or the **exhaustion** stage, of the stress response occurs. In this final stage, the body has depleted all of its energy resources by continually trying, but failing, to recover from the initial alarm stage. Research shows that prolonged periods of stress can contribute to numerous emotional and physiological disorders including depression, anxiety, heart disease, stroke, hypertension and immune system disturbances that increase susceptibility to infections (American Psychological Association, n.d.).

Signs of the exhaustion stage include:

Physiological Signs and Symptoms:
- Hypertension
- Elevated cholesterol
- Atherosclerosis
- Heart disease
- Stroke

Psychological Signs and Symptoms:
- Irritability
- Depression
- Anxiety
- Paranoia

Male vs. Female Response to Stress

Research shows that males respond to stress differently, and more aggressively, than females do. Interestingly, the difference in the stress response between genders may be a result of a particular gene that males have but females do not: the sex-determining region Y (SRY) gene. The SRY gene is located on the Y chromosome, which directs male development, may promote aggression and the fight-or-flight response to stress. Additionally, since females do not have the SRY gene, their responses to stresses are different and generally less aggressive. (Lee & Harley, 2012). Research conducted by Dasgupta (2018) suggests gender differences to stress are necessary as the fight-or-flight response is not appropriate for females with offspring. Dasgupta argues that as the primary caregiver, it is not appropriate for females to leave their offspring. Instead, women tend to form close bonds with other females so that during times of stress they can help each other. This approach to stress is referred to as the **tend-and-befriend** response.

According to Taylor et al. (2000), hormonal differences between males and females also contribute to variations in the response to stress. For example, oxytocin (a hormone secreted by the pituitary gland as part of the stress response), promotes nurturing and social contact and is enhanced by the hormone estrogen. The interaction between oxytocin and estrogen may contribute to the tend-and-befriend stress response in females while simultaneously inhibiting the fight-or-flight response. Conversely, the hormone testosterone inhibits the release of oxytocin. The inhibition of oxytocin by testosterone may in turn contribute to the fight-or-flight response, while simultaneously preventing the tend-and befriend response, in males (Taylor et al., 2000).

The American Psychological Association (n.d.) has reported other differences between males and females with dealing with stress. For example, males tend to be more reluctant to believe that stress is having an impact on their health and thus place less emphasis on the need to manage their stress than females do. Additionally, males are less likely to see psychologists and make lifestyle and/or behavior changes. As a result, males tend to be at a slightly higher risk for emotional and physiological disorders associated with high stress levels and unhealthy lifestyles and behaviors.

Stress and the College Student

The college experience is a major source of stress for most students. Respondents to the American College Health Association survey (2018) reported various factors which negatively affected their academic performance. Some of the factors mentioned include stress, anxiety, depression, concern for a troubled friend, relationship problems, financial problems, and/or death of a family member.

For many students, college is the first time living away from home and on their own. Interestingly, stress for college students seems to be most prevalent during the freshman and senior years. For freshmen, the stress comes from being in a totally new physical and social setting as well as new and more challenging academic expectations. For seniors, the stress comes from the anticipation of life beyond college to include work, marriage, and finances (Johnson & Morris, 2012).

Ironically, the stress associated with college seems to be similar between Christian and secular schools. According to researchers, the top five stressors for all college students include (Fahey et al., 2011; Walter et al., 2006):

1. Academics. The majority of students surveyed rated academics as the leading cause of stress, higher than any other stressor associated with college life.

2. Relationships. Many college students have lives beyond just that of school and/or have roommates. Some are in a dating relationship, while others are married and/or have children. Managing these relationships, in addition to academics, can be a major source of stress, especially if other individuals involved are less than supportive.

3. Future concerns. As college life comes to an end, many students struggle with concerns regarding their future including finding a spouse and a career.

4. Time management. Keeping up with different class schedules and due dates for assignments can be a major source of stress. However, these pressures can be drastically compounded when combined with poor time management skills and family and/or work responsibilities.

5. Financial matters. College is expensive, and as a result, the majority of college students need some form of financial aid to afford it. In order to cover costs, many college students need to work or take out loans. Often work and college loans become additional stressors as they compete with academics and other responsibilities.

Though not listed in the top five, procrastination and technology are other common sources of stress for college students. Moser (2014) associates fear (e.g., feeling overwhelmed), overconfidence and laziness as some of the underlying culprits of procrastination. To combat procrastination, Moser (2014) proposes four possible strategies: *Analyze* (Am I wasting time?); *Prioritize* (Am I investing my time wisely?); *Biblicize* (Is my time spent on what truly matters biblically?); and *Exercise* (Am I being disciplined with my time?).

Chapter 4: Stress Management and Sleep

Another useful tool in helping to prioritize tasks by urgency and importance is the Eisenhower Matrix (Moser, 2014). This tool is also useful in helping to sort out less urgent and important tasks that should either be delegated or deleted. An example of the Eisenhower Matrix is provided in **Figure 4.5**.

Figure 4.5. The Eisenhower Matrix for Time Management

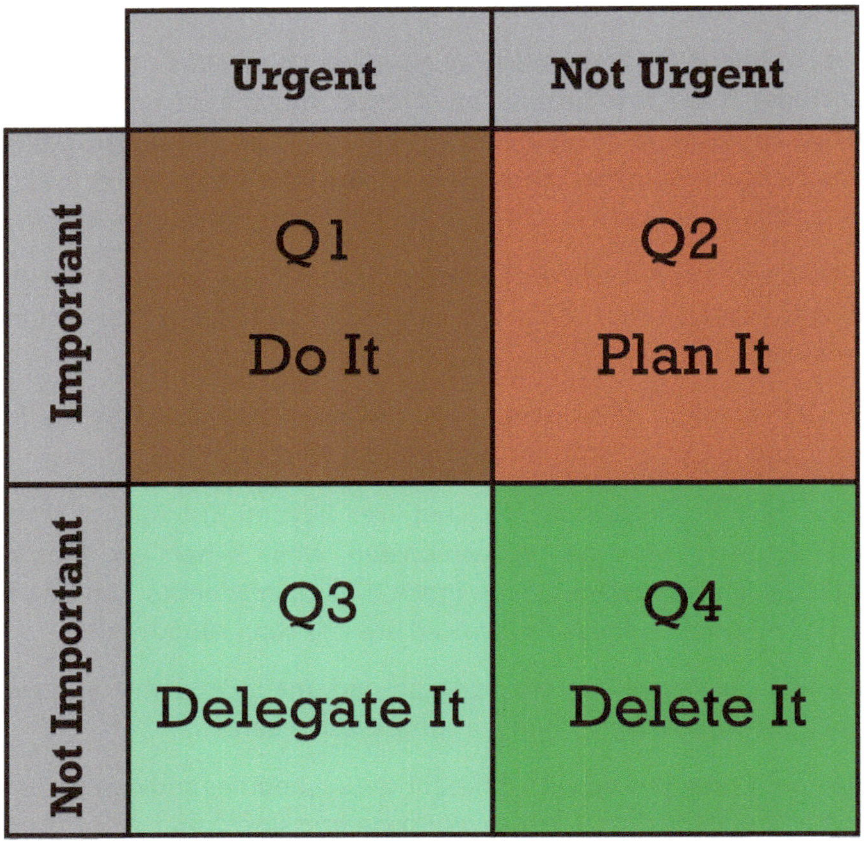

	Urgent	**Not Urgent**
Important	Q1 Do It	Q2 Plan It
Not Important	Q3 Delegate It	Q4 Delete It

Although technology has dramatically improved the college experience in many ways, it can also be a significant source of stress. If not careful, college students can spend too much time on social media, which, similar to work, can start to compete with academics and other responsibilities. A more extensive listing of common stressors for college students is provided in **Table 4.1** (Anderson, 1972).

Table 4.1. Common Stressful Events Among College Students

Point Value	Life Event	Point Value	Life Event
87	Death of a spouse	50	Change to a different line of work
77	Marriage	50	Change to a new school
77	Death of close family member	48	Major change in social activities
76	Divorce	47	Major change in responsibilities at work
74	Marital separation	46	Major change in the use of alcohol
68	Death of a close friend	45	Revision of personal habits
68	Pregnancy or fathering a child	44	Trouble with school administration
65	Major personal injury or illness	43	Work at a job while attending school
62	Fired from work	42	Trouble with in-laws
60	Broken marital engagement or steady relationship	42	Change in residence or living conditions
58	Sex difficulties	41	Change in or choice of a major field of study
58	Marital reconciliation	41	Change in dietary habits
57	Major change in type and/or amount of recreation	40	Outstanding personal achievement
57	Major change in self-concept or self-awareness	38	A lot more or a lot less trouble with your boss
56	Major change in the health of a family member	36	Major change in church activities
54	Engaged to be married	34	Major change in sleeping habits
53	Major change in financial state	33	Trip or vacation
52	Mortgage or loan for purchase of less than $10,000	30	Major change in eating habits
50	Enter college	26	Major change in the number of family get-togethers
50	Gain of new family member	22	Found guilty of minor violations of the law
50	Major conflict in or change in values		

Emotional Intelligence and Relational Wisdom

Emotional intelligence refers to the ability to manage one's own emotions, communicate emotional states to others, and pick up on the emotional conditions of others (Walters & Byl, 2021; Goleman, 2005). Possessing these abilities help to improve productivity, life satisfaction, and relationships in the workplace, school, and at home (Sande, 2020). **Relational wisdom** refers to the ability to discern the emotions, interests, and abilities both in yourself and others; to interpret them in the light of Scripture; and to use this insight to manage your responses and relationships successfully (Sande, 2020a; Sande 2020b). In essence, relational wisdom is the

CHAPTER 4: STRESS MANAGEMENT AND SLEEP

desire and ability to live out the two Great Commandments outlined by Jesus. Specifically, to love God with all your heart, soul and mind and to love your neighbor as yourself (Matthew 22:37-39).

Effective Ways to Manage Stress

Research shows that some individuals are able to deal with and manage their stress better than others. Individuals who are able to manage their stress well are less likely to develop stress-related emotional and physiological disorders. Some of the characteristics of individuals with successful **stress management** include those who view situations and events optimistically, exercise on a regular basis, eat well and receive adequate rest, and have a strong faith. Furthermore, these individuals tend to have an emotional support system in place by forming strong friendships and maintaining ties with family (Johnson & Morris, 2012).

Provided below are 10 effective ways for managing stress (Swenson, 1992; Thygerson & Thygerson, 2016; Walters & Byl, 2013):

1. Regular exercise. Participating in regular exercise, even low-intensity exercise, has been shown to substantially reduce stress and anxiety levels.

2. Proper nutrition. Eating a well-balanced diet can help to reduce the risks associated with chronic stress and physiological disorders associated with poor nutrition.

3. Adequate sleep. Tired individuals do not manage stress well. Adequate sleep helps to improve resiliency and reduce stress.

4. Prayer / Meditation on Scripture. Praying regularly helps to lower agitation and loneliness as well as improving morale and the ability to cope. In addition to prayer, meditating on Scripture can help to put temporary circumstances into an eternal perspective. Some pertinent passages to consider include Matthew 11:28-30; Romans 8:18, 26-39; Philippians 4:4-9; and James 1:2-7.

5. Sense of humor. Laughter releases muscle tension, promotes deep breathing and triggers a relaxation response. Research suggests it may be physiologically impossible to be both stressed and laughing at the same time.

6. Support system. Individuals with a positive support system fare better when faced with stressful situations. Conversely, negative relationships can be more harmful than helpful.

7. Establishing margins. It is important to set boundaries in terms of your energy, time and resources so not to overextend.

8. Listening to music. Listening to music can lower heart rate, blood pressure, and muscle tension. Exposure to soothing, lyrical music can help to lessen the effects of depression and anxiety.

9. Time management. Learning to effectively manage your time can significantly reduce

stress and anxiety. Overcommitting and procrastination are significant stressors for many individuals. Here are a few strategies for improving time management skills: set priorities; budget enough time; consider doing least favorite tasks first; consolidate tasks when possible; and delegate when appropriate and/or possible.

10. Avoid **self-induced stressors**. Sometimes we are our own source of stress as poor personal habits can often lead to stress. Here are a few strategies for avoiding self-induced stressors: don't procrastinate; don't over-commit your time; set time limits on social media; establish a daily routine; and deal appropriately with anger.

Anxiety, Depression, and Hope

As previously mentioned, chronic stress, if left unchecked, can lead to severe anxiety and/or depression. According to a 2018 American College Health Association survey tailored to college students, they reported feeling:

- Very sad (68.7%)
- Overwhelming anxiety (63.4%)
- Overwhelming anger (4.12%)
- So depressed that it was difficult to function (41.9%)

Similarly, according to the 2020 Healthy Minds Study, 37% of college students experienced depression and an additional 31% experienced generalized anxiety disorder (Eisenberg & Lipson, 2020).

Anxiety is a state characterized by a feeling of worry, nervousness or unease as a result of an event that is either imminent or uncertain. Some of the different categories of anxiety include social anxiety disorder, post-traumatic stress disorder, generalized anxiety disorder, panic disorders, and various phobias. Physiological symptoms of these disorders include increased heart rate, sweating, nausea, panic attacks, nightmares or flashbacks, fatigue, and headaches (Walters & Byl, 2021). These disorders are usually treated through counseling and medications.

Depression is a mental illness characterized by a state of extreme sadness and/or low spirits. Depression is not a character flaw or a sign of weakness. Researchers believe that depression results from a combination of physiological, psychological and social factors such as genetics, chemical imbalance, stress, inadequate social support, and/or negative and/or irrational thoughts.

Some of the more common symptoms of depression, assuming they persist for two weeks or more, include (American Psychiatric Association, 2000):

- Feeling sad or depressed
- Loss of interest in activities once enjoyed
- Trouble concentrating, remembering and/or making decisions

- Persistent fatigue
- Feelings of guilt, worthlessness and/or hopelessness
- Inability to sleep or sleeping too much
- Irritability
- Restlessness
- Binge eating or loss of appetite
- Headaches
- Digestive problems
- Suicidal thoughts and/or attempts

If you are severely depressed, or know someone who is, getting help from a mental health professional is essential. Fortunately, treatment for depression can be highly effective (Fahey et al., 2011).

Unrelenting suffering, personal failure, and/or failed dreams often lead to anxiety, depression, and/or suicide (Powlison, 2010). However, Scripture provides us with hope (Psalm 31, Psalm 32, Psalm 33:18-19, Romans 8:15-35). It is important to remember that our lives matter to God, that he cares for us, and that we can bring our hopelessness to him (Psalm 86:7; 1 Peter 1:3-5).

What to Do if Someone is Suicidal

If you are severely depressed, or know someone who is, getting expert help from a mental health professional is essential. Fortunately, treatment for depression can be highly effective (Fahey et al., 2011). However, if chronic depression is left unchecked, it can lead to thoughts or attempts of suicide. Provided below are the recommended steps to take if someone you know is contemplating suicide:

- Take suicidal talk seriously
- Show genuine concern
- Urge the individual to seek professional help

If you are suicidal, or know someone who is, it is important to know you are not alone and that help is available. If the threat of suicide is immediate, seek help immediately (e.g., call 911 or campus safety at (937) 766-7992 or 999 from a campus phone). Additionally, the National Suicide Prevention Lifeline is open 24/7 at 988 and provides free and confidential talk with trained counselors. Additional resources are available on their website (suicidepreventionlifeline.org).

Some of the warning signs of suicide include:

- Taking about killing or harming one's self
- Expressing strong feeling of hopelessness or being trapped
- An unusual preoccupation with death or dying
- Acting recklessly (as if they have a death wish)
- Calling or visiting people to say goodbye
- Getting personal affairs in order
- Saying things like "Everyone would be better off without me" or "I want out"
- A sudden change from being extremely depressed to acting calm and/or happy

Dealing with issues like anxiety, depression, hopelessness, and suicidal thoughts requires a team approach to include family members and qualified mental health professionals. Examples of qualified mental health professionals include certified or licensed counselors, psychologists, and psychiatrists. In addition to seeking help, a thorough physical exam may be necessary to determine if an undiagnosed physical illness is contributing to these issues.

Cedarville University (CU) Counseling Services provides a variety of individual and small group therapies aimed at helping students with their emotional and spiritual needs. Although there is a waiting list for appointments, students at risk of self-harm can be seen right away. For more information, or to schedule an appoint, contact CU Counseling Services at:

- http://www.cedarville.edu/Offices/Counseling-Services.aspx
- counseling@cedarville.edu
- (937) 766-7855
- SSC Rm 163

In addition to CU Counseling Services, other resources to consider for help include dorm resident directors and resident assistants, CU faculty and staff and local church leadership.

Sleep

As mentioned previously, the amount of sleep an individual gets on a regular basis plays an integral role in their ability to cope with and manage stress. According to the Center for Disease Control and Prevention, only one third of U.S. adults are getting the recommended amount of sleep per night. Unfortunately, loss of sleep has been linked to many health problems and chronic diseases as well as motor vehicle crashes or errors leading to injury or death (CDC, 2020). Although the Bible does not prescribe a specific amount of sleep a person should be getting per night, it does stress the importance of sleep for good physical, mental and spiritual health. In fact, Genesis 2:2-3 says that God himself rested on the seventh day. Obviously, being omnipotent, the act of creation did not cause God to be tired nor did he need to rest. Instead, because man was made in God's image, he used this opportunity to demonstrate the need for and importance of rest.

Some theologians argue that the ability to sleep, or not sleep, may be a reflection of our faith, trust and obedience in God (BibleMesh, 2013). For example, Psalm 4:8 says that David was able to sleep soundly even amid his different trials as he knew his life and circumstances were secure in the Lord. Psalm 127:1-2 teaches us not to "put off "sleep because what ultimately happens in life is a result of God's sovereignty and not the result of our own labor. Finally, Proverbs 3:24 says when we place our trust in God, and lean not on our own understanding, that when we lie down, we will not be afraid and our "sleep will be sweet". There will undoubtedly be times in life when it is hard, if not impossible to sleep; however, frequent insomnia may be an indication that we need to worry less and trust God more.

Sleep Regulation

Sleep is regulated by two systems: sleep-wake homeostasis and internal circadian biological clock. **Sleep-wake homeostasis** creates a balance between sleep and wakefulness. After long periods of being awake the need for sleep accumulates and signals to the body that it is time to sleep. Sleep-wake homeostasis also helps to ensure enough sleep is accumulated at night to account for the hours of wakefulness. The internal **circadian biological clock**, also known as circadian rhythm, regulates feelings of sleepiness and wakefulness over a 24-hour period. The internal circadian biological clock fluctuates and causes you to feel more alert and sleepier at certain points throughout the day (Dement & Vaughan, 1999). The internal circadian biological clock prefers consistency. Significant disruptions to normal sleeping patterns, such as when traveling to different time zones, can result in excessive sleepiness, loss of concentration, poor motor control, increased irritability, slowed reflexes, and nausea (Smolensky & Lamberg, 2000). This condition is commonly referred to as **jet lag**.

Interestingly, the circadian clock is not constant but changes throughout life. For example, the circadian clock is significantly different during adolescence than it is during childhood and adulthood. Research has shown that increases in **melatonin** (a hormone released at night to promote sleep) levels occur later at night for adolescents than it does for children and adults. This delayed release of melatonin can cause adolescents to feel more alert at night thus making it difficult for them to fall asleep before 11:00 p.m. (Walters & Byl, 2021). This problem is compounded when they must get up early for school and/or other commitments thereby making it difficult for them to get the necessary amount of sleep (9.25 hours per night on average, 8.5 hours per night minimum).

To help combat this, the National Sleep Foundation recommends dimming the lights as bedtime approaches to help boost melatonin levels thereby making it easier for adolescents to fall asleep earlier. Additionally, exposing them to bright lights as soon as possible in the morning may help them wake up and feel more alert sooner (National Sleep Foundation, n.d.; National Sleep Foundation, 2010).

Sleep Architecture

Sleep phases can be classified into two primary categories: nonrapid eye movement (NREM) and rapid eye movement (REM). In normal adults, NREM accounts for approximately 75 percent of sleep and REM accounts for approximately 25 percent of sleep (National Sleep Foundation, 2006).

NREM is a deeper state of sleep, as compared to REM sleep, and is where most of physical restoration associated with sleep occurs. NREM can be further classified into three stages: stage I, stage II, and stage III. Stage I is a transitory phase of sleep lasting only about 10 minutes. During this phase, individuals are easily awakened. In fact, individuals who are awakened from stage I sleep often claim they were not yet asleep (Coren, 1996).

Stage II is where actual sleep begins as serves as a transition period between light sleep and deep sleep. This stage of sleep usually lasts between 5-20 minutes. Individuals who are awakened during this phase would admit to being asleep.

Stage III is the deepest stage of sleep and where the majority of physical restoration occurs. In fact, research has shown that chronic lack of stage III sleep can permanently stunt growth (Dement & Vaughan, 1999). During this phase, the blood supply to the brain is decreased and all but the essential bodily functions are shut down (Walters & Byl, 2021). Stage III sleep generally lasts from 10 minutes to one hour.

REM sleep begins at the end of Stage III sleep (i.e., approximately one hour after falling asleep). REM sleep is similar to being awake in that it is a period of intense brain activity. In fact, REM sleep is when most dreams occur. During REM sleep, heart rate and blood pressure increases; breathing becomes more rapid, irregular, and shallow; the eyes rapidly move in various directions (thereby coining the term REM); and the skeletal muscles relax (Walter & Byl, 2021). One cycle of REM sleep lasts between 1-20 minutes. A complete sleep cycle (i.e., stage I, stage II, stage III, REM) lasts about 90 minutes and is repeated several times per night. In subsequent cycles, the amount of time spent in deep sleep gets shorter and the amount of time spent in REM sleep gets longer. A brief description of the various categories of sleep are provided in **Table 4.2**.

Table 4.2 Stages of Sleep.

	NREM			REM
	Stage I	Stage II	Stage III	-
Description	Light Sleep	Transitory Period	Deep Sleep	Dreams Occur
Duration	10 minutes	5-20 minutes	10-60 minutes	1-20 minutes

Sleep Deprivation

Studies have shown that the majority of Americans are sleep deprived (Murphy & Delanty, 2007). **Sleep deprivation** is a condition where the amount of sleep received fails to meet the physiological needs of the body and mind. Although, occasional sleep deprivation is inevitable, chronic sleep deprivation is problematic. Research shows that chronic sleep deprivation can have major consequences on one's emotional, mental, and physical wellbeing (Walters & Byl, 2013). Some of the symptoms of chronic sleep deprivation include:

- General fatigue
- Emotional irritability
- Cognitive impairment
- Physical impairment
- Psychosis (a mental disorder characterized by a disconnection from reality)

How Much Sleep Is Recommended?

As depicted in **Figure 4.6**, sleep requirements fluctuate significantly based on age (Condor, 2001). For most adults (i.e., ages 18-64), the general recommendation is about 8 hours of sleep each night. However, individual sleep needs can vary significantly (Dement & Vaughan, 1999). In addition to age, gender and genetics may affect sleep needs as well. Ironically, too much sleep can also be problematic. Research has shown increased mortality rates for those who routinely get substantially less than 7 hours of sleep per night as well as those who routinely get 9 hours or more (Ferrie et al., 2007; Gallicchio & Kalesan, 2009; Hublin et al., 2007).

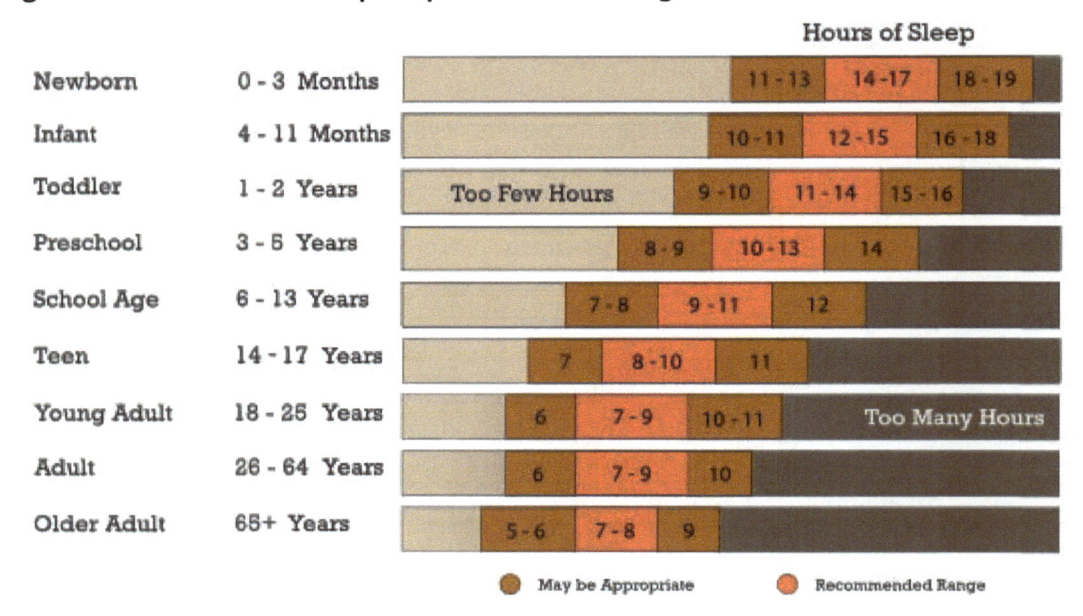

Figure 4.6. Amount of Sleep Required Based on Age

Age Group	Age Range	Too Few Hours	May be Appropriate	Recommended Range	May be Appropriate	Too Many Hours
Newborn	0 - 3 Months		11-13	14-17	18-19	
Infant	4 - 11 Months		10-11	12-15	16-18	
Toddler	1 - 2 Years	Too Few Hours	9-10	11-14	15-16	
Preschool	3 - 5 Years		8-9	10-13	14	
School Age	6 - 13 Years		7-8	9-11	12	
Teen	14 - 17 Years		7	8-10	11	
Young Adult	18 - 25 Years		6	7-9	10-11	Too Many Hours
Adult	26 - 64 Years		6	7-9	10	
Older Adult	65+ Years		5-6	7-8	9	

There are several different methods to determine whether an individual is getting enough sleep and how much sleep one needs. The University Center for the Diagnosis and Treatment of Sleep Disorders has developed a sleep deprivation quiz (Maas, 1999) to determine whether an individual receives enough sleep. To take the quiz, simply answer "yes" or "no" to the following five questions based on the sleep behavior performed over the past six months.

1. Do you frequently fall asleep if given a sleep opportunity (i.e., at least 10 minutes in a cool, dark, and quiet environment)?
2. Do you frequently need an alarm clock to wake up?
3. Do you frequently catch up on sleep during weekends?
4. Do you frequently take naps during the day?
5. When you wake up, do you feel tired most mornings?

If an individual answered yes to two or more of the questions, they need more sleep. To determine how much sleep one needs, first establish a regular bedtime each night to stabilize the internal circadian biological clock. Additionally, ensure that there are no disturbances that would cause one to be awakened early. Individuals typically report sleeping 10-12 hours the first night, 9-10 hours the next several nights, and then progressively less over time until their sleep schedule stabilizes. Most individuals can stabilize their sleep schedule within two weeks and report needing somewhere between 7-9 hours per night (Walters & Byl, 2013).

Factors That Affect Sleep

Research shows that the average college student only receives around six hours of sleep per night, which is significantly less than the average U.S. adult (Maas, 1998; Walters, 2005). **Figure 4.7** compares the self-reported averages of sleep per night between college students and those reported by the average U.S. adult. According to Walters (2009), the top three factors that negatively affect sleep for college students are academics, social activities, and technology (e.g., social media, streaming video, video games).

Figure 4.7. Percent of College Students and U.S. Adults Receiving 8 Hours or More of Sleep per Night

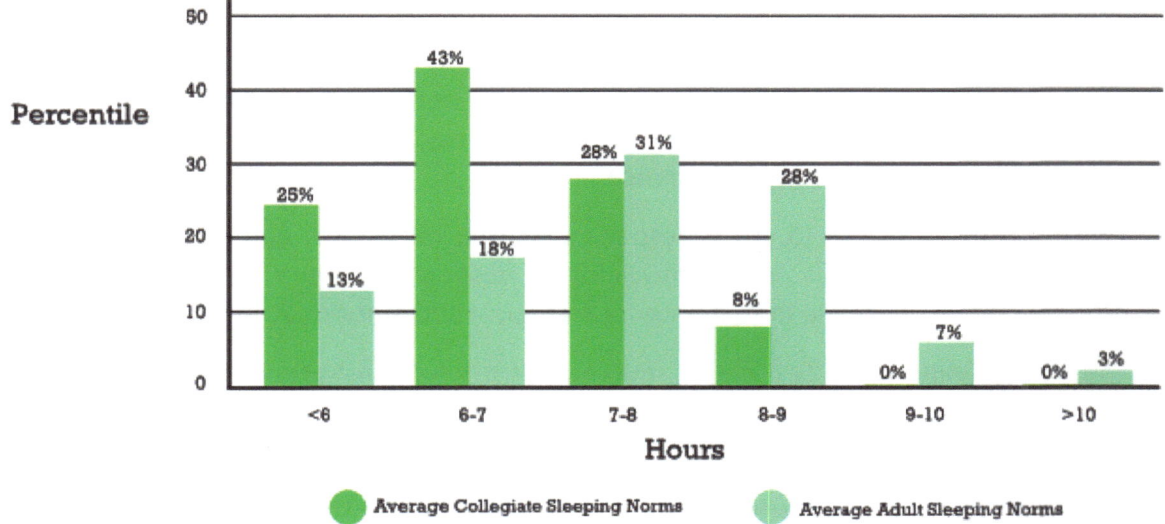

Tips for Getting a Good Night's Sleep

As previously mentioned, sleep plays a vital role in effective stress management as well as the prevention and recovery of various emotional and physiological conditions. Provided below are six recommendations for improving your **sleep hygiene** (i.e., quality sleep habits):

1. Create a quality sleep environment. A quality sleep environment means that the bedroom should be quiet, dark, and cool. In terms of temperature, most individuals prefer their room to be around 65°F (Maas, 1999).

2. Establish a consistent bedtime and nighttime routine. Constantly changing one's bedtime will affect the internal circadian biological clock thereby making one's sleep cycle unbalanced and more difficult to regulate.

3. Whenever possible, use the bed just for sleeping. Using one's bed to perform other activities such as eating, studying or watching tv sends mixed signals to the subconscious thus potentially making falling asleep more difficult.

4. Keep the cellphone out of sight and out of reach. The tendency for most individuals is to check their phone every time there is a notification of an email, text or social media post. Keeping the cellphone away from the nightstand can help to reduce or eliminate this temptation.

5. If possible, avoid looking at bright screens for at least 2-3 hours before bed. The blue light emitted from electronics can block the sleep-inducing hormone melatonin making it harder to fall and stay asleep. Although abstinence from screen time is preferred, the use of blue light filters can help minimize the impact that electronic devices have on melatonin levels.

6. Exercise regularly. Research shows that individuals who exercise regularly go to sleep faster and sleep longer than sedentary individuals (Kubitz et al., 1996).

Summary

- There is a strong correlation between stress and performance and depending upon how we perceive that stress and the body's response to it, we can either positively or negatively impact personal performance.

- There are three stages to stress response: alarm, resistance, and exhaustion which collectively induce a cascade of physiological responses within the body and if not properly managed, can lead to deleterious physical and emotional harm.

- The college experience is a major source of stress for most students, where the top five stressors experienced include: academics, relationships, future concerns, time management, and financial matters.

- Individuals who engage in successful stress management (those who view situations optimistically, exercise regularly, eat well and receive adequate rest) are less likely to develop stress-related emotional and physiological disorders.

- College students are prone to become or be diagnosed with depression which results from a combination of physiological, psychological and social factors.

- Chronic (persistent) depression can lead to thoughts or attempts of suicide; however, treatment for depression can be highly effective and support is made readily available for students through various campus services.

- Approximately one-third of U.S. adults receive adequate sleep which is vital for establishing balance in the body's natural sleep-wake homeostasis and internal circadian rhythm.

- Understanding how much sleep one needs and the factors which affect sleep are essential for maintaining one's emotional, mental, and physical wellbeing.

References

1. American College Health Association. (2011). *National College Health Assessment.* Retrieved from www.acha-ncha.org/data_highlights.html.

2. American College Health Association. (2018). *American College Health Association-National College Health Assessment II: Reference Group Executive Summary.* Silver Spring, MD: American College Health Association.

3. American Psychological Association. (n.d.). *Stress in America: Stress and Gender.* Retrieved from https://www.apa.org/news/press/releases/stress/2011/gender.pdf.

4. Anderson, G. E. (1972). *College Schedule of Recent Experience.* Fargo, ND: North Dakota State University.

5. BibleMesh (2013, September 24). Does the Bible Say Anything About Sleep Habits? Retrieved from https://biblemesh.com/blog/does-the-bible-say-anything-about-sleep-habits/.

6. Center for Disease Control and Prevention (2020, April 15). *Sleep and Sleep Disorders.* Retrieved from https://www.cdc.gov/sleep/index.html.

7. Condor, B. (2001, September 9). *Early to bed.* Chicago Tribune: 1, 6.

8. Coren, S. (1996). *Sleep Thieves: An Eye-Opening Exploration into the Science and Mysteries of Sleep.* New York: The Free Press.

9. Dasgupta, A. (2018). The Science of Stress Management: A Guide to Best Practices for Better Well-Being. Lanham, MD: Rowman & Littlefield.

10. Dement, W., & Vaughan, C. (1999). *The Promise of Sleep.* New York, NY: Delacorte Press.

11. Eisenberg, D., & Lipson, S. (2020). *The Healthy Mind Study 2020 Winter/Spring Data Report. University of Michigan Counseling and Psychological Services.* Retrieved from The Healthy

Chapter 4: Stress Management and Sleep

Minds Study (healthymindsnetwork.org).

12. Fahey, T., Insel, P., & Roth, W. (2011). Fit & Well: Core Concepts and Labs in Physical Fitness and Wellness. (9th Ed.). New York, NY: McGraw Hill.

13. Ferrie, J.E., Shipley, M.J., Cappuccio, F.P., Brunner, E., Miller, M.A., Kumari, M., et al. (2007). *A prospective study of change in sleep duration: Associations with mortality in the Whitehall II cohort.* Sleep, 30(12), 1659–66.

14. Gallicchio, L., & Kalesan, B. (2009). *Sleep duration and mortality: A systematic review and meta-analysis.* Journal of Sleep Research, 18, 148–58.

15. Hanin, Y., Speilberger, C., & Diaz-Guerrero, R. (1986). *State-Trait Anxiety Research on Sports in the USSR in C.D.* Cross-Cultural Anxiety, 3:45-64.

16. Hill, W. (1957). *Comments on Taylor's Drive Theory and Manifest Anxiety.* Psychological Bulletin, 54(6):490-3.

17. Hublin, C., Partinen, M., Koskenvuo, M., Kaprio, J. (2007). *Sleep and mortality: A population-based 22-year follow- up study.* Sleep Journal, 30(10), 1245–53.

18. Johnson, P., and Morris, L. (2012). *Physical Fitness and the Christian* (5th Ed.). Dubuque, IA: Kendall Hunt.

19. Kubitz, K.A., Landers, D.M., Petruzzello, S.J., & Han, M. (1996). *The effects of acute and chronic exercise on sleep: A meta-analytic review.* Sports Medicine, 21, 277–91.

20. Lee, J., & Harley, V. (2012). *The Male Fight-Flight Response: A Result of SRY regulation of Catecholamines?* Bioessays, 34(6):454-7.

21. Maas, J.B. (1998). *Asleep in the Fast Lane: Our 24-hour Society.* Ithaca, NY: Cornell University Psychology Film Unit.

22. Maas, J.B. (1999). *Power Sleep.* New York, NY: Harper Perennial.

23. Moore-Ed, M., & Levert, S. (1998). *The Complete Idiot's Guide to Getting a Good Night's Sleep.* New York: Alpha.

24. Moser, P. (2014). *Taking Back Time: Biblical Strategies for Overcoming Procrastination.* Mullica Hill, NJ: Biblical Stretegies, LLC.

25. Murphy, K., & Delanty, N. (2007). *Sleep deprivation: A clinical perspective.* Sleep and Biological Rhythms, 5(1), 2–14.

26. National Sleep Foundation (n.d.). *Sleep Drive and Your Body Clock.* www.sleepfoundatin.org/article/sleep-topics/sleep-drive-and-your-body-clock.

27. National Sleep Foundation (2006). *Sleep-Wake Cycle: Its Physiology and Impact on Health.* www.sleepfoundation.org/sites/default/files/sleepwakecycle.pdf.

28. National Sleep Foundation (2010). *How Much Sleep Do We Really Need?* www.sleepfoundation.org/articles/how-much-sleep-do-we-realy-need.

29. Powlison, D. (2010). *Help for the Suicidal*. Glenside, PA: Christian Counseling and Educational Foundation.

30. Sande, K. (2004). *The Peacemaker: A Biblical Guide to Resolving Personal Conflict* (3rd ed.) Grand Rapids, MI: Baker Books.

31. Sande, K. (2020a). *Discover Relational Wisdom*. Retrieved from https://rw360.org.

32. Sande, K. (2020b). *Discover RW*. Retrieved from https://rw360.org/discover-rw/.

33. Selye, H. (1974). *Stress Without Distress*. New York, NY: J.B. Lippincott.

34. Smolensky, M., & Lamberg, L. (2000). *The body clock guide to better health*. New York: Henry Holt & Co.

35. Swenson, Richard A. (1992). *Margin: Restoring Emotional, Physical, Financial and Time Reserves to Overloaded Lives*. Colorado Springs, CO: Navpress.

36. Taylor, S., Cousino, K., Lewis, B., Gruenewald, T., Gurung, R., & Updegraff, J. (2000). *Biobehavioral Responses to Stress in Females: Tend-and Befriend, Not Fight-or Flight*. Psychological Review, 107(3):411-429.

37. Thygerson, A., & Thygerson, S. (2016). *Fit to be Well: Essential Concepts*. (4th Ed.). Burlington, MA: Jones & Bartlett Leaning.

38. Walters, P. (2005). *Sleep: The forgotten factor: Part II*. Paper presented at the annual National Wellness Conference, Stevens Point, WI.

39. Walters, P. (2009). *Sleep thieves: College students identify what they do instead of sleep*. (Oral presentation.) Wheaton College.

40. Walters, P., & Byl, J. (2013). *Christian Paths to Health and Wellness* (2nd Ed.). Champaign, IL: Human Kinetics.

41. Walters, P., & Byl, J. (2021). *Christian Paths to Health and Wellness* (3nd Ed.). Champaign, IL: Human Kinetics.

42. Yerkes, R., & Dodson, J. (1908). *The Relation of Strength of Stimulus to Rapidity of Habit-Formation*. Journal of Comparative and Neurological Psychology, 18:459-82.

Chapter 4: Stress Management and Sleep

Chapter 5
Training for Endurance

Key Terms:

Aerobic metabolism
Adenosine triphosphate
Anaerobic metabolism
APMHR equation
Cardiovascular fitness
Creatine phosphate
Cross-training shoe
Exercise economy
Fartlek training
Glycolysis
High-intensity interval training

Interval training
Lactate
Lactate threshold
Long slow distance training
Maximal lactate steady state
Maximum heart rate
Motion control shoe
Muscle fiber type
Neutral shoe
Oxidative system
Pace / tempo training

Phosphagen system
Pyruvate
Rate of perceived exertion
Road-running shoe
Stability shoe
Talk test
Trail-running shoe
Treadmill tempo run
VO_2max
Work:Rest ratio
Zero-drop shoe

Learning Objectives:

- Recognize the importance of cardiovascular health and the three basic energy systems used to replenish levels of adenosine triphosphate (ATP)

- Define VO_2max, lactate threshold, muscle fiber type and exercise economy and describe how each relates to endurance performance

- List the five types of endurance training and discuss some of the physiological benefits associated with each

- Define rate of perceived exertion (RPE) and the Talk Test and describe how they relate to MHR

- List the different types of running shoes and discuss techniques for selecting a running shoe

CHAPTER 5: TRAINING FOR ENDURANCE

Introduction

Cardiovascular fitness is the ability of the heart and lungs to efficiently deliver oxygenated blood to the working muscles as well as the muscle's ability to extract and use the oxygen provided. Endurance training is a specific method of training used to improve cardiovascular fitness.

Regular participation in endurance training has been shown to improve longevity (life expectancy), blood pressure, blood cholesterol, and body composition. Additional benefits associated with regular endurance training include a decreased risk for certain diseases such as heart disease, diabetes, and cancer. Research shows that the risk factors associated with coronary heart disease often begin in childhood or early adolescence and the majority of young adults aged 18-24 already have at least one risk factor. Research also shows that having at least one risk factor in young adulthood increases an individual's risk of developing long-term coronary heart disease (Arts et al., 2014). Finally, endurance training may be especially advantageous for college students as it also helps to improve sleep quality, mental health and cognitive function (Walters & Byl, 2021).

Table 5.1 depicts some of the specific physiological adaptations associated with chronic endurance training (Haff & Triplett, 2016).

Table 5.1. Physiological Adaptations Associated with Chronic Endurance Training

↑ Aerobic power (VO$_2$max)	↓ Percent body fat
↑ Oxygen carrying capacity	↓ Resting and maximal heart rate
↑ Mitochondrial and capillary density	↓ Resting and maximal blood pressure
↑ Maximal cardiac output and stroke volume	-
↑ Resting stroke volume	-
↑ Arteriovenous oxygen difference	-
↑ Cardiac muscle strength	-
↑ Connective tissue strength	-
↑ Metabolic enzyme number and activity	-
↑ Fat-burning capacity	-
↑ Metabolic energy stores (e.g., ATP, CP, glycogen, triglycerides)	-

When performing endurance training, it is important to personalize the training regime to the individual instead of using a program found online or designed for another athlete. According to Baechle & Earle (2008):

> A common trend with many endurance athletes is to adopt and embrace the training practices of other highly successful or well-known endurance athletes. Although this strategy may be effective for a few, most endurance athletes would be better served by constructing their own training regimen based on a good working knowledge of the sound principles and an understanding of their own physical limitations and needs. (p. 490)

The purpose of this chapter is to introduce some of the key principles necessary in order to design and implement a safe and effective personalized endurance training program. However, before designing such a program, it is important to first understand the different biological energy systems used by the body to produce energy.

Biological Energy Systems

There are three basic energy systems used to replenish levels of **adenosine triphosphate (ATP)**, the energy used to power muscle contractions: **phosphagen, glycolytic** and **oxidative**. The phosphagen system produces ATP primarily for an extremely short duration (≤ 10 seconds) and very high intensity activities such as heavy resistance training and short distance sprints (≤ 100 meters). The glycolytic system produces ATP for short duration (> 10 seconds - < 2 minutes) and high intensity activities such as high-rep resistance training and long-distance sprints (e.g., 200-m, 400-m, 800-m sprints). In contrast, the oxidative system produces ATP for long duration (> 2 minute) and low to moderate intensity activities such as walking, jogging and riding a bike.

The phosphagen and glycolytic systems are anaerobic systems (not requiring the presence of oxygen) that occur in the sarcoplasm of muscle cells. The oxidative system is an aerobic system (requiring the presence of oxygen) that occurs in the mitochondria of muscle cells. All three macronutrients (i.e., carbohydrates, protein, fat) can be used to produce ATP, but only carbohydrates can be metabolized without the presence of oxygen. As a result, carbohydrate availability is crucial during **anaerobic metabolism**. **Table 5.2** depicts the characteristics of the three biological energy systems (Haff & Triplett, 2016; Walters & Byl, 2013).

Table 5.2. Characteristics of the Phosphagen, Glycolytic and Oxidative Energy Systems

	PHOSPHAGEN	**GLYCOLYTIC**	**OXIDATIVE**
Exercise Duration	0-10 sec.	11-120 sec.	> 2 min.
Exercise Intensity	Very High	High	Low to Moderate
Rate of ATP Production	Immediate	Rapid	Slow
Fuel	ATP	Muscle Glycogen / Blood Glucose	Stored Carbohydrate and Fat
Oxygen Used?	No	No	Yes

It is important to emphasize that all three energy systems are always active. The extent to which each system is active and contributing to ATP production is dependent upon exercise duration and intensity. **Table 5.3** depicts the percent contribution of anaerobic and **aerobic metabolism** based on exercise duration (Haff & Triplett, 2016).

Table 5.3. Percent Contributions of Anaerobic and Aerobic Metabolism

	0-5 SEC.	**30 SEC.**	**60 SEC.**	**90 SEC.**	**150 SEC.**	**200 SEC.**
Anaerobic	96	75	50	35	30	22
Aerobic	4	25	50	65	70	78

Phosphagen system. The phosphagen system is involved at the beginning of all activity regardless of exercise intensity and provides energy by breaking down ATP and **creatine phosphate (CP)** (an important compound that donates its phosphate to adenosine diphosphate (ADP) in order to make ATP) stored in the muscle cell. This process continues until exercise stops or the intensity is low enough to allow glycolysis or the oxidative system to take over. The amount of ATP and CP stored in the muscle is relatively small, which explains why the phosphagen system can only provide energy for a short period of time. The ability to store more ATP and CP in the muscle is likely one of the reasons why some individuals are able to sprint faster and longer than others.

Glycolytic system. The process of breaking down carbohydrates involves multiple catabolic reactions and thus is why the glycolytic system is not as fast at producing ATP as the phosphagen system. However, because there is greater supply of glycogen and glucose in the muscle as compared to ATP and CP, the duration of energy production in the glycolytic system is significantly longer than that of the phosphagen system. The end result of glycolysis is **pyruvate**. Depending on exercise intensity and the availability of oxygen, pyruvate will either be converted to **lactate** (substance created when glucose is broken down for energy during intense exercise) or shuttled into the mitochondria of the muscle cell and enter the **Krebs cycle** (next step after glycolysis used in the production of ATP). If the energy demand is great, such as with resistance training and sprinting, then pyruvate is converted into lactate. If the energy demand is not as great and oxygen is available in sufficient quantities, such as with walking, jogging, and riding a bike, then pyruvate is shuttled from the sarcoplasm to the mitochondria where it enters the Krebs cycle. It is sometimes mistakenly said that lactic acid is formed from pyruvate during high intensity exercise. However, due to the pH in the muscle as well as some of the previous steps in the glycolysis process, lactate – not lactic acid – is produced (Haff & Triplett, 2016).

Oxidative system. The oxidative system is the primary source of ATP production during rest and low-intensity activities. Although carbohydrates and fats are the preferred substrates, the oxidative system can also metabolize protein. At rest, roughly 70% of the ATP production comes from fat and 30% from carbohydrates. As exercise intensity increases, however, there is a shift from fats to carbohydrates. In fact, during high-intensity activity virtually all of the ATP produced comes from carbohydrates. During long duration low activity exercise, both fats and carbohydrates are used to produce ATP. The percentage of contribution coming from carbohydrates and fat is based on exercise intensity, duration, and substrate availability.

As mentioned previously, all three energy pathways are always active and contributing to some extent to the overall production of ATP. Therefore, it is recommended to train and develop each of the different energy systems individually. Short distance sprints will help to develop the phosphagen system; longer distance sprints will help to develop the glycolytic system; and long duration, low-intensity exercise will help to develop the oxidative system. **Figure 5.1.** depicts when the different biological energy systems are used as well as the ATP production capacity of each. **Table 5.4** provides recommendations for how to train each of the different energy systems.

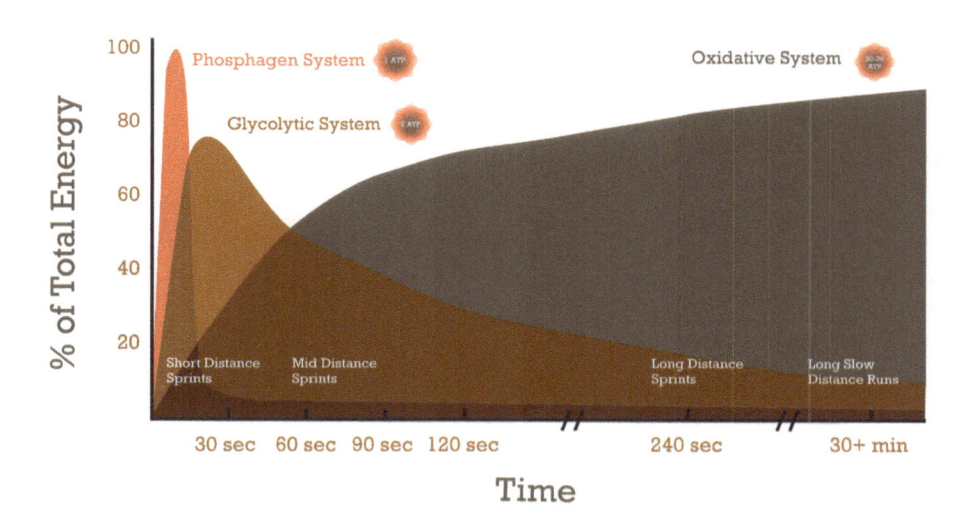

Figure 5.1. The 3 Biological Energy Systems Used During Exercise

Table 5.4. Training the Three Energy Systems

Energy System	Ways to Train
Phosphagen	Short Distance Sprints (e.g., 40-yd dash, 100-m sprints)
Glycolytic	Mid-Distance Sprints (e.g., 200-m sprints, 400-m sprints) Shuttle Runs (e.g., 300-yd shuttle)
Oxidative	Long-Distance Sprints (e.g., 800-m sprints) Pace-Tempo Training (e.g., 5-min easy, 10-min hard repeats, 1-mile repeats) Long Slow Distance Runs (e.g., run 3+ miles, run 20+ minutes)

Factors Related to Endurance Performance

There are four major factors that influence endurance performance: VO_2max (aka maximal aerobic power), lactate threshold, exercise economy and muscle fiber type.

VO_2max is the maximum amount of oxygen the body can take in and utilize during one minute of high intensity exercise. VO_2max is expressed mathematically as the amount of O_2 consumed by the body in a minute divided by body weight in kilograms (kg).

$$VO_2\text{max} = \frac{\text{ml of } O_2 \text{ consumed}}{\text{Body Weight (kg)}}$$

A higher VO_2max correlates to an increased ability of the muscles to extract and utilize oxygen, which allows the individual to train harder and longer. Additionally, a higher VO_2max also correlates to an increased ability of the muscles to buffer lactate production and delay the onset of fatigue. Elite level VO_2max scores for males are in the upper 70s into the 80s ml/kg/min and in the mid-60s to low 70s ml/kg/min for females. Conversely, VO_2max scores for the average college age male are somewhere between the upper 30s to low 40s ml/kg/min and in the mid-30s ml/kg/ml for the average college age female. After the age of 40, VO_2max decreases by roughly 10% per

Chapter 5: Training for Endurance

decade until it gets down to 20 ml/kg/min. **Table 5.5** provides VO_2max score classification based on gender and age (McCardle et al., 2015). Participation in regular endurance training is shown to increase the VO_2max of untrained individuals (up to 25-30%). However, significant improvements in well-trained endurance athletes are less likely.

Table 5.5. VO_2max Score Classification Based on Gender and Age

	≤ 29		30 - 39		40 - 49		50 - 59		60 -69	
	Male	Female	Male	Female	Male	Female	Male	Female	Male	Female
Excellent	≥ 53	≥ 49	≥ 50	≥ 45	≥ 45	≥ 45	≥ 43	≥ 40	≥ 41	≥ 37
Good	44 - 52.9	39 - 48.9	42 - 49.9	37 - 44.9	39 - 44.9	37 - 44.9	38 - 42.9	34 - 39.9	36 - 40.9	33 - 36.9
Average	34 - 43.9	31 - 38.9	31 - 41.9	28 - 36.9	27 - 38.9	28 - 36.9	25 - 37.9	22 - 33.9	23 - 35.9	21 - 32.9
Fair	25 - 33.9	24 - 30.9	23 - 30.9	20 - 27.9	20 - 26.9	20 - 27.9	18 - 24.9	15 - 21.9	16 - 22.9	13 - 20.9
Poor	≤ 24.9	≤ 23.9	≤ 22.9	≤ 19.9	≤ 19.9	≤ 19.9	≤ 17.9	≤ 14.9	≤ 15.9	≤ 12.9

Numerous studies have shown that run time of various endurance events (e.g., 1.0-mile, 1.5-mile) correlates extremely well to VO_2max (Haff & Triplett, 2016). This correlation proves to be very useful because if you know one variable then you can accurately predict the other. For example, an individual who ran a mile in 7 minutes and 30 seconds would have an estimated VO_2max score of 38 ml/kg/min. Similarly, an individual who had their VO_2max measured in a human performance lab and achieved a VO_2max score of 48 ml/kg/min should be able to run a mile in just over 6 minutes. **Table 5.6** provides estimated VO_2max scores based on run times of various distances (Cooper, 1968; Daniels, 2014).

Table 5.6. Estimated VO$_2$max Score Based on Various Run Distances (min:sec)

VO$_2$max	1-Mile	1.5-Mile	2-Mile	5-km	10-km	½ Marathon	Marathon
30	9:11	16:20	19:19	30:40	63:46	2:21:04	4:49:17
32	8:41	15:38	18:18	29:05	60:26	2:13:49	4:34:59
34	8:14	14:50	17:24	27:39	57:26	2:07:16	4:22:03
36	7:49	13:54	16:34	26:22	54:44	2:01:19	4:10:19
38	7:27	13:12	15:49	25:12	52:17	1:55:55	3:59:35
40	7:07	12:36	15:08	24:08	50:03	1:50:59	3:49:45
42	6:49	12:14	14:31	23:09	48:01	1:46:27	3:40:43
44	6:32	11:35	13:56	22:15	46:09	1:42:17	3:32:23
45	6:25	11:22	13:40	21:50	45:16	1:40:20	3:28:26
46	6:17	11:07	13:25	21:25	44:25	1:38:27	3:24:39
47	6:10	10:53	13:10	21:02	43:36	1:36:38	3:21:00
48	6:03	10:40	12:55	20:39	42:50	1:34:53	3:17:29
49	5:56	10:24	12:41	20:18	42:04	1:33:12	3:14:06
50	5:50	10:17	12:28	19:57	41:21	1:31:35	3:10:49
51	5:44	10:01	12:15	19:36	40:39	1:30:02	3:07:39
52	5:38	9:53	12:02	19:17	39:59	1:28:31	3:04:36
53	5:32	9:44	11:50	18:58	39:20	1:27:04	3:01:39
54	5:27	9:35	11:39	18:40	38:42	1:25:40	2:58:47
55	5:21	9:26	11:28	18:22	38:06	1:24:18	2:56:01
56	5:16	9:18	11:17	18:05	37:31	1:23:00	2:53:20
57	5:11	9:09	11:06	17:49	36:57	1:21:43	2:50:45
58	5:06	9:02	10:56	17:33	36:24	1:20:30	2:48:14
59	5:02	8:51	10:46	17:17	35:52	1:19:18	2:45:47
60	4:57	8:43	10:37	17:03	35:22	1:18:09	2:43:25
61	4:53	8:32	10:27	16:48	34:52	1:17:02	2:41:08
62	4:49	8:25	10:18	16:34	34:23	1:15:57	2:38:54
63	4:45	8:12	10:10	16:20	33:55	1:14:54	2:36:44
64	4:41	8:09	10:01	16:07	33:28	1:13:53	2:34:38
65	4:37	8:02	9:53	15:54	33:01	1:12:53	2:32:35
66	4:33	7:55	9:45	15:42	32:35	1:11:56	2:30:36
67	4:30	7:48	9:37	15:29	32:11	1:11:00	2:28:40
68	4:26	7:43	9:30	15:18	31:46	1:10:05	2:26:47
69	4:23	7:38	9:23	15:06	31:23	1:09:12	2:24:57
70	4:19	7:30	9:16	14:55	31:00	1:08:21	2:23:10
71	4:16	7:23	9:09	14:44	30:38	1:07:31	2:21:26
72	4:13	7:16	9:02	14:33	30:16	1:06:42	2:19:44
73	4:10	7:08	8:55	14:23	29:55	1:05:54	2:18:05
74	4:07	7:00	8:49	14:13	29:34	1:05:08	2:16:29
75	4:04	6:53	8:43	14:03	29:14	1:04:23	2:14:55
76	4:02	6:47	8:37	13:54	28:55	1:03:39	2:13:23
77	3:58	6:36	8:31	13:44	28:36	1:02:56	2:11:54
78	3:56	6:28	8:25	13:35	28:17	1:02:15	2:10:27
79	3:53	6:20	8:20	13:26	27:59	1:01:34	2:09:02
80	3:51	6:10	8:14	13:17	27:41	1:00:54	2:07:38

CHAPTER 5: TRAINING FOR ENDURANCE

By understanding the relationship between VO$_2$max and run time, it is also possible to manipulate the VO$_2$max equation in order to determine a specific VO$_2$max score to be attained. The numerator of the equation, which is expressed in ml of O$_2$ consumed, can be manipulated to calculate how much fitness someone would need to gain to attain a particular VO$_2$max score. The denominator, which is expressed in kg, can be manipulated to calculate how much weight would need to be lost to attain a specific VO$_2$max score. For example, say you have a 165 lb. (75 kg) female who currently runs the mile in 7 minutes and 45 seconds but whose goal is to run a mile in 7 minutes. Assuming her current fitness level (numerator) remained the same, we could manipulate the VO$_2$max formula to determine what her body weight (denominator) would need to be in order to achieve a VO$_2$max score of 41 (which equates to a 7:00 1.0-mile run time).

$$\frac{??? \text{ ml O}_2}{75 \text{ kg}} = 36 \text{ ml O}_2/\text{kg} \quad \rightarrow \quad 36 \text{ ml O}_2/\text{kg} \times 75 \text{ kg} = 2{,}700 \text{ ml O}_2$$

$$\frac{2{,}700 \text{ ml O}_2}{??? \text{ kg}} = 41 \text{ ml O2}/\text{kg} \quad \rightarrow \quad 2{,}700 \text{ ml O}_2 \div 41 \text{ ml O}_2/\text{kg} = 65.8 \text{ kg}$$

$$75 \text{ kg} - 65.8 \text{ kg} = 9.2 \text{ kg} \quad \rightarrow \quad 9.2 \text{ kg} \times 2.2 \text{ lbs.}/\text{kg} = 20.2 \text{ lbs.} \quad \rightarrow \quad 165 \text{ lbs.} - 20.2 \text{ lbs.} = 144.8 \text{ lbs.}$$

From the above calculations, we see that she would need to lose a little over 20 lbs. in order to improve her VO$_2$max score from 36 to 41 ml/kg/min. Again, this example assumed that her current level of fitness (numerator) remained the same. Additionally, losing weight may not always be the best approach to improving VO$_2$max scores. For example, it would be contraindicated for individuals who already have a low percentage of body fat to lose weight, as the majority of weight lost would come from either water and/or fat free mass (muscle). Instead, it would be better for those individuals to perform regular speed and pace/tempo training in an effort to improve their level of fitness (numerator). In most cases, VO$_2$max scores are improved by increasing one's level of physical fitness (numerator) while simultaneously decreasing body weight (denominator). Recommendations for improving VO$_2$max consist of performing high-intensity interval training 1-2 times per week (Haff & Triplett, 2016).

Lactate threshold (LT) is the point in exercise at which lactate starts to accumulate in the blood above resting levels. Many researchers believe lactate threshold to be a better predictor of cardiovascular fitness than VO$_2$max (Haff & Triplett, 2016). An individual's LT defines the upper limit of a sustainable pace that can be maintained during training and/or competition. After blood lactate starts to accumulate above resting levels, it becomes impossible for the body to sustain that pace thereby resulting in fatigue. Running at paces below LT will allow the body to reach a steady state in which lactate production no longer increases and remains relatively stable. Ideally, athletes would be able to find and run at their **maximal lactate steady state (MLSS)** as this would allow them to run at the fastest possible pace without causing fatigue.

Ironically, athletes with the same VO$_2$max can have significant differences in their lactate threshold. For example, assume we have two athletes preparing for a 1-mile run and both have the same or similar VO$_2$max scores. However, the LT for the first athlete occurs at 70% of their VO$_2$max; whereas, the LT for the second athlete occurs at 60% of their VO$_2$max. Because the first athlete is able to run at and sustain a pace at higher percentage of their VO$_2$max, he/she will be able to run 1.0-mile faster than the second athlete. In untrained individuals, LT generally occurs around 60-70% of their VO$_2$max. In well-trained endurance athletes, LT generally occurs around 75-80% of their VO$_2$max. In elite endurance athletes, LT can occur at 90% or more of their VO$_2$max (McCormick, n.d.). Recommendations for increasing LT include high-intensity interval training and/or interval training 1-2 times per week as well as pace / tempo training 1-2 times per week (Haff & Triplett, 2016).

Exercise economy is the amount of energy required to maintain a consistent pace. Although not to the same extent as VO$_2$max or LT, research suggests exercise economy to be another important factor in predicting endurance performance and may explain some of the performance differences between individuals (Peterson & Rittenhouse, 2019). Some of the factors that influence exercise economy include neuromuscular coordination, muscle fiber type, joint stability, and flexibility (Training 4 Endurance, 2017). Recommendations for improving exercise economy include regular participation in drills aimed at improving overall run technique (e.g., skipping, bounding, double and single-leg hops, sprinting). Other recommendations include lower body resistance and plyometric training, especially single-leg exercises (e.g., Bulgarian split squats, lunges), as well as exercises aimed at strengthening the torso (e.g., plank, side plank, back hyperextensions).

Muscle fiber type is another, albeit small, factor that can influence endurance performance. Individuals with higher percentages of slow-twitch (type I) muscle fibers tend to perform better at slower, longer endurance events (e.g., 5-km, 10-km, ½ marathon, marathon); whereas individuals with higher percentages of fast-twitch (type II) muscle fibers tend to perform better at faster, shorter endurance events (e.g., 100-m, 200-m, 400-m, 800-m). Although the majority of slow-twitch muscle fibers seem to be set at birth, a small percentage of fast-twitch fibers can become more aerobic in nature with chronic endurance training (a process called fiber type transition). **Figure 5.2** depicts the differences in muscle fiber type percentages for long, middle, and short distance endurance athletes. The red cells represent slow-twitch (type I) muscle fibers; whereas, the white cells represent fast-twitch (type II) muscle fibers.

Figure 5.2. Fiber Type Differences between Endurance Athletes

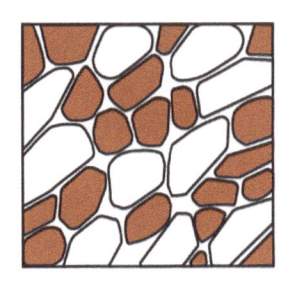

Long Distance Events
(e.g., 5-km, 10-km)

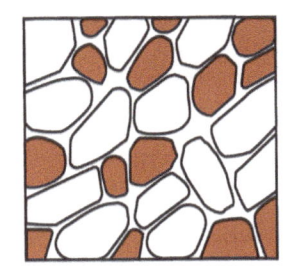

Mid Distance Events
(e.g., 1-mi, 1.5-mi)

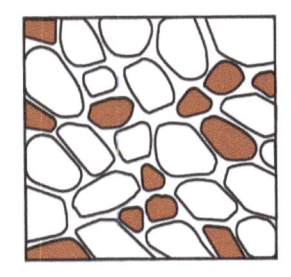

Short Distance Events
(e.g., 100-m, 200-m)

Types of Endurance Training

Now that we understand the different biological energy systems and factors affecting endurance performance, let's explore some of the different ways in which to train to improve endurance performance. There are five different types of endurance training programs: long slow distance (LSD) training, pace / tempo training, interval training, high-intensity interval training and Fartlek training. Each type of endurance has its own specific guidelines regarding exercise frequency, intensity, duration, and progression. **Table 5.7** outlines the training guidelines for the five different types of endurance training (Haff & Triplett, 2016).

Table 5.7. The Five Types of Endurance Training

Endurance Type	Intensity	Duration	Frequency	Work : Rest Ratio
Long Slow Distance	70-80% MHR	6-7 RPE	30-120 min	1+	-
Pace / Tempo	80-90% MHR	7-8 RPE	20-30 min	1-2	-
Interval	> 90% MHR	8-9 RPE	3-5 min	1-2	1:1
High-Intensity Interval	≤ 100% MHR	9-10 RPE	30-90 sec	1	1:5
Fartlek	70-90% MHR	6-8 RPE	20-60 min	1	-

MHR = Maximum heart rate

RPE = Rate of perceived exertion (quantitative measure of perceived exertion during physical activity)

Long slow distance (LSD) training, aka low-intensity steady state training, is a type of endurance training that employs a constant pace at low to moderate intensity over an extended distance or period of time. Due to the low to moderate intensities used, LSD is effective in improving VO_2max scores in untrained or moderately trained individuals, however, less effective in improving VO_2max scores in well-trained individuals. Generally speaking, more run mileage per week is almost always better than less mileage in terms of improving LSD performance. However, some researchers suggest that running more than 60 miles per week may increase an individual's risk for overtraining and/or injury (Prevost, 2015). The physiological adaptations associated with LSD training include improved cardiovascular function, oxidative capacity, thermoregulation, mitochondrial energy production and fat utilization (Haff & Triplett, 2016).

Pace / tempo training, aka lactate threshold training, is another type of endurance training that employs intensities at or slightly higher than race pace intensity. The primary function of pace / tempo training is to develop a sense of running pace as well as improve the body's ability to sustain that pace. There are two types of pace / tempo training: steady and intermittent. Steady pace / tempo training involves employing training intensities equal to lactate threshold (LT) consistently for 20-30 minutes. Intermittent pace / tempo training also employs training intensities equal to LT but through a series of intervals with brief rest periods in between. With either type (i.e., steady or intermittent), training intensities should not go above LT. In fact, it is recommended to increase training distance rather than intensity. The physiological adaptations associated with pace/tempo training include: improved running economy, improved LT, increased mitochondrial density, increased number and activity of oxidative enzymes and an aerobic shift in the type II muscle fibers (Haff & Triplett, 2016).

Interval training is a type of endurance training that employs training intensities close to VO$_2$max. In order to account for, and recover from, the amount of lactate being produced with this type of training, sufficient time should be afforded between intervals. The recommended **work-to-rest (work:rest) ratio** for interval training is 1:1. Specifically, work intervals should last between 3-5 minutes with similar amount of time afforded for rest in between (e.g., 3 minutes of running followed by 3 minutes of slow walking). The physiological adaptations associated with interval training include increased VO$_2$max and anaerobic metabolism (Haff & Triplett, 2016).

High-intensity interval training (HIIT), previously referred to as repetition training, is another type of endurance training used to develop speed and endurance. High-intensity interval training employs short bouts of speed training at intensities above VO$_2$max. The recommended work:rest ratio for HIIT is 1:5. Specifically, work intervals should last between 30-90 seconds with 2.5-7.5 minutes of rest in between. Both interval training and HIIT are very taxing on the body and thus should not be performed more than 1-2 times per week. The physiological adaptations associated with HIIT include increased VO$_2$max and anaerobic metabolism as well as increases in running speed and economy, capillary density, left ventricle size, maximal cardiac output, resting and maximal stroke volume, blood volume and hemoglobin (Haff & Triplett, 2016).

Fartlek, which is Swedish for "speed play", is the last type of endurance training that combines low slow distance (LSD) training with several of the other types of endurance training (e.g., pace / tempo, interval). Examples of Fartlek training include running the straightaways and walking the curves on a standard 200-m or 400-m track, running the distance between 4 telephone poles then walking the distance between 2 telephone poles, or performing back-to-front sprints (i.e., type of team jogging where all of the participants are in a single file line where the last person in line sprints to the front, which is repeated for the duration of the exercise). Due to its variability and versatility, Fartlek training may also help to reduce the boredom and monotony often associated with long-term endurance training. The physiological adaptations associated with Fartlek training include enhanced VO$_2$max, lactate threshold, running economy and fuel utilization (Haff & Triplett, 2016).

Although there are five distinct types of endurance training, categorization can be reduced to three: long slow distance training, pace / tempo training and speed training. Since Fartlek training is a combination of several of the other types of endurance training (e.g., LSD, pace / tempo, interval), inclusion in an endurance training program is not necessary as long as all of the other types are already being performed.

Additionally, since both interval and HIIT utilize the same energy pathways and result in similar physiological adaptations, the two types of training could be used interchangeably. For example, if your endurance training program calls for one day per week of speed training, you could alternate back and forth between interval and HIIT training. **Table 5.8** provides some sample workouts for LSD, pace / tempo and speed (i.e., interval, HIIT) training.

CHAPTER 5: TRAINING FOR ENDURANCE

Table 5.8. Sample Workouts for Each Type of Endurance Training

LSD	PACE / TEMPO	SPEED	
		INTERVAL	HIIT
Run 3-5 miles	5-min Easy / 10-min Hard Repeats	4-6x 400m Sprints	8-10x 100m Sprints
Run 30+ minutes	Treadmill Tempo Run	2-3x 800m Sprints	6-8x 200m Sprints
		1-mile Repeats	6-8 x 300yd Shuttle

The above recommendations illustrate how to train the different types of endurance training (i.e., LSD, pace / tempo, interval, high-intensity interval training, Fartlek) through various running-specific drills and activities. However, it is worth mentioning that the different types of endurance training can also be trained using non-running activities as well such as walking, swimming, biking, rowing and elliptical training. **Table 5.9** provides some sample workouts for LSD, pace / tempo and speed training for non-running activities.

Table 5.9. Sample Workouts for Non-Running Activities

LSD	PACE / TEMPO	SPEED	
		INTERVAL	HIIT
Exercise 30+ min.	5-min Easy / 10-min Hard Repeats	3-5 min. high-intensity repeats coupled with 3-5 min. of low-intensity recovery periods	30-90 sec. high-intensity repeats coupled with 2.5-5 min. of low-intensity recovery periods

Treadmill Tempo Run

As mentioned previously, pace / tempo training is an effective method for improving lactate threshold (LT). Additionally, traditional approaches to pace / tempo training include either steady or intermittent training. Another, more recent, option to training pace /tempo, and improving LT, is the **treadmill tempo run**. This approach to pace / tempo is best used when training for mid distance endurance events (e.g., 1.0-mile, 1.5-mile, 2.0-mile, 3.0-mile, 5-km). Provided below are the required steps for how to perform the treadmill tempo run for the mile.

Step 1: Subtract 10-20 seconds from last 1.0 mile run time to determine desired run time

Step 2: 60 ÷ desired run time = required miles per hour (MPH)

Step 3: Run 1.0-mile at required MPH at 0% incline and walk as required. However, only the distance ran counts toward the 1.0-mile distance

Step 4: When able to run the entire 1.0-mile without stopping, increase incline to 0.5% and repeat

Step 5: When able to run the entire 1.0-mile at 0.5% incline without stopping, increase incline to 1.0% and repeat

Step 6: When able to run the entire 1.0-mile at 1.0% incline without stopping, subtract 10-20 seconds from current desired run time and repeat the entire process

Let's perform a sample calculation using our example from earlier. Let's use 7 minutes and 45 seconds as our current 1.0-mile run time. For **Step 1**, let's subtract 15 seconds (halfway between 10 and 20), which equates to a desired run time of 7 minutes and 30 seconds. For **Step 2**, we need to convert the number of seconds to a numeric. For example, as a numeric 30 seconds = 0.5, not 0.3. To convert to a numeric, divide the number of seconds by 60 (i.e., 30 ÷ 60 = 0.5). So, our required miles per hour would be 8 mph (i.e., 60 ÷ 7.5 = 8).

In terms of determining how many seconds to subtract, faster runners should be more conservative (subtracting less time) with the number of seconds to subtract whereas novice or slower runners should be more liberal (subtracting more time). For example, individuals capable of running a 1.0-mile run time of 6 minutes or faster should only subtract 10 seconds whereas someone capable of running a 1.0-mile run time of 8 minutes and 45 seconds or slower should subtract 20 seconds. A good way to gauge whether you need to subtract more or less time is by counting how many times you had to stop and walk. If you had to stop more than two times in a session, then you likely subtracted too many seconds. Conversely, if you did not have to stop at all, then you likely did not subtract enough seconds. If performed correctly and consistently 1-2 time per week, most individuals are able to achieve their desired run time in about 4-6 weeks. **Table 5.10** provides the required miles per hour (mph) for several possible 1.0-mile run times.

Table 5.10. Desired Run Times and Required Miles Per Hour (MPH) for the 1.0-Mile Run

Desired Run Time	Required MPH	Desired Run Time	Required MPH	Desired Run Time	Required MPH
12:00	5.0	8:34	7.0	6:40	9.0
11:40	5.1	8:27	7.1	6:35	9.1
11:32	5.2	8:20	7.2	6:31	9.2
11:20	5.3	8:13	7.3	6:27	9.3
11:07	5.4	8:07	7.4	6:23	9.4
11:00	5.5	8:00	7.5	6:20	9.5
10:40	5.6	7:53	7.6	6:15	9.6
10:32	5.7	7:47	7.7	6:11	9.7
10:20	5.8	7:40	7.8	6:07	9.8
10:10	5.9	7:35	7.9	6:04	9.9
10:00	6.0	7:30	8.0	6:00	10.0
9:50	6.1	7:24	8.1	5:56	10.1
9:40	6.2	7:20	8.2	5:53	10.2
9:31	6.3	7:14	8.3	5:50	10.3
9:20	6.4	7:08	8.4	5:46	10.4
9:14	6.5	7:04	8.5	5:43	10.5
9:05	6.6	7:00	8.6	5:40	10.6
9:00	6.7	6:54	8.7	5:37	10.7
8:49	6.8	6:49	8.8	5:34	10.8
8:40	6.9	6:44	8.9	5:30	10.9

As mentioned previously, the treadmill tempo run is a very effective way of training for mid distance endurance events (e.g., 1.0-mile, 1.5-mile, 2.0-mile, 3.0-mile, 5-km). Although this method of training can be used for race distances greater than a 10-km (6.2-mi.), it may not prove as effective, as it does for mid-distance events, due to the pace being too slow to produce the physiological adaptations associated with LT training. Even so, pace / tempo training may still be beneficial for ultra-endurance athletes as it has been shown to increase both running economy and lactate threshold (LT), which can result in improved run times for longer distance events.

As depicted above, the number 60 is the dividend used to calculate the desired run time for 1.0-mile. **Table 5.11** provides the required dividend and recommended seconds or minutes to subtract for several other mid-distance and long-distance endurance events.

Table 5.11. Required Dividend and Recommended Seconds to Subtract for Various Endurance Events

RACE DISTANCE (MI.)	REQUIRED DIVIDEND	SECONDS TO SUBTRACT	MINUTES TO SUBTRACT
1.0	60	10-20	-
1.5	90	15-30	-
2.0	120	20-45	-
3.0	180	30-60	-
3.1 (5-km)	180.6	30-60	-
6.2 (10-km)	361.2	60-90	-
13.1 (½ Marathon)	786	-	3-5
26.2 (Marathon)	1,572	-	10-20
50	3,000	-	45-60
100	6,000	-	90-120

Measuring Intensity for Endurance Training

As depicted in **Table 5.7**, the intensity used for the different types of endurance training is typically based on **maximum heart rate (MHR)**. However, unless you have a heart rate monitor, it can be difficult to accurately assess heart rate while exercising. Additionally, research has shown that MHR can vary significantly between individuals regardless of fitness level or age thereby calling into question the accuracy of using prediction equations to determine MHR (Prevost, 2015).

A study by Robergs (2002) demonstrates the variability of the **age-predicted maximum heart rate (APMHR) equation** (i.e., 220 - Age = MHR). The green dots in **Figure 5.3** represent measured MHR for individuals of various ages. The red line represents estimated MHR for each age group as calculated by the APMHR equation. As demonstrated in the figure, the APMHR equation over-predicted MHR for some individuals and under-predicted MPR for others. This means that if the APMHR equation was used to prescribe exercise intensity that some individuals would be undertraining while others would be overtraining.

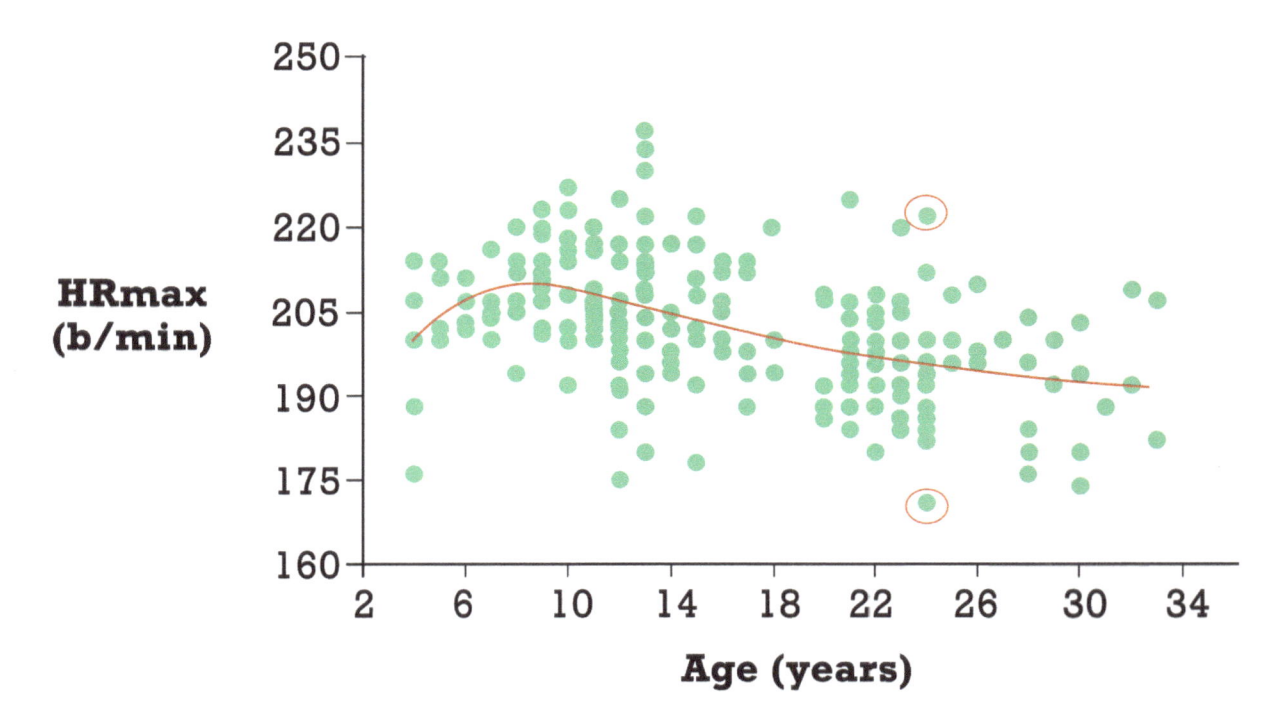

Figure 5.3. Accuracy of the Age-Predicted Maximum Heart Rate (APMHR) Equation

As a result of the limitations associated with MHR, other methods are often used for accessing exercise intensity including **rate of perceived exertion (RPE)** and the **talk test**. The RPE is a quantitative measure of how an individual perceives exertion during physical activity. The talk test is another easy way to estimate exercise intensity. For example, exercise is classified as moderate-intensity if an individual can talk, but not sing, during the activity. As demonstrated in **Table 5.12**, research shows a strong collection correlation between MHR, RPE, and the talk test (U.S. Navy Command Fitness Leader Course, n.d.). In other words, if you do not have the ability to measure your MHR or access to a heart rate monitor, using RPE or the talk test is an easy and reliable means of monitoring exercise intensity.

Table 5.12. Correlation between Maximum Heart Rate (MHR), Rate of Perceived Exertion (RPE) and the Talk Test

	RPE	TALK TEST	% MHR
1	Very Light Activity	Minimal effort required	< 40
2-3	Light Activity	Breathing is easy, can sing	40-49
4-6	Moderate Activity	Can carry a conversation	50-69
7-8	Vigorous Activity	Short of breath, can only speak a sentence or two	70-85
9	Very Hard Activity	Can only speak one word at a time	86-92
10	Maximum Effort Activity	Completely out of breath, unable to talk	> 92

Developing a Personalized Endurance Training Program

Several factors need to be considered when developing a personalized endurance training program. Some of the factors include the fitness level and injury status of the individual as well as the distance and/or duration of the event. For example, individuals training for endurance events lasting roughly 30 minutes or less (e.g., 1.5-mile, 2.0-mile, 3.0-mile, 5-km runs) would benefit more from an endurance training program consisting of pace / tempo, speed and some long slow distance (LSD) work. Whereas, individuals training for endurance events lasting longer than 30 minutes (e.g., 10-km, ½ marathon, marathon, 50-miler) would benefit more from an endurance training program consisting predominantly of LSD and possibly some pace / tempo work.

Provided below is a sample 9-week "Couch to 5-km" running program (c25k, n.d.). As depicted in **Table 5.13**, this program consists primarily of LSD training, which may be suitable for novice runners or those individuals interested more in the health benefits associated with regular endurance training than in performance. However, if the goal is to maximize endurance performance, then both interval training and high-intensity interval training (HIIT) should also be performed regularly in order to improve VO_2max and lactate threshold (LT). **Table 5.14** provides a sample 9-week endurance training that may be better suited for individuals interested in improving performance as it consists of LSD, pace / tempo, and speed training.

Table 5.13. Sample Couch to 5-km Running Program

Week	Session 1	Session 2	Session 3
1	Brisk 5-min. walk, then alternate 60-sec. of jogging and 90-sec. of walking for 20 min.	Brisk 5-min. walk, then alternate 60-sec. of jogging and 90-sec. of walking for 20 min.	Brisk 5-min. walk, then alternate 60-sec. of jogging and 90-sec. of walking for 20 min.
2	Brisk 5-min. walk, then alternate 90-sec. of jogging and 2-min. of walking for 20 min.	Brisk 5-min. walk, then alternate 90-sec. of jogging and 2-min. of walking for 20 min.	Brisk 5-min. walk, then alternate 90-sec. of jogging and 2-min. of walking for 20 min.
3	Brisk 5-min. walk., then Jog 200-yds (or 90-sec.), walk 200-yds (or 90-sec.), jog 400-yds (or 3-min.), walk 400-yds (or 3-min.)	Brisk 5-min. walk., then Jog 200-yds (or 90-sec.), walk 200-yds (or 90-sec.), jog 400-yds (or 3-min.), walk 400-yds (or 3-min.)	Brisk 5-min. walk., then Jog 200-yds (or 90-sec.), walk 200-yds (or 90-sec.), jog 400-yds (or 3-min.), walk 400-yds (or 3-min.)
4	Brisk 5-min. walk., then Jog ¼-mi. (or 3-min.), walk ⅛-mi. (or 90-sec.), jog ½-mi. (or 5-min.), walk ¼ mi. (or 2.5-min.), jog ¼-mi. (or 3-min.), walk ⅛-mi. (or 90-sec.), jog ½-mi. (or 5-min.)	Brisk 5-min. walk., then Jog ¼-mi. (or 3-min.), walk ⅛-mi. (or 90-sec.), jog ½-mi. (or 5-min.), walk ¼ mi. (or 2.5-min.), jog ¼-mi. (or 3-min.), walk ⅛-mi. (or 90-sec.), jog ½-mi. (or 5-min.)	Brisk 5-min. walk., then Jog ¼-mi. (or 3-min.), walk ⅛-mi. (or 90-sec.), jog ½-mi. (or 5-min.), walk ¼ mi. (or 2.5-min.), jog ¼-mi. (or 3-min.), walk ⅛-mi. (or 90-sec.), jog ½-mi. (or 5-min.)
5	Brisk 5-min. walk., then Jog ½-mi. (or 5-min.), walk ¼-mi. (or 3-min.), jog ½-mi. (or 5-min.), walk ¼-mi. (or 3-min.), Jog ½-mi. (or 5-min.)	Brisk 5-min. walk., then Jog ¾-mi. (or 8-min.), walk ½-mi. (or 5-min.), jog ¾-mi. (or 8-min.)	Brisk 5-min. walk., then Jog 2.0-mi. (or 20-min.) with no walking
6	Brisk 5-min. walk., then Jog ½-mi. (or 5-min.), walk ¼-mi. (or 3-min.), jog ¾-mi. (or 8-min.), walk ¼-mi. (or 3-min.), Jog ½-mi. (or 5-min.)	Brisk 5-min. walk., then Jog 1-mi. (or 10-min.), walk ¼-mi. (or 3-min.), jog 1-mi. (or 10-min.)	Brisk 5-min. walk., then Jog 2¼-mi. (or 25-min.) with no walking
7	Brisk 5-min. walk., then Jog 2½-mi. (or 25-min.)	Brisk 5-min. walk., then Jog 2½-mi. (or 25-min.)	Brisk 5-min. walk., then Jog 2½-mi. (or 25-min.)
8	Brisk 5-min. walk. Jog 2¾-mi. or 28-min.	Brisk 5-min. walk. Jog 2¾-mi. or 28-min.	Brisk 5-min. walk. Jog 2¾-mi. or 28-min..
9	Brisk 5-min. walk, then Jog 3-miles. or 30-min.	Brisk 5-min. walk, then Jog 3-miles. or 30-min.	Brisk 5-min. walk, then Jog 3-miles. or 30-min.

Chapter 5: Training for Endurance

Table 5.14. Sample 9-Week Endurance Training Program

Week	ET Type	Frequency	Duration	Sets	Rest Interval
1	LSD	3	20	N/A	N/A
	Pace / Tempo	N/A	N/A	N/A	N/A
	Speed	N/A	N/A	N/A	N/A
2	LSD	3	22	N/A	N/A
	Pace / Tempo	N/A	N/A	N/A	N/A
	Speed	N/A	N/A	N/A	N/A
3	LSD	3	25	N/A	N/A
	Pace / Tempo	1	15	N/A	1:1
	Speed	N/A	N/A	N/A	N/A
4	LSD	3	27	N/A	N/A
	Pace / Tempo	1	17	N/A	1:1
	Speed	N/A	N/A	N/A	N/A
5	LSD	3	30	N/A	N/A
	Pace / Tempo	1	20	N/A	1:1
	Speed	N/A	N/A	N/A	N/A
6	LSD	2-3	30	N/A	N/A
	Pace / Tempo	1	20	N/A	1:1
	Speed	1	N/A	3-4	1:5
7	LSD	2-3	30	N/A	N/A
	Pace / Tempo	1-2	20	N/A	< 1:1
	Speed	1	N/A	3-4	1:5
8	LSD	2	30	N/A	N/A
	Pace / Tempo	1-2	20	N/A	< 1:1
	Speed	1-2	N/A	3-4	1:5
9	LSD	2	30	N/A	N/A
	Pace / Tempo	1-2	20	N/A	< 1:1
	Speed	1-2	N/A	4-5	< 1:5

How to Choose a Running Shoe

Whether you're running for pleasure or to compete, finding the right pair of running shoes is important as it helps to prevent running-related injuries as well as make the overall experience of running more enjoyable. Provided below are some recommendations to help find the correct running shoe for you (REI.com, n.d.). Although the below guidelines are intended for running shoes, they also apply to shoes used just for walking as well.

1. **Determine where you plan on running.** There are three basic types of running shoes: road-running, trail-running and cross-training shoes. **Road-running shoes** are designed for

runs on pavement, sidewalks, treadmills and tracks. **Trail-running shoes** are designed for off-road runs that may include the presence of rocks, mud, roots and/or other obstacles. **Cross-training shoes** are designed for strength training, cross-training and/or other activities where thinner sole shoes are preferred.

2. **Determine the desired level of cushioning.** The degree of cushioning provided by shoes is determined by two factors: foam firmness and sole thickness. The extent of firmness and thickness is a matter of personal preference. There are five major types of shoe cushioning: maximum cushion, moderate cushion, minimal cushion, barefoot and zero-drop.

   - **Maximum cushion** *shoes offer the thickest and softest foam and may be best suited for runners participating in long distance or multi-day runs.*

   - **Moderate cushion** *shoes offer a degree of cushioning between that of maximum and minimal cushion shoes.*

   - **Minimal cushion** *shoes offer a minimal amount of cushioning and may be best suited for runners who prefer the ability to feel the ground under them.*

   - **Barefoot** *shoes offer no or minimal cushion and provide a very thin layer (e.g., 3-4 mm) of material between foot and ground. It is important to note that barefoot shoes provide no arch support or stability features.*

   - **Zero-drop** *shoes provide an equal amount of cushioning from the heel to the toes. Conversely, traditional running shoes typically have more cushioning under the heel and less under the midfoot and toes - which results in the heel striking the ground first when running. Zero-drop shoes, on the other hand, have the same amount of cushioning throughout the sole - which results in the midfoot striking the ground first when running. It is important to note that zero-drop shoes place greater stress on the Achilles tendon, as compared to traditional running shoes, and therefore may require an adjustment period.* **Figure 5.4** *depicts the differences between a traditional running shoe and a zero-drop running shoe.*

Figure 5.4. Traditional Running Shoe vs. Zero-Drop Running Shoe

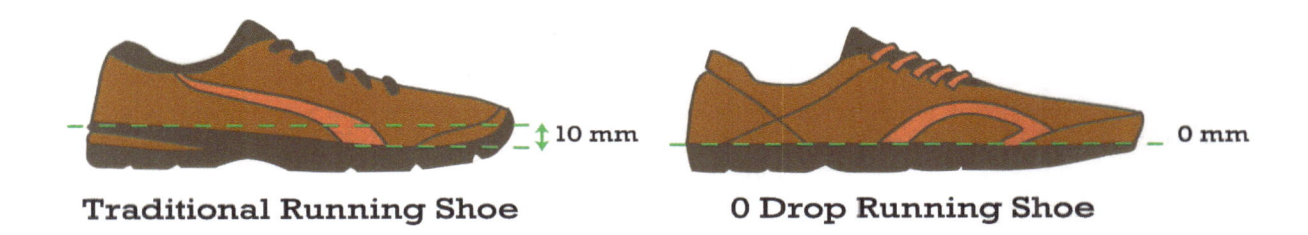

Traditional Running Shoe — 10 mm

0 Drop Running Shoe — 0 mm

Chapter 5: Training for Endurance

3. **Determine the desired level of support.** Once the desired level of cushioning has been determined, the next step is to determine the desired level of support as running shoes can be used to help limit and control the amount of foot pronation (i.e., the degree to which the foot rolls inward after striking the ground).

   There are three categories of support for running shoes: neutral, stability and motion control. **Neutral shoes** typically do not have any motion control features (e.g., medial posts to reinforce the arch side of each midsole) and are best suited for neutral runners or those who supinate (i.e., foot rolls outward). **Stability shoes** have stability devices embedded that help control pronation and are best suited for runners who exhibit mild to moderate overpronation. **Motion control** have stiffer heels and firm posts embedded that reinforce the arch side of each midsole and are best suited for runners who exhibit moderate to severe overpronation.

   Just as there are three categories of running shoe support, there are also three patterns of pronation: normal (or neutral) pronation, overpronation, and supination. One way to determine which pattern of pronation you have is to examine the wear pattern on a well-used pair of running shoes. **Table 5.15** can be used to determine support category to consider based on an individual's gait pattern and shoe wear pattern.

Table 5.15. Recommended Shoe Support Type Based on Gait and Wear Pattern

	Gait Pattern	Wear Pattern	Recommended Shoe Support Type
Normal Pronation (foot rolls inward a typical amount)			Neutral shoes or stability shoes with light structure
Supination (foot rolls outward excessively)			Neutral shoes
Overpronation (foot rolls inward excessively)			Stability shoes with structured support or motion control shoes

Tips for Selecting the Right Running Shoe for You

Once shoe type (i.e., road-running, trail-running, cross-training), level of cushioning (i.e., maximum cushion, moderate cushion, minimal cushion, barefoot, zero-drop), and level of support (i.e., neutral, stability and motion control) have all been the determined, the next and final step is purchase the right pair of running shoes. Provided below are five recommendations to help find the right running shoe for you (REI.com, n.d.).

1. **Try shoes on at the end of the day.** It is important to note that your feet swell throughout the day and will be largest at the end of the day. Trying shoes on in the morning may result in buying shoes that are too small.

2. **Try on both shoes.** Some individuals have one foot that is larger than the other. With that in mind, be sure to try on both the right and left shoe and select a pair that fits the larger foot.

3. **Allow for a thumbnail's length of space in the toe box.** A properly fitted shoe will allow you to wiggle your toes. Additionally, the width should be snug but still allow the foot to move without rubbing.

4. **Bring insoles, running socks and/or orthotics (if used) with you.** Socks, inserts and/or orthotics will undoubtedly affect how shoes fit. With that in mind, be sure to bring everything you plan on wearing in the shoes with you when trying on a new pair of shoes.

5. **Make sure they're comfortable.** Running shoes do not need to be broken in. Instead, they should be comfortable and provide a proper fit right out of the box.

Although not included in the above recommendations, how individuals lace their shoes can also have a profound impact on their fit and feel. For example, using the **runner's loop** can help secure your heel and keep it from slipping. Similarly, using **window lacing** can help relieve pressure points on the top of your foot, and the **reef knot** can help secure the laces and keep them from coming undone. **Table 5.16** depicts some of the common lacing techniques used with running shoes.

Table 5.16. Common Lacing Techniques Used with Running Shoes

Runner's Loop (secures heel and prevents toes from sliding forward)	Window Lacing (alleviates pressure points on the top of the foot)	Reef Knot (holds laces more securely)

When to Replace Your Running Shoes

Researchers recommend that running shoes be replaced after accumulating between 350-500 miles (Cook et al., 1985). While walking is not as hard on shoes as running, it is still unlikely they are able to provide adequate support and cushioning after 500 miles. Individuals who average 30 minutes per day of walking (or 3-4 hours per week) should consider replacing their shoes every six months. Individuals who average 60 minutes per day of walking (or 7-8 hours per week) should consider replacing their shoes every three months.

In addition to mileage, body weight is another important factor to consider. The more an individual weighs, the faster the support and cushioning will wear out. Individuals weighing over 200 pounds may want to consider replacing their shoe even more often than the aforementioned recommendations.

Summary

- Cardiovascular fitness is the ability of the heart, lungs, and organs to consume, transport, and utilize oxygen.

- There are three basic energy systems simultaneously at work during exercise: the phosphagen, glycolytic, and oxidative systems. They are used to replenish levels of adenosine triphosphate (ATP), the energy used to power muscle contractions.

- VO_2max is the maximum amount of oxygen that the body can take in and utilize in one-minute of high-intensity exercise. Knowing what your VO_2max score is and how to effectively train to improve it is important as VO_2max correlates well to certain distance run times (e.g., 1.5-mile).

- Lactate threshold (LT) is the point in exercise where lactate production starts to exceed lactate removal in the blood. Research has shown LT to be a better predictor of one's cardiovascular fitness than VO_2max.

- Exercise economy is the amount of energy required to maintain a particular running speed or generate a specific amount of power. Although not to the same extent as VO_2max and LT, exercise economy does have a significant impact on endurance performance.

- High-intensity interval training (HIIT) is a type of endurance training that utilizes repeated short to long bouts of high-intensity exercise combined with short recovery periods. Research has shown that the benefits of HIIT are almost identical to that of traditional endurance training.

- There are five distinct types of endurance training (i.e., long slow distance (LSD), pace/tempo, interval, repetition, Fartlek) each with their own specific training guidelines in terms of exercise intensity, duration, frequency, and rest.

- Although an easy and popular method to use, maximum heart rate (MHR) prediction equations have been shown to be an unreliable means of assessing and prescribing exercise intensity. In contrast, the rate of perceived exertion (RPE) and the Talk Test are easy and reliable measures of assessing exercise intensity that can be readily adapted to help develop a personalized endurance training program.

References

1. Arts, J., Luz Fernandez, M., & Lofgren, I. (2014). *Coronary Heart Disease Risk Factors in College Students*. Advances in Nutrition, 5(2):177-187.

2. Baechle, T. R., & Earle, R. W. (Eds.). (2008). *Essentials of Strength Training and Conditioning*. (3rd ed.). Champaign, IL: Human Kinetics.

3. C25k. (n.d.). *Couch to 5k*. Retrieved from http://www.c25k.com/.

4. Command Fitness Leader Certification Course. *Exercise Principles and Programming* (S5620612A) [PowerPoint Presentation]. Navy Physical Readiness Program, Millington, TN.

5. Cook, S., Kester, M., & Brunet, M. (1985). *Shock Absorption Characteristics of Running Shoes*. Am J Sports Med, 13(4):248-253.

6. Daniels, J. (2014). *Daniels' Running Formula*. (3rd Ed.). Champaign, IL: Human Kinetics.

7. Haff, G., & Triplett, N. (Eds.). (2016). *Essentials of Strength Training and Conditioning*. (4th ed). Champaign, IL: Human Kinetics.

8. Ivy, J. Exercise Training and Conditioning: What Works and Why. Nutrition for Sports, Exercise and Weight Management Workshop. 05-06 February, 2016. Arlington, VA.

9. McArdle, W., Katch, F., & Katch, V. (2015). *Exercise Physiology: Nutrition, Energy and Human Performance*. (8th Ed.). Baltimore, MD: Wolters Kluwer Health.

10. McCormick, W. (n.d.). Aerobic Training [PowerPoint Presentation]. Loyola Marymount University, Los Angeles, CA.

11. Prevost, M. (2015). Built to Endure [eBook]. Retrieved from http://built-to-endure.blogspot.com/.

12. REI.com. (n.d.) *How to Choose Running Shoes*. Retrieved from https://www.rei.com/learn/expert-advice/running-shoes.html.

13. Roberts, R. A. (2002). The Surprising History of the HRmax = 220 - age equation. Journal of Exercise Physiology, 5(2).

14. Training 4 Endurance. (2017). Exercise Economy / Economy of Motion. Retrieved from http://training4endurance.co.uk/physiology-of-endurance/exercise-economy/.

15. Walters, P., & Byl, J. (2021). *Christian Paths to Health and Wellness* (3rd ed). Champaign, IL: Human Kinetics.

Chapter 6
Training for Strength

Key Terms:

Accommodation	Fiber type transition	Repetition
Agonist muscle	General physical preparedness	Repetition method
Antagonist muscle	Henneman's size principle	Reversibility
Assistance exercise	Individuality	Sarcopenia
Bands	Intermediate muscle fiber	Sarcoplasmic hypertrophy
Bone density	Linear periodization	Set
Chains	Load	Slow-twitch muscle fiber
Compound exercise	Max effort method	Specific physical preparedness
Compression exercise	Myofibril	Specificity
Concentric contraction	Myofibrillar hypertrophy	Stabilizer muscle
Conjugate method	Non-linear periodization	Strength training
Deload	Olympic lifting	Structural exercise
Directed adaptation	Osteoporosis	Tempo
Dynamic effort method	Partials	Time under tension
Eccentric contraction	Periodization	Traction exercise
Eccentric training	Power exercise	Volume
Fast-twitch muscle fiber	Progressive overload	

Learning Objectives:

- List and discuss the foundational terms necessary to understand strength training
- Address the impact and significance of strength training on overall body composition and bone density
- Discuss the physiological differences in regard to muscle hypertrophy between males and females
- Describe the association between various load and rep range assignments associated with different strength training goals

Chapter 6: Training for Strength

- Examine the differences and benefits associated with both linear and non-linear periodization models
- Define and differentiate between compound, assistance, and power exercises and provide example exercises for each
- List some of the additional training considerations for intermediate / advanced lifters

Introduction

Some individuals are intimidated by strength training. With the wide array of exercises, equipment and programs available, the thought of where and how to start strength training can be overwhelming. The purpose of this chapter is to introduce basic strength training concepts and programming recommendations.

Strength training (aka resistance training) is a method of training which uses resistance in order to produce gains in muscular endurance, size, strength and power. Some of the benefits associated with regular strength training include increased muscular strength, power, fat metabolism, functional capacity and bone density, improved body composition and decreased risk of falling and/or injury. **Table 6.1** provides some additional physiological adaptations associated with regular strength training (Rainey & Murray, 2005; Haff & Triplett, 2016)

Table 6.1. Physiological Adaptations Associated with Chronic Strength Training

↑ Rate of force production	↓ Percent body fat
↑ Fiber cross-sectional area	Slows down the aging process
↑ Volume of muscle proteins	-
↑ Metabolic enzyme activity	-
↑ Metabolic energy stores (e.g., ATP, CP, glycogen)	-
↑ Strength of connective tissue (tendons, ligaments)	-

Basic Strength Training Terms and Concepts

Similar to sports and other types of training, strength training has its own vocabulary. In order to better understand how to perform strength training, it is important to first understand some of the basic strength training terms and concepts.

An **agonist muscle** is a muscle that contracts and causes movement. An **antagonist muscle** is a muscle that opposes the agonist muscle and causes movement in the opposite direction. A **stabilizer muscle** is a muscle that contracts but results in no significant movement (e.g., to maintain posture and/or immobilize a joint). For example, when performing a standing barbell curl, the biceps are the agonist muscle, the triceps are the antagonist muscle, and the rectus abdominis and erector spinae serve as stabilizer muscles.

A **repetition**, also referred to as a rep, refers to the complete motion of a particular exercise or movement pattern. For example, one rep of the bench press occurs when you lower the bar until it contacts the chest and then press the bar back up until the arms are fully extended.

A **set** is the specific number of reps performed sequentially prior to resting. For example, two sets of 10 on the bench press means you completed 10 reps on the bench press, two separate times.

Load, also referred to as intensity, refers to the amount of weight being lifted. For example, say you used a standard Olympic bar, which weighs 45 lbs., and had a 25 lb. plate on each side for your two sets of 10 reps on the bench press; your load would be 95 lbs. (45 lb. bar + 25 lb. plate + 25 lb. plate).

Volume refers to the total number of exercises, sets, and reps you complete in a particular workout. Generally speaking, volume and intensity are inversely related. In other words, as intensity (e.g., load) increases, volume should decrease and vice versa.

Concentric contraction is a type of muscle contraction in which the force generated by the muscle is greater than the force of the resistance thereby resulting in the muscle shortening.

Eccentric contraction is a type of muscle contraction in which the force of the resistance is greater than the force generated by the muscle thereby resulting in the muscle elongating (lengthening).

Isometric contraction is a type of muscle contraction in which the force generated by the muscle equals the force of the resistance thereby resulting in no change in the length of the muscle.

Compound exercise, also referred to as a **core exercise,** is a movement that recruits one or more major muscle groups (e.g., pectoralis major, latissimus dorsi, quadriceps) and involves two or more joints. Examples of compound exercise include the bench, row, press, squat and deadlift. Due to their direct application to sport, compound exercises should receive training priority.

Assistance exercise is a movement that recruits smaller muscle groups (e.g., biceps, triceps), involves only one joint, and is considered less important in terms of improving sport performance. Examples of assistance exercises include biceps curls, triceps extensions, leg curls and leg extensions.

Power exercise is a movement that is performed very quickly or explosively. Examples of a power exercise include the power clean, snatch, and clean and jerk. When all three exercises are performed in one training session, the recommended order for execution is power exercises → compound exercises → assistance exercises. Although the sport of powerlifting (which includes the bench press, squat, and deadlift) includes the word "power" in its name, a more fitting name would be strength-lifting since success in the sport is based on the amount of weight lifted rather than the speed in which the weight is lifted.

Structural exercise is a movement that either directly or indirectly loads the spine. Examples of a structural exercise include the back squat, standing overhead press and deadlift.

Compression exercise is a movement that directly loads the spine thereby causing compression of the intervertebral discs. Examples of a structural exercise include back squat, shoulder-loaded calf raises and standing overhead press.

Traction exercise is a movement in which the range of motion unloads the spine by expanding the space between the intervertebral discs. Examples of a traction exercise include the belt squat, lying leg curl and lat pull-down. It is recommended that individuals with low back pain or injury perform more traction exercises, as compared to compression exercises, whenever possible.

Tempo refers to the pace or rhythm at which a movement is performed. **Table 6.2** provide tempo recommendations based on different strength training goals (ACEFitness.org, 2014).

Table 6.2. Tempo Recommendations

Training Goal	Concentric Phase (sec.)	Eccentric Phase (sec.)
Endurance	1-2	2-6+
Size	1-2	2-4
Strength	1-2	1-2
Power	Explosive	Explosive

Time under tension (TUT) refers to how long the muscle is under strain during a set. For maximal hypertrophy (increase in muscle size), it is recommended to use lighter weights with a TUT of between 45 - 60 seconds.

Deload is a short pre-planned period of recovery built into an exercise regime in which both exercise intensity and volume are purposely reduced. A typical deload period is scheduled every 3-6 weeks and lasts for a week.

General physical preparedness (GPP) refers to any training method used to improve general conditioning such as strength, power, endurance, speed and flexibility. GPP is meant to lay the foundation for SPP and, according to Simmons (2007), roughly 80% of your overall training should come by way of GPP.

Specific physical preparedness (SPP), also referred to as **sports-specific physical preparedness,** refers to training of specific movements in a specified activity, usually a sport. For example, in the sport of powerlifting, this would entail training the bench press, squat and deadlift. According to Simmons (2007), roughly 20% of your overall training should come by way of SPP.

The **maximal effort method** is a method of strength training used by powerlifters to develop muscular strength. This method uses heavy loads for sets of either 5 reps, 3 reps or 1 rep.

The **dynamic effort method** is a method of strength training used by powerlifters to develop muscular contraction speed. This method uses lighter loads (e.g., 30% of 1 repetition maximum (RM), 35% of 1RM or 40% of 1RM) for sets of 3 reps. The recommended speed of contraction is between 0.9 – 1.2 meters per second (Wenning, n.d.).

The **repetition method**, also referred to as **repeated effort training**, is a method of strength training used by powerlifters to develop muscular size. This method uses both a higher volume of sets (≥ 6 sets per muscle group) and number of reps per set (e.g., 8-12 reps per set). Because the focus is on size (hypertrophy), and not strength or speed, this method is also used by bodybuilders.

The **principle of specificity** states that in order to get better at a specific task or movement, you must practice and perform the skill regularly. In other words, although the bench press and squat are both strength training exercises, they employ completely different muscles. As a result, each exercise must be performed separately in order to yield the desired training effect.

The **principle of directed adaptation,** a subset of the principle of specificity, states that a similar stimulus must be presented in sequence for some time in order for the physiological adaptations associated with that stimulus to be retained long term. In essence, this principle states that the same exercises and rep schemes should be used for several weeks consistently before transitioning to a different set of exercises and rep schemes.

The **principle of accommodation** states the body's response to a constant stimulus decreases over time. While performing two sets of 10 reps with 90 lbs. on the bench press may be an appropriate stimulus initially, if the stimulus does not change, the body will eventually adapt and thereby prevent further physiological adaptations from occurring (e.g., increased muscular size and strength). Herein lies the dilemma, not using a specific set of exercises and rep schemes long enough violates the principle of directed adaptation. However, using a specific set of exercises and rep schemes for too long violates the principle of accommodation. To prevent either scenario from occurring, it is recommended to change up the exercises and rep schemes used about every 3-6 weeks.

The **principle of progressive overload** states that the training stimulus needs to increase over time in order for progress to continue. These increases can include changes in intensity (e.g., % 1RM), volume (e.g., number of sets and reps) and/or frequency (e.g., number of training days per week).

The **principle of 72 hours** states that at least three days, assuming appropriate exercise intensity and volume were used, should be afforded between workout sessions using the same compound lift(s). For example, if the individual performed bench press on Monday, he/she could perform squats on Tuesday but would have to wait until at least Thursday before performing bench press again.

The **principle of individuality** states that each individual has unique strengths and weaknesses and will respond to training differently. There are several factors that influence strength training potential such as age, gender, training experience, injury status, muscle fiber type, tendon insertion points and hormonal balance.

The **principle of reversibility** states that the physiological adaptations associated with training are lost when training is stopped; however, detraining effects can be reversed when training is resumed.

Impact of Strength Training on Body Composition and Bone Density

Research has shown that strength training has a larger impact on body composition than endurance training (Boutcher, 2011). Additionally, regular strength training has been proven to decrease fat mass, increase fat-free mass and lessen the effects of **sarcopenia** (age-related loss of muscle mass and strength). Between the ages of 30 and 65, the average American loses a half-pound of muscle and gains one pound of fat each year (Walters & Byl, 2013). **Figure 6.1** depicts a magnetic resonance imaging (MRI) scan of the upper leg. The scan shows some of the body composition changes associated with aging. Although the circumference of the thigh remained relatively unchanged, there is a significant increase in the amount of subcutaneous fat as well as a notable decrease in muscle mass. Additionally, there is a significant amount of bone loss, thereby increasing the risk of fractures and/or osteoporosis.

Figure 6.1. Impact of Aging on Body Composition

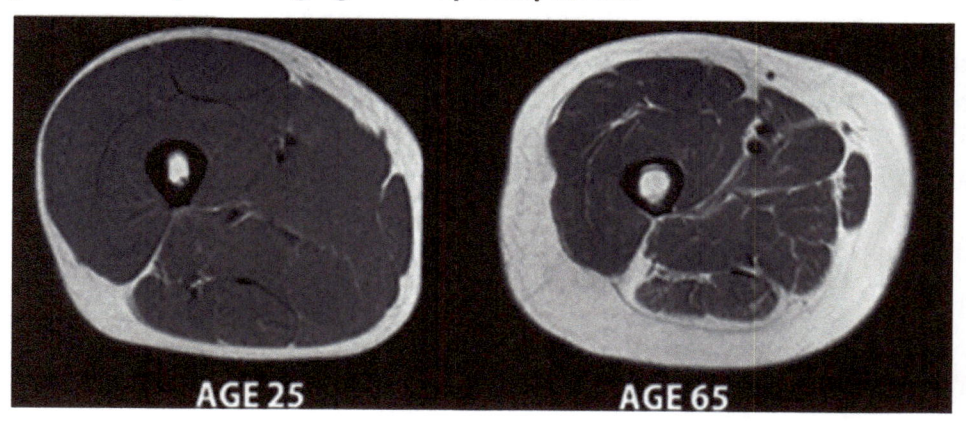

Fortunately, participation in regular strength training can help prevent both fat gain and muscle loss. **Figure 6.2** depicts changes in body composition after one year of strength training. The green line represents changes in fat mass, whereas, the orange line represents changes in fat-free mass. As you can see from the figure, this individual lost over 5 lbs. of fat and gained 3.5 lbs. of muscle.

Figure 6.2. Impact of Strength Training on Body Composition

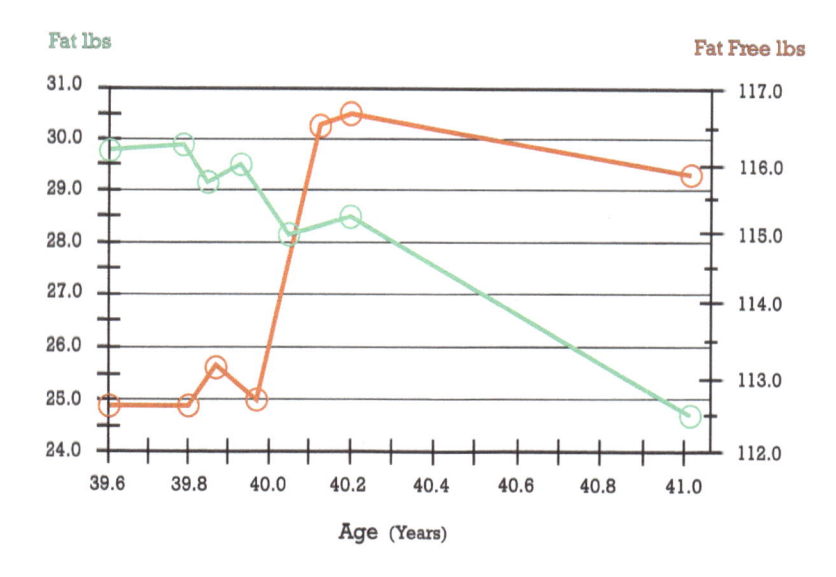

In addition to improving body composition, regular strength training can also help to improve **bone density** (amount of bone mineral in bone tissue) and reduce the risk of **osteoporosis** (disease in which the density and quality of bone are reduced). Research shows that bone density peaks around the age of 25 for most individuals and then begins to deteriorate (Walters & Byl, 2013). These findings depict the importance of regular participation in strength training early (e.g., late teens to mid-20s) in order to establish sufficient bone density and help prevent or delay the onset of osteoporosis. **Figure 6.3** depicts bone density scans, as taken by *dual-energy* x-ray *absorptiometry* (*DEXA*), of two active duty servicemembers. The graph on the left

Chapter 6: Training for Strength

depicts a 40-year old female who regularly performed endurance training (e.g., running, rowing), but rarely performed strength training. The graph on the right depicts a 43-year old male who has performed strength training for over 20 years. As depicted in the below graphs, the female servicemember is currently at the 10th percentile for bone density for her age. Conversely, the male servicemember is well above the 90th percentile for bone density for his age. Higher percentiles represent higher levels of bone density and a reduced risk of osteoporosis and fracture.

Figure 6.3. Impact of Strength Training on Bone Density

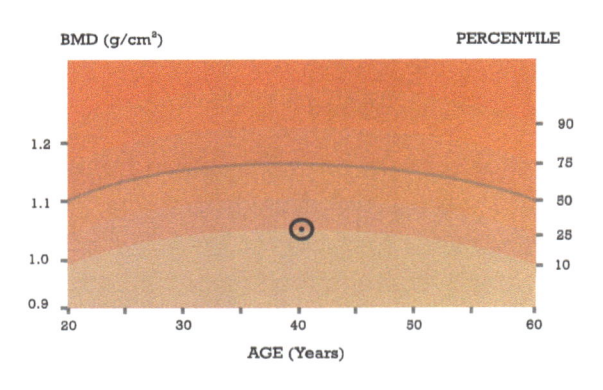

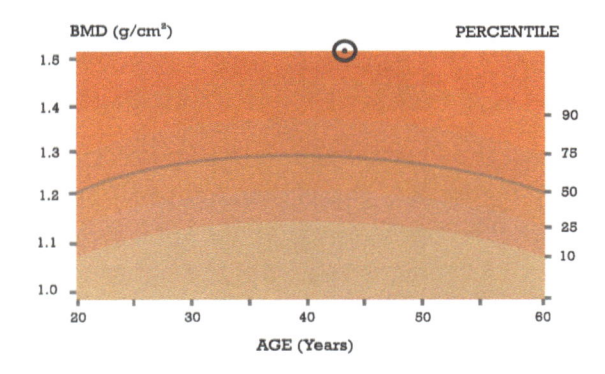

Subject A: 40-year old Female with Limited ST Experience

Subject B: 43-year old Male with > 20 years of ST Experience

Figure 6.4 depicts the changes in bone density for the female servicemember after one year of strength training. Although her bone density did improve, it was not statistically significant. The takeaway message is that strength training can help to improve bone density regardless of age, but the earlier you start strength training the better. Strength training not only reduces the risk of osteoporosis, but it also reduces the risk of fracture as well. Research shows that risk for fracture increases significantly when bone density is *less than 1 g/cm² (Doroudinia & Colletti, 2015).*

Figure 6.4. Changes in Bone Density with Regular Strength Training

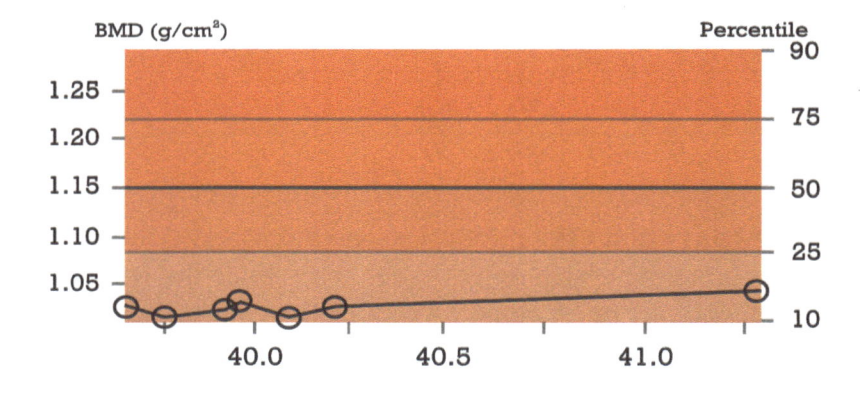

Major Muscle Groups and Fiber Types

Approximately two-thirds of the muscles in the body are skeletal muscles. In fact, there are over 600 skeletal muscles within the body, which account for roughly 40 percent of overall body weight (Rainey & Murray, 2005). **Figure 6.5** depicts some of the major muscle groups.

Figure 6.5. Major Muscle Groups

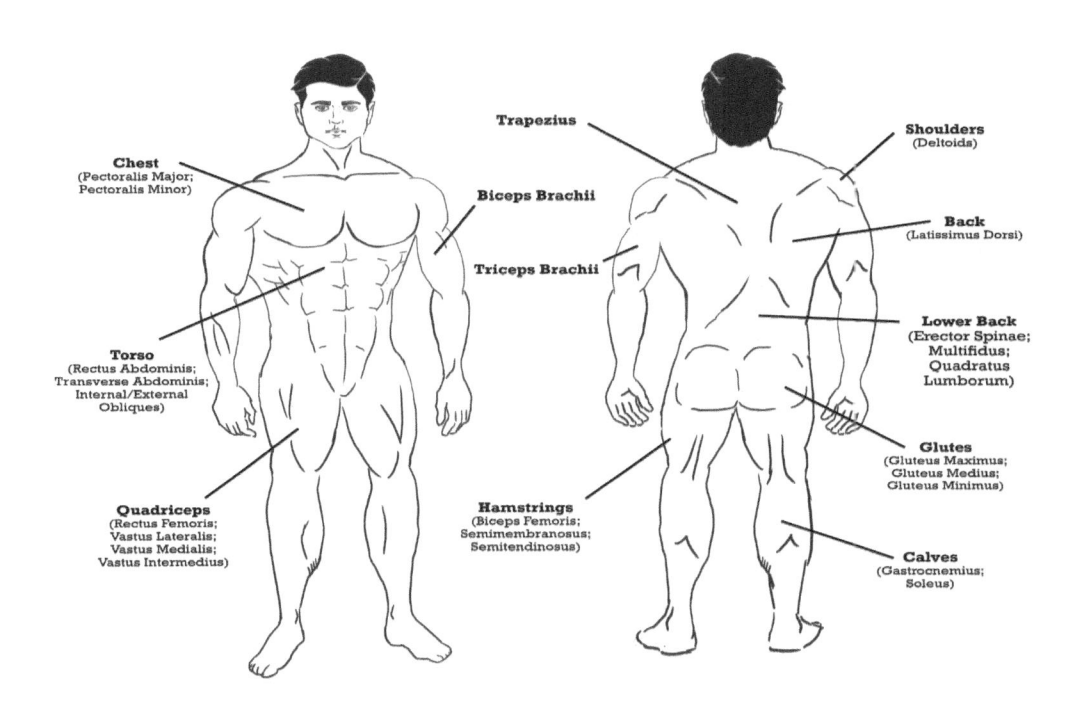

Each muscle group is comprised of individual muscle fibers. There are two basic types of muscle fibers: **slow-twitch** (aka slow oxidative or type I) and **fast-twitch** (aka type II). Similarly, there are two basic subtypes of fast twitch muscle fibers: fast oxidative (aka type IIa) and fast glycolytic (aka type IIx). Fast oxidative are sometimes referred to as **intermediate fibers** because they possess characteristics of both slow twitch and fast twitch muscle fibers (Betts et al., 2017).

Although the percentages of muscle fibers are genetically determined, transitions between subtypes can occur with regular strength training (Haff & Triplett, 2016). This process is referred to as **fiber type transition** (i.e., change in a fiber's subtype classification as a result of chronic training). As previously mentioned, transitions between subtypes of the same fiber type can occur with training; however, transitions from one fiber type to another do not occur regardless of training. In other words, slow-twitch muscle fibers cannot transition to become fast-twitch muscles fibers nor can fast-twitch muscle fibers transition to become slow-twitch muscle fibers.

In addition to fiber type transition, the **Henneman's size principle** states that under load, muscle fibers are recruited from smallest to largest. In other words, type I fibers are activated before type II fibers. To ensure all muscle fibers are recruited, it is recommended to train across a wide spectrum of repetition ranges. Lighter loads with high repetitions will target and develop the type I fibers; whereas higher loads with few repetitions will target and develop the type II fibers. Therefore, it is recommended to train at a variety of load and repetition assignments in order to target and develop each muscle fiber type individually and maximize hypertrophy. **Figure 6.6.** depicts some of the physiological differences between type I and type II muscle fibers.

Figure 6.6. Slow-Twitch vs. Fast-Twitch Muscle Fibers

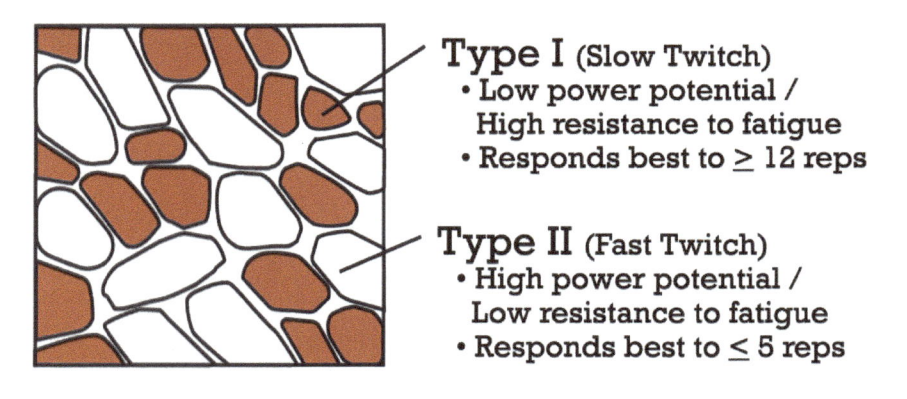

Type I (Slow Twitch)
• Low power potential / High resistance to fatigue
• Responds best to ≥ 12 reps

Type II (Fast Twitch)
• High power potential / Low resistance to fatigue
• Responds best to ≤ 5 reps

Muscle Hypertrophy

The process of hypertrophy involves an increase in the number of **myofibrils** (long filaments that comprise a muscle fiber) as well as the number of contractile proteins (i.e., actin and myosin) within the myofibrils. The extent of hypertrophy is largely based on muscle fiber type. Although both type I and type II muscle fibers adapt and enlarge with chronic strength training, type II fibers generally manifest greater increases in size than type I fibers. Ultimately, an individual's potential for hypertrophy is likely correlated to the relative percentage of type II muscle fibers (Haff & Triplett, 2016).

Research suggests there are two ways in which the muscle get bigger: sarcoplasmic hypertrophy and myofibrillar hypertrophy (Zatsiorsky & Kraemer, 2006). As the name suggests, **sarcoplasmic hypertrophy** is characterized by growth of the **sarcoplasm** (cytoplasm of a muscle fiber that contains ATP, phosphagens and various metabolic enzymes) and noncontractile proteins. **Myofibrillar hypertrophy** is characterized by an increased number of myofibrils as well as actin and myosin filaments. Although heavy strength training will lead to both sarcoplasmic and myofibrillar hypertrophy, Olympic weightlifting and powerlifting tend to promote more myofibrillar hypertrophy; whereas, bodybuilding tends to promote more sarcoplasmic hypertrophy. **Figure 6.7** depicts the anatomy of skeletal muscle. **Figure 6.8** depicts the differences between sarcoplasmic and myofibrillar hypertrophy within a muscle fiber.

Figure 6.7. Anatomy of Skeletal Muscle

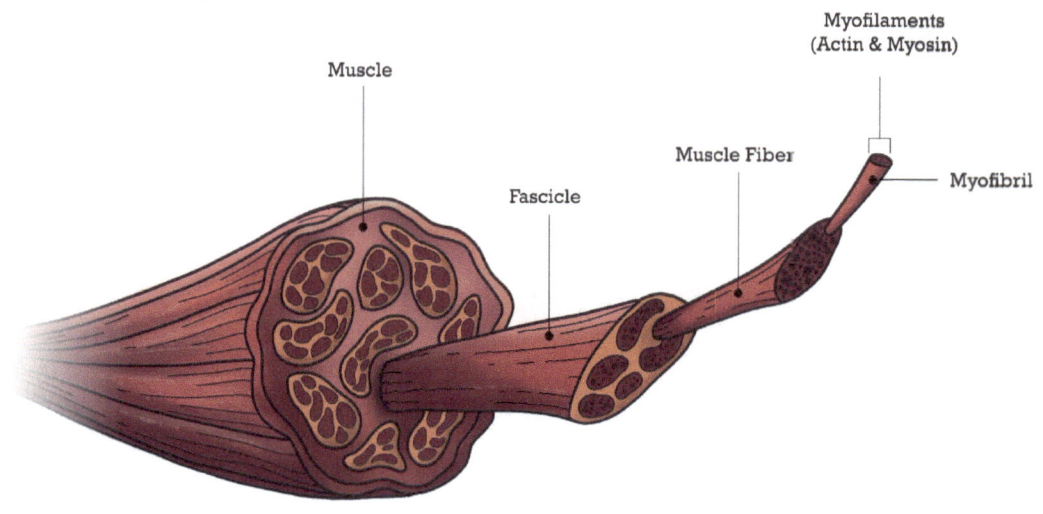

Figure 6.8. Sarcoplasmic vs. Myofibrillar Hypertrophy

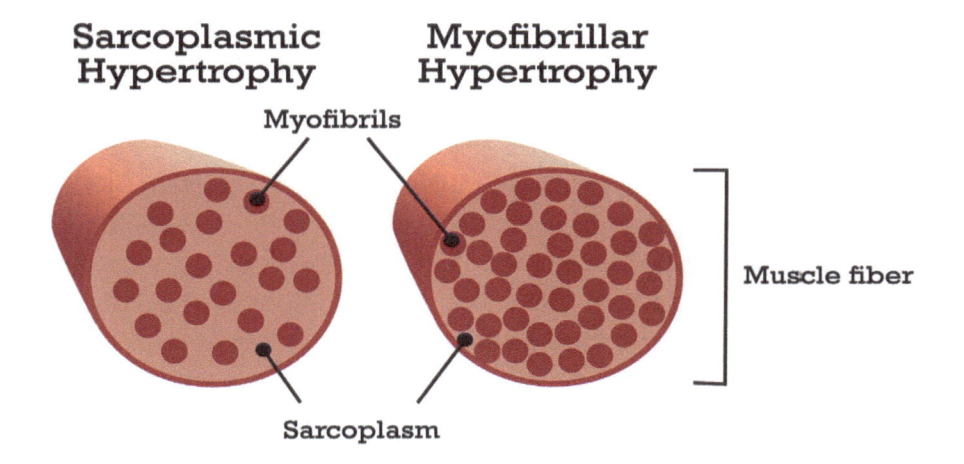

Physiological Differences Between Males and Females

There are numerous physiological differences between males and females which can result in significant disparities in their response to strength training. For example, females have fewer and smaller muscle fibers than males. Even so, females have the same array of muscle fiber types as males, both type I, type II and all of their sub-types (Zatsiorsky & Kraemer, 2006). Seventy five percent of untrained females have slow-twitch fibers that are larger than the fast-twitch fibers. The average female's maximal mean total body strength is about 60% of the average male's maximal total body strength. Average upper body strength of females ranges from 25-55 % of male's average upper body strength. Average lower body strength of females ranges from 70-75% of male's average lower body strength (Fleck & Kraemer, 2004).

Chapter 6: Training for Strength

Finally, resting circulatory concentrations of testosterone are 10-20 times lower in females than in males (Kraemer & Ratamess, 2003). According to Zatsiorsky & Kraemer (2006), females, especially basketball players, have higher incidences of anterior cruciate ligament (ACL) injury due to a narrower trochanteric notch and other anatomical factors such as broader hips and a greater Q-angle of the knee. With this in mind, females, especially athletes, can help to reduce the risk of injury and improve performance through regular strength training and proper technique.

Load and Repetition Assignments Based on Training Goal

Like endurance training, there are several different types of strength training programs: endurance size, strength and power. Each type of strength training has its own specific guidelines in terms of load, goal reps, goal sets and rest intervals. **Table 6.3** depicts the training guidelines for the four different types of strength training (Haff & Triplett, 2016).

Table 6.3. Load and Volume Assignments based on Training Goal

Training Goal	Load (% 1RM)	Goals Reps	Goal Sets	Rest
Endurance	≤ 67	≥ 12	2-3	≤ 30 sec.
Hypertrophy	67-85	6-12	3-6	30-90 sec.
Strength	≥ 85	≤ 6	2-6	2-5 min.
Power	75-90	1-5	3-5	2-5 min.

Each type of strength training is associated with specific physiological adaptations. For example, if an individual's primary training goal is hypertrophy, he/she should perform multiple sets of 6-12 reps at a moderate load (i.e., 67-85% 1RM). However, if an individual's primary training goal is explosiveness (power), then he/she would be better suited for multiple sets of 1-5 rep at a heavy load (i.e., 75-90% 1RM). Knowing how the body responds to different types of strength training is important in order to produce the desired physiological adaptations. This is an important consideration for individuals who wish to benefit from strength training without necessarily putting on a significant amount of muscle mass. Choosing the wrong load and volume assignments for your primary training goal can result in unintended or undesired physiological adaptations. **Figure 6.9** depicts some of the specific physiological adaptations associated with bodybuilding, powerlifting and Olympic weightlifting. Specifically, bodybuilding (which employs load and volume assignments for hypertrophy), produces the greatest gains in muscle size but not in muscle strength or power. Powerlifting (which employs load and volume assignments for strength) produces the greatest gains in strength but not in size or power. Olympic weightlifting (which employs load and volume assignments for power) produces the greatest gains in power but not in muscle size or strength.

Figure 6.9. Differences in Physiques for Various Types of Strength Training

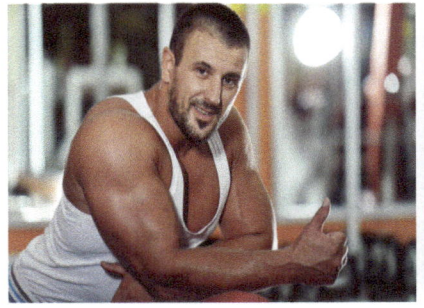

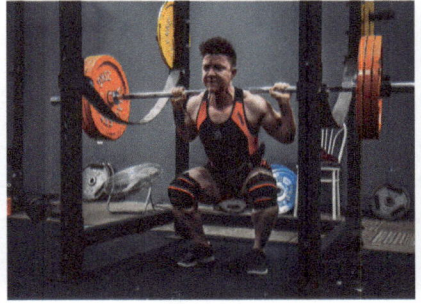

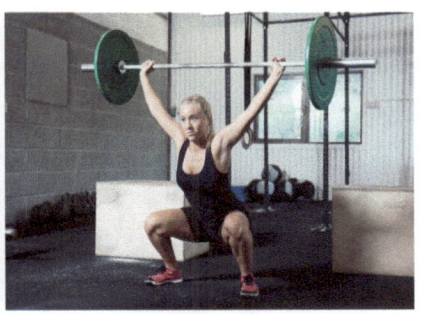

Bodybuilding   **Powerlifting**   **Olympic Weightlifting**

Figure 6.10 depicts the relationship between the number of reps performed and the various strength training goals. This information will benefit individuals who have multiple strength training goals. For example, individuals interested in producing gains in both muscular strength and size would benefit from using sets of 6 repetitions. Similarly, individuals interested in gaining both size and endurance would benefit from using sets of 12 repetitions. This approach would not work, however, for individuals interested in producing simultaneous gains in both strength and endurance as the rep ranges associated with these two goals do not overlap. Cosgrove (2019) recommends that individuals "surf the repetition continuum" in order to promote gains in all four strength training goals as well as reduce the risk of overtraining and/or injury associated with prolonged use of heavy loads. One strategy that uses a variety of repetition ranges in order to improve performance and prevent overtraining and injury is periodization.

Figure 6.10. Repetition Continuum

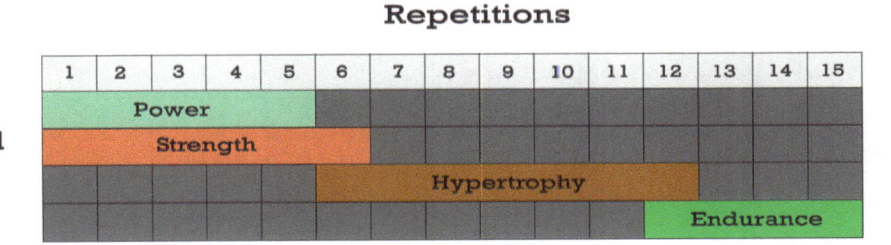

Periodization

Periodization, also referred to as **phase potentiation,** is the strategic sequencing of programming variables within an overall program in order to promote long-term training and performance improvements. Periodization uses preplanned and systematic variations in training specificity, intensity, and volume throughout the different phases (cycles). There are two basic types of periodization: linear (aka traditional) and non-linear (aka undulating). **Linear periodization** uses a systematic approach to programming by dividing training into various phases (i.e., preparatory, first transition, competition, second transition) or seasons (i.e., off-season, pre-season, in-season, post-season) that transitions from high-volume / low-intensity to low-volume / high-intensity

Chapter 6: Training for Strength

training. Because of this unique scheduling of phases, linear periodization is sometimes referred to as **block training**. An example of the linear periodization model is provided in **Table 6.4** (Haff & Triplett, 2016).

Table 6.4. Linear (Traditional) Periodization Model

Phase	Preparatory --------------------------------> First Transition			Competition		Second Transition
Season	Off-Season		Pre-Season	In-Season		Post-Season
Phase	Endurance and Hypertrophy	Basic Strength	Strength / Power	Peaking OR	Maintance	Active Rest
Intensity	Low to Moderate	High	High	Very High	Moderate	Recreational Activities
	50-75% 1RM	80-90% 1RM	75-95% 1RM	≥ 93% 1RM	80-85% 1RM	
Volume	High to Moderate	Moderate	Low	Very Low	Moderate	
	3-6 sets	3-5 sets	3-5 sets	1-3 sets	2-3 sets	
	10-20 reps	4-8 reps	2-5 reps	1-3 reps	6-8 reps	

Non-linear periodization, on the other hand, does not divide training up into various phases or blocks but rather uses weekly fluctuations in training volume and intensity. An example of the non-linear periodization model is provided in **Table 6.5** (Simmons, 2007). The Westside-Barbell **Conjugate Method**, developed by powerlifter and strength coach Louie Simmons, is a popular example of the non-linear periodization model.

Table 6.5. Non-Linear (Undulating) Periodization Model

	Day 1	Day 2	Day 3	Day 4	Day 5
	Max Effort: Lower Body	**Max Effort: Upper Body**	Off	**Dynamic Effort: Lower Body**	**Dynamic Effort: Upper Body**
Week 1	Work up to 1RM	Work up to 1RM		10 x 2 @ 50% 1RM	9 x 3 @ 50% 1RM
Week 2				10 x 2 @ 55% 1RM	9 x 3 @ 55% 1RM
Week 3				10 x 2 @ 60% 1RM	9 x 3 @ 60% 1RM
Repetition Method (Repeated Effort Training): 2-3 Assistance Exercises * (3 sets of 10-25 reps) + 1 Back Exercise (3 sets of 10-25 reps) + 2 Ab Exercises (3 sets of 10-25 reps) + Reverse Hypers (3-5 sets of 10-50 reps) * Pick exercises that address weak areas					

Both the linear and non-linear models of periodization have proven to be effective at developing muscle size, strength, and power. With that in mind, it comes down to personal preference as to which model of periodization an individual should use. Regardless of which model of periodization is used, the two most important training variables to produce optimal results are exercise intensity and volume (Zatsiorsky & Kraemer, 2006).

The above examples of linear and non-linear periodization can be convoluted and confusing for some individuals, especially those new to strength training. With that in mind, alternative examples of both types of periodization that are easier to understand, and follow are provided below. An example of an alternate linear periodization model is provided in **Table 6.6**. An example of an alternate non-linear periodization model is provided in **Table 6.7**.

Table 6.6. Alternate Linear (Traditional) Periodization Model

ENDURANCE			HYPERTROPHY			STRENGTH			POWER		
Week	Reps	Sets	Week	Reps	Sets	Week	Reps	Sets	Week	Reps	Sets
1	≥ 12	2	5	6-12	3	10	≤ 6	3	15	1-5	3
2	≥ 12	3	6	6-12	4	11	≤ 6	4	16	1-5	4
3	≥ 12	4	7	6-12	5	12	≤ 6	5	17	1-5	5
4	Deload		8	6-12	6	13	≤ 6	6	18	Deload	
			9	Deload		14	Deload				

Table 6.7. Alternate Non-Linear (Undulating) Periodization Model

	SETS OF 12	SETS OF 10	SETS OF 8	SETS OF 6	SETS OF 4	SETS OF 2	TOTAL SETS
Week 1	2	1	1	1	1	-	6
Week 2	-	2	1	1	1	1	6
Week 3	-	1	2	1	1	1	6
Week 4	-	1	1	2	1	1	6
Week 5	-	1	1	1	2	1	6
Week 6	-	1	1	1	1	2	6
Week 7	Deload						

Developing a Personalized Strength Training Program

As with programming for endurance training, individuals should develop their own strength training program based on their own physical limitations and needs. Yet, knowing where and how to start strength training can be intimidating. The purpose of this section is to provide some recommendations as to which strength training exercises to perform and when.

The common practice for some individuals is to target and train specific muscles. Although this approach can be effective, the extent of the results is largely based on which exercises are selected. For example, compound exercises produce greater results in terms of muscle size and strength gains than assistance exercises. As a result, compound exercises (lifts) should form the foundation of any strength training program. The five compound lifts are the bench press, bent over row, shoulder press, squat and deadlift. **Figure 6.11** illustrates the five compound lifts. **Figure 6.12** depicts which muscles are utilized for each of the five compound lifts. Performance standards for each of the five compound lifts are provided in **Appendix F**. Adjustment procedures for various pieces of Nautilus equipment are provided in **Appendix H**. Examples of free-weight, machine, resistance band, and bodyweight exercises for each of the compound lifts are provided in **Appendix I**.

CHAPTER 6: TRAINING FOR STRENGTH

Figure 6.11. The Five Compound Lifts

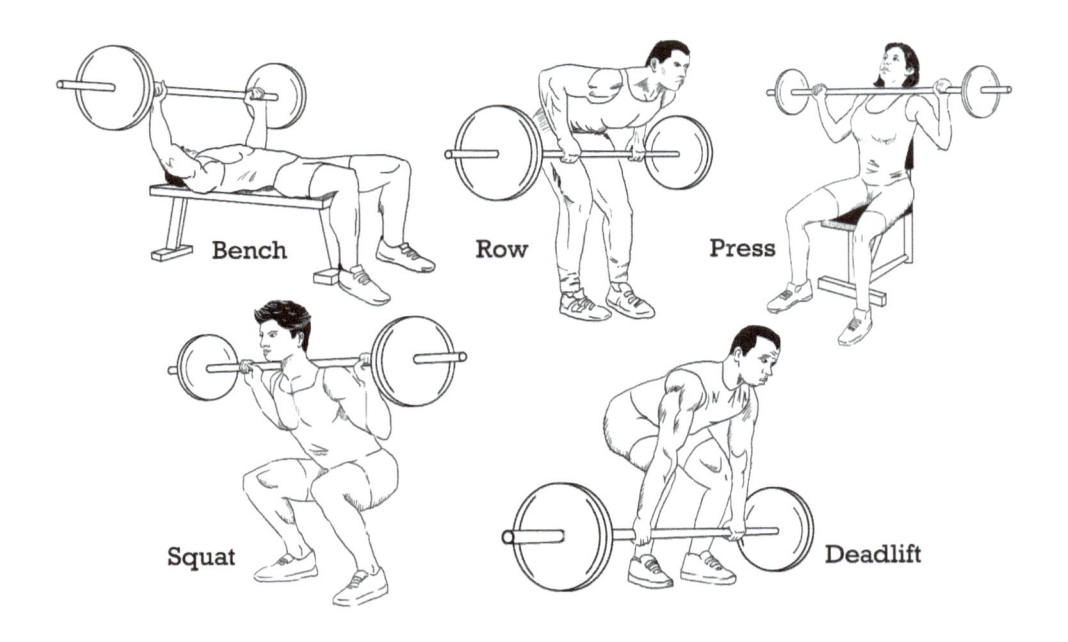

Figure 6.12. Muscles Used by the Five Compound Lifts

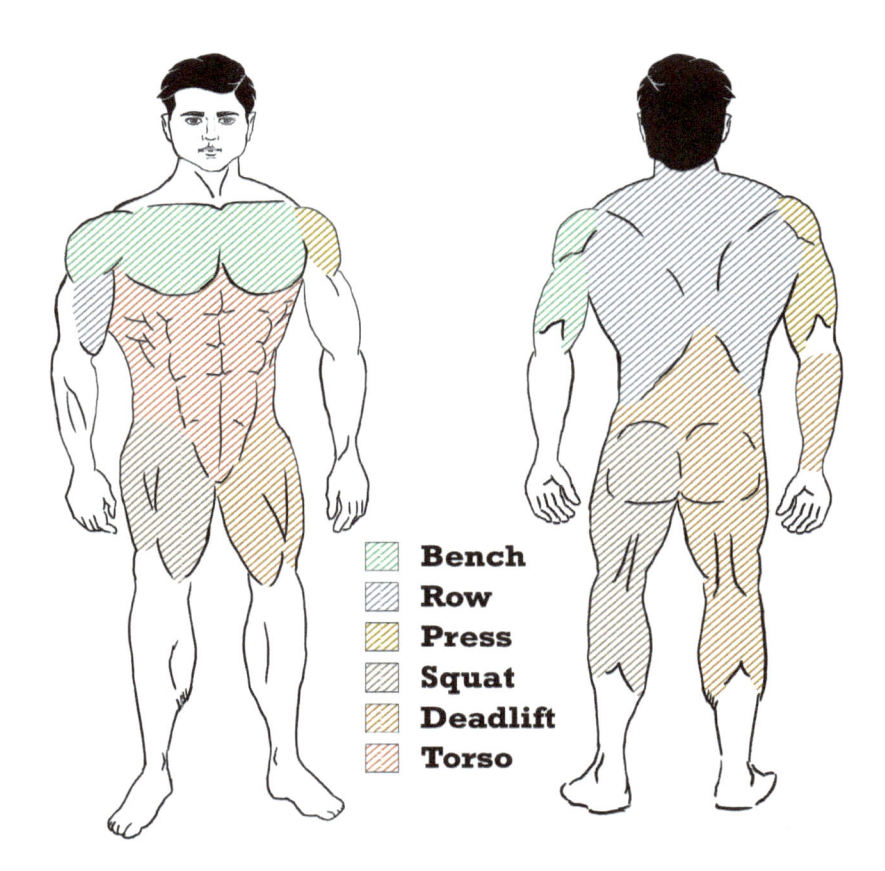

128

Table 6.8 provides frequency, set (per muscle group), rep and rest interval recommendations for the compound lifts and whether assistance exercises are appropriate based on training status (Israetel et al., 2015). For example, a novice (beginner) lifter is anyone with six months or less of strength training experience. An intermediate lifter is anyone between six months and two years of strength training experience. An advanced lifter is anyone with two years or more of strength training experience. Although it is a good idea to advance from beginner to intermediate when appropriate, it is not necessary to advance from intermediate to advanced unless the goal is to maximize strength and size gain. Additionally, as long as all five compound lifts are being performed, assistance exercises are not necessary for beginner and intermediate lifters. For example, since the bench press includes elbow extension, there is no need to perform a separate exercise(s) for the triceps. Similarly, since the bent-over row includes elbow flexion, there is no need to perform a separate exercise(s) for the biceps.

Table 6.8. Programming Recommendations for the 5 Compound Lifts

Training Experience	Frequency	No. of Sets	No. of Reps	Rest between Sets	Assistance Exercises?
Beginner (≤ 6 months)	2 - 3	1-5	• Strength: ≤ 6 • Size: 6 - 12 • Endurance: 12+	• Strength: 2 - 3 min. • Size: 30 - 90 sec. • Endurance: 30 sec.	No
Intermediate (6 mo. - 2 yrs.)	3 - 4	2-10	• Strength: ≤ 6 • Size: 6 - 12 • Endurance: 12+	• Strength: 2 - 3 min. • Size: 30 - 90 sec. • Endurance: 30 sec.	Optional
Advanced (≥ 2 years)	4 - 7	3-12	• Strength: ≤ 6 • Size: 6 - 12 • Endurance: 12+	• Strength: 2 - 3 min. • Size: 30 - 90 sec. • Endurance: 30 sec.	Yes

Table 6.9 provides a list of recommended exercises for each of the different compound lifts. Also provided is a list of options for the assistance lifts that can be used to help target and train the primary muscles used in the compound lifts. To use the table, select one compound exercise, one to two assistance exercises and one torso exercise. For example, if the desired compound lift was bench, the individual could select barbell bench, pec flyes, triceps pushdowns and the plank. [*Please note that each exercise listed in Table 6.9 is hyperlinked to an instructional video on how to safely perform the exercise.*]

Using the information from **Tables 6.8** and **6.9**, we can now design a workout for each of the different compound lifts. For example, let's use an individual who is an intermediate lifter (i.e., between six months and two years of lifting experience) and whose primary strength goal is to gain strength. A possible workout for the bench could be as follows:

- Barbell bench, 5 sets of 6 reps
- Pec Fly, 3 sets of 6 reps
- Triceps Pushdowns, 3 sets of 6 reps
- Plank, 4 sets of 1-min. holds

Chapter 6: Training for Strength

Table 6.9. Programming Recommendations for the 5 Compound Lifts

		Compound Lifts (Pick One) Sets: ≥ 3 - 6+	Assistance Lifts (Pick One to Two) Sets: 0 - 4+	Torso Exercises (Pick One) Sets: 3 - 4+
Bench	●	Barbell (BB) Bench Dumbbell (DB) Bench BB Incline DB Incline	Cable Cross-Overs Pec Fly Skull Crushers Triceps Pushdowns	Plank Side Plank
Row	▲	Pendlay / Bent-Over Row Seated Row 1-Arm Row Lat Pulldowns / Pull-Ups	Lat Pushdowns Gravitron Pull-Ups BB / DB Shrugs Preacher Curls	Isometric Sit-up Back Hypers
Press	■	BB Standing Military Press DB Standing Military Press BB Seated Military Press DB Seated Military Press	Lateral Raises Front Raises Bent-Over (Rear) Raises Arnold Press	Reverse Hypers Pallof Press
Squat	★	Back Squat Front Squat Goblet Squat Bulgarian Split Squat	Leg Press Leg Extensions Stiff Leg Deadlift Leg Curls	Vertical Knee Raise Bird Dogs Dead Bugs
Deadlift	⬟	Conventional Deadlift Sumo Deadlift Hex-Bar Deadlift Romanian Deadlift	Glute Press Good Mornings Hip Thrusters Glute Bridges	Single-Arm Suitcase Hold

In most cases, individuals will be performing more than one compound lift per training session. **Table 6.10** provides recommendations on how to appropriately pair the different compound lifts. For example, the bench press can be paired with either the press or the row. Similarly, the deadlift can be paired with either the row or the squat.

Table 6.10. Pairing Recommendations for the 5 Compound Lifts

	BENCH	ROW	PRESS	SQUAT	DEADLIFT
BENCH	-	X	X	-	-
ROW	X	-	-	-	X
PRESS	X	-	-	X	-
SQUAT	-	-	X	-	X
DEADLIFT	-	X	-	X	-

As mentioned previously, it is recommended that each compound lift be performed weekly. **Table 6.11** provides recommendations on when to perform each compound lift based on the number of available training days per week. If you recall from **Table 6.9**, ● = bench; ▲ = row; ■ = press; ★ = squat; and ⬟ = deadlift.

A Christian Guide to Body Stewardship, Diet and Exercise

Table 6.11. Sample 2-, 3-, 4-, 5-, 6- and 7-Day Strength Training Programs

	Mon	Tues	Wed	Thurs	Fri	Sat	Sun
2-Days / Week	● ■ ★			▲ ⬟			
3-Days / Week	● ■		★ ⬟		▲		
4-Days / Week	● ■ ★	▲ ⬟		● ■ ★	▲ ⬟		
5-Days / Week	● ■	▲	★ ⬟	● ■	▲		
6-Days / Week	● ■	★ ⬟	▲	● ■	★ ⬟	▲	
7-Days / Week	▲	★	● ■	⬟	▲	★	● ■

Provided below is a proposed workout for an intermediate lifter wanting to perform both the bench and press compound lifts in the same training session.

- Barbell bench, 5 sets of 6 reps
- Pec Fly, 3 sets of 6 reps
- Triceps Pushdowns, 3 sets of 6 reps
- Plank, 3 sets of 1-min. holds
- BB Standing Military Press, 5 sets of 6 reps
- Lateral Raise, 3 sets of 6 reps
- Bent-Over Raise, 3 sets of 6 reps

If a torso exercise is also performed, this would equate to a total of 25 working sets, which may seem like a lot, but is necessary and appropriate for their training goal. In terms of training volume, Israetel et al. (2015) recommends that no more than 15 total sets be performed for high-fatiguing exercises (e.g., compound lifts) and no more than 25 total sets be performed for low-fatiguing exercises (e.g., assistance lifts) per training session. Additionally, Israetel et al. (2015) suggests that performing less than 9 total sets per training session may result in a training stimulus that is too low to facilitate maximal gains in muscle size and/or strength. Zatsiorsky & Kraemer (2006) suggest that as much as 20-25 sets can be performed for each muscle group per training session. Remember, these are just recommendations. The prescribed number of sets should be tailored to the individual based on their ability to recover, current level of fitness, time availability, fitness goals and training / injury status.

Training Considerations for Advanced Lifters

Some additional methods of strength training for advanced lifters to consider include eccentric training, also referred to as negative training, partials, chains, bands and Olympic lifts. Partials, chains and bands are commonly employed by competitive powerlifters, especially for lifts like the bench press, squat and deadlift.

Research indicates that up to 20% more weight can be lifted eccentrically, where the muscle contracts while being lengthened, than can be concentrically, where the muscle contracts and is shortened (Kelly et al., 2015). The recommended tempo for **eccentric training** is between 3-5 seconds. Due to the heavy loads and slow tempos used, there is generally more muscle damage and soreness associated with this type of training.

Similar to eccentric training, **partials** allow for the use of heavier loads due to a reduced or limited range of motion. Although this type of training can be used for a variety of lifts, it is most often used for the bench press and deadlift. For safety reasons, partials are best performed in a power rack with adjustable pin holes.

Another popular training option is the use of **chains**. When using chains, it is recommended that one to two links of the chain be in contact with the floor when in the starting and/or lockout position. As the bar is lowered, the links of the chain begin to pile on the floor thereby reducing the load on the bar. Conversely, as the bar is raised, more links of the chain become suspended thereby increasing the load on the bar. If used properly, the use of chains can help to improve the lockout phase of the lift being trained.

Similar to chains, **bands** apply increasing tension to the bar as the individual approaches the lockout position. It is recommended that bands substitute no more than 20-35% of the total load used (Haff & Triplett, 2016). It is important to note that composition and tension can vary significantly between bands, thereby affecting balance and load distribution. With that in mind, when employing multiple bands, it is important to select and use bands of similar construction and tension.

Another option for advance lifters to consider is the Olympic lifts (e.g., snatch, clean and jerk, power cleans). Although the Olympic lifts can produce gains in muscular size and strength, they are primarily used to develop muscular power. Because Olympic lifts are more technique orientated (requiring a certain amount of skill to perform safely and correctly), they do have a slightly higher risk for injury and thus may not be well suited for everyone. While incorporating the Olympic lifts may be a good option for those individuals interested in developing and maximizing explosive power, incorporation of these lifts is not necessary for individuals only interested in developing general fitness, hypertrophy and/or strength.

Summary

- There are four distinct training goals (i.e., endurance, hypertrophy, strength, power) associated with strength training with each having their own specific training guidelines in terms of load assignments, goal sets, goal reps, and rest.

- Research has shown that engaging in regular strength training has a significant impact on body composition including decreased fat mass, increased fat-free mass, improved bone density and reduced effects of age-related loss of muscle mass and strength.

- During consistent strength training, muscle fiber types naturally transition. It is recommended to train across a wide spectrum of repetition ranges to include lighter loads with high repetitions and higher loads with few repetitions. There is some overlap among the different training goals in terms of the recommended rep ranges, which allows for some physiological adaptations to occur simultaneously.

- Gains in muscular size, strength, and power are possible with all three types of strength training (i.e., bodybuilding, powerlifting, Olympic lifting). However, bodybuilding is tailored more to developing size; powerlifting is tailored more to developing strength; and Olympic lifting is tailored more to develop power.

- Periodization is a strategy used to promote long-term training and performance improvements through the implementation of preplanned, systemic variations in training specificity, intensity, and volume. There are two basic types of periodization: traditional (linear) and undulation (non-linear) and each have shown to improve muscle size, strength, and power.

- Compound exercises (aka lifts) should form the foundation of any strength training program and include the bench, row, press, squat and deadlift.

- An effective strength training program regime incorporates all of the compound lifts and clearly outlines appropriate frequency, set, rep, and rest intervals based on training status.

- Individuals who are seeking additional methods of strength training for advanced lifting should consider including eccentric training (also referred to as negative training), partials, chains, bands and Olympic lifts.

References

1. ACEFitness.org. (2014, July 03). *Weightlifting Tempo & Sets: How to Select the Right Sets for Your Clients*. Retrieved from https://www.acefitness.org/education-and-resources/professional/expert-articles/4931/weight-lifting-tempo-amp-sets-how-to-select-the-right-sets-for-your-clients/.

2. Betts, J., Young, K., Wise, J., Johnson, E., Poe, B., Kruse, D., Korol, O., Johnson, J., Womble, M., & DeSaix, P. (2017). *Anatomy and Physiology*. Houston, TX: OpenStax.

3. Boutcher, S. (2011). *High-Intensity Intermittent Exercise and Fat Loss*. Journal of Obesity. DOI: 10.1155/2011/868305.

4. Cosgrove, A. (2019, August). *Unlocking Fat Loss*. Seminar presented at Perform Better Functional Training Summit, Providence, RI.

5. Doroudinia, A., & Colletti, P. (2015). *Bone Mineral Measurements*. Clinical Nuclear Medicine, 40(8): 647-57.

6. Fleck, S., & Kraemer, W. (2004). *Designing Resistance Training Programs*. (3rd ed). Champaign, IL: Human Kinetics.

7. Haff, G., & Triplett, N. (Eds.). (2016). *Essentials of Strength Training and Conditioning*. (4th ed). Champaign, IL: Human Kinetics.

8. Israetel, M., Hoffmann, J, & Smith, C. (2015). *Scientific Principles of Strength Training*. Renaissance Periodization.

9. Kelly, S., Brown, L., Hooker, S., Swan, P., Buman, M., Alvar, B., & Black, A. (2015). *Comparison of Concentric and Eccentric Bench Press Repetitions to Failure*. J Stength Cond Res, 29(4):1027-32.

10. Kraemer, W., & Ratamess, N. (2003). *Endocrine Responses and Adaptations to Strength and Power Training*. In Komi, P. (Ed.), *Strength and Power in Sport*. (2nd ed.), p. 361-386.

11. Rainey, D., & Murray, T. (2005). *Foundations of Personal Fitness*. Woodland Hills, CA: McGraw Hill.

12. Simmons, L. (2007). *The Westside Barbell Book of Methods*. Columbus, OH: Westside Barbell.

13. Wenning, M. (n.d.). *Matt Wenning's Conjugate Training Secrets: Volume 2*. Wenning Strength Media, Columbus, OH.

14. Zatsiorsky, V., & Kraemer, W. (2006). *Science and Practice of Strength Training* (2nd ed). Champaign, IL: Human Kinetics.

Chapter 7
Training for Mobility

Key Terms:

Active stretch	Mobility	Stability
Balance	Muscle spindle	Stretch reflex
Cartilaginous joints	Passive stretch	Synovial joints
Cool-down	Phasic muscles	Tonic muscles
Compression force	Plasticity	Torsion force
Elasticity	Prehab	Valsalva maneuver
Fibrosis	Range of motion	Venous return
Fibrous joints	Referred pain	Warm-up
Flexibility	Shear force	
Golgi tendon organ	Spinal stenosis	

Learning Objectives:

- List and discuss the factors affecting mobility and flexibility
- Discuss the benefits of performing a thorough warm-up and cool down
- List the three different planes of movement
- Describe and address the benefits of the four types of stretching
- Define some of the different prehab techniques to help improve flexibility and mobility
- List and discuss some of the different causes and treatment options for low back pain

CHAPTER 7: TRAINING FOR MOBILITY

Introduction

It is no secret that Americans have become more sedentary in recent years (Owens et al., 2010). Vallance et al. (2018) found that the average American adult spends 9 hours per day sitting, with older adults spending 10 hours or more sitting. Numerous improvements in technology have decreased the amount of manual labor required for performing both work- and leisure-related tasks. Even items such as skateboards, which have the potential for expending some physical exertion, have become motorized thereby reducing or eliminating the potential exercise-related benefits. As a result of this sedentary shift, some fitness advocates are promoting that being sedentary, specifically prolonged sitting, is the new smoking. In essence, prolonged sitting shares similar long-term consequences to smoking.

Is it true? Does prolonged sitting really elicit the same potential long-term health risks as smoking? According to Vallance et al. (2018), the health-related comparison between smoking and prolonged sitting is not even close. Smoking, by far, possesses a significantly higher risk for certain metabolic disorders and diseases as well as a higher mortality risk. Even so, research suggests that individuals who sit for longer than 7 hours per day have a 10 - 20% increased risk of mortality. Additionally, prolonged sitting increases the risk for type 2 diabetes, high blood pressure and depression, decreases aerobic efficiency, and reduces mobility - especially of the hip and lower back.

Vallance et al. (2018) reported that at least 60 - 75 minutes per day of moderate to vigorous intensity activity was necessary to fully reduce the mortality risk associated with prolonged sitting. Starrett (2015) recommends individuals get up and stand every 10-15 minutes and allocate at least four minutes of mobility work for every 30 minutes of continuous sitting, in order to avoid the negative health effects of prolonged sitting. Unfortunately, Vallance et al. (2018) also reported that the majority of Americans currently do not attain at least 30 minutes of physical activity per day, thus making the possibility of eliminating the health-related risks associated with prolonged sitting unattainable for most.

Collectively these findings provide compelling evidence and rationale for performing regular, if not daily, mobility training. Doing so will not only help to reduce the risk of certain health-related diseases and loss of mobility, but also serve as another opportunity to be good stewards of the body God has given us.

Common Mobility-Related Terms and Concepts

Mobility is the ability of a joint to move unhindered through its range of motion. **Flexibility** is the ability of a muscle, or group of muscles, to passively lengthen through its range of motion. **Balance** is the ability to control the body's position while stationary. **Stability** is the ability to control the body's position during movement or return to a desired position following a disturbance. Individuals with poor mobility, flexibility, stability and/or balance are at greater risk of falling.

However, individuals who participate in regular mobility, flexibility, balance and stability training have a lower incidence of low back pain, reduced risk of injuries, increased **range of motion** (ROM) and improved posture (Gordon & Bloxham, 2016).

An **active stretch** involves actively moving one muscle group in order to stretch another. Active stretching not only helps to improve the flexibility of the target muscle but also prepares it for the physical activity to follow. A **passive stretch**, on the other hand, uses some type of external force (e.g., stretching strap, partner) to stretch the target muscle without any muscular contraction from the individual being stretched.

Factors Influencing Mobility and Flexibility

There are several anatomical and training-related factors that can influence an individual's mobility and flexibility (Haff & Triplett, 2016). Some of these factors include:

- **Neural Control.** The central nervous system (CNS) plays a major role in determining the overall ROM an individual is able to attain. If the CNS perceives a particular ROM as either unfamiliar or unsafe, it will prevent the muscle from relaxing and thus reaching its full-length capacity. Regularly performing mobility and flexibility exercises will expose the CNS to positions of new or greater ROM, thereby reducing or eliminating the protective response and allow for greater ROM to be obtained.

- **Joint structure.** Joint type largely determines the ROM surrounding a joint. There are three basic types of joints in the body: fibrous, cartilaginous, and synovial. **Fibrous joints** (e.g., sutures of the skull) allow for little to no movement; **cartilaginous joints** (e.g., intervertebral disks) allow for limited movement; and **synovial joints** (e.g., elbow, knee) all for the greatest amount of movement.

- **Connective tissue.** The **elasticity** (ability to return to resting length) and **plasticity** (ability to assume a new or greater length) of tendons, ligaments, and joint capsules can also affect ROM. Regularly performing mobility and flexibility exercises can help improve the elastic and plastic connective potential of the various connective tissues.

- **Gender.** Generally speaking, females are more flexible than males. These gender-related differences are most likely due to structural and anatomical differences (e.g., pelvis width, amount of fat-free mass). Regardless of these differences, significant improvements in ROM can be achieved by both genders with regular mobility and flexibility training.

- **Age.** Generally speaking, younger individuals are more flexible than older individuals. These age-related differences are most likely due to increased inactivity with age and **fibrosis** (a condition in which fibrous connective tissue replaces degenerating muscle fibers). As long as mobility and flexibility training are performed regularly, full ROM can be maintained throughout all phases of life (e.g., adolescence, adulthood, old age). However, a substantial amount of ROM can be gradually lost if mobility and flexibility training are not performed regularly. **Figure 7.1** depicts how mobility and full ROM can be maintained with age. **Figure**

Chapter 7: Training for Mobility

7.2 depicts how lifting technique can be comprised if mobility is lost and full ROM cannot be maintained. In essence, the lack of regular mobility and flexibility training can result in reduced ROM over time, which in turn can significantly increase an individual's risk for injury when performing everyday tasks and activities (e.g., lifting a box off the floor).

Figure 7.1. Mobility Can Be Maintained w/ Age

Figure 7.2. Good vs. Bad Lifting Technique

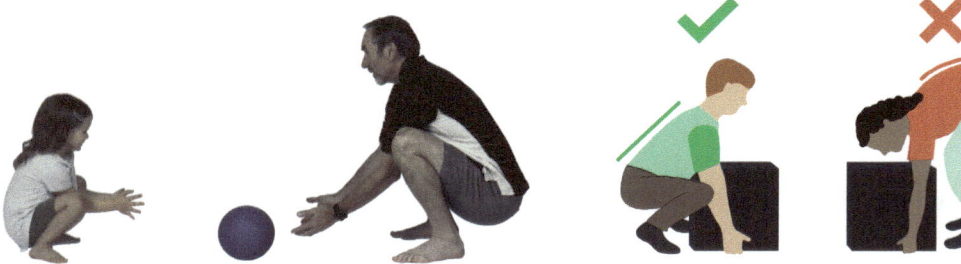

- **Activity level.** Generally speaking, active individuals are more flexible than inactive (sedentary) individuals. However, activity by itself does not necessarily improve mobility and/or flexibility, rather only if it involves movement through a joint's and/or muscle's full ROM.

- **Strength training with limited ROM.** Regularly performing strength training exercises through a full ROM can help to improve an individual's mobility and flexibility. However, regularly performing strength training exercises with partial or limited ROM can actually decrease an individual's mobility and flexibility.

- **Extreme muscle hypertrophy.** One of the primary goals of strength training is muscle hypertrophy. However, excessive amounts of muscle hypertrophy can affect ROM. In some cases, the desire for muscle mass may supersede the need for full ROM (e.g., bodybuilding, powerlifting, strongman). **Figure 7.3** depicts the relationship between flexibility and injury risk. As depicted in the figure, either extreme of flexibility increases an individual's risk for injury. The takeaway message is that individuals with extremely poor flexibility would likely benefit from some amount of flexibility training. Conversely, individuals who are hyperflexible would likely benefit from some amount of strength training.

Figure 7.3. Relationship between Flexibility and Injury Risk

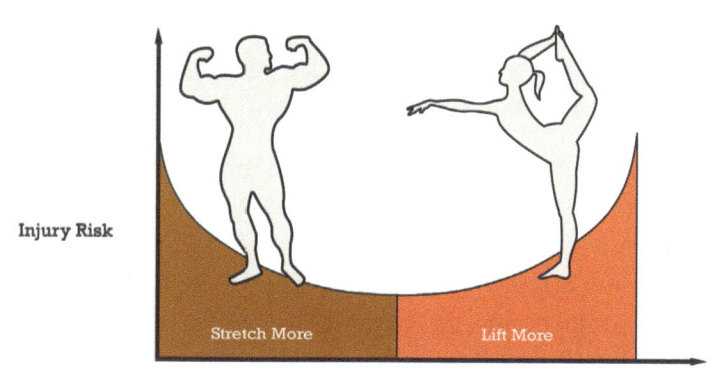

Warm-Up and Cool-Down Purpose and Recommendations

It is recommended that each training session begin with a proper warm-up and end with a proper cool-down. The purpose of a **warm-up** is to prepare the body for the more intense and demanding activity to follow. A proper warm-up increases the temperature of and the blood flow to the muscles thereby improving their elasticity and plasticity. Collectively, these actions help to improve ROM and decrease the risk of injury. In addition to improved muscle elasticity and plasticity, performing a proper warm-up has also been shown to increase force and power development, coordination and reaction time (Peterson & Rittenhouse, 2019).

A proper warm-up should begin with gentle movements focusing on ROM then gradually progress to movements that are more dynamic (e.g., jumping, bounding, plyometric). Additionally, movements in all three movement planes (i.e., sagittal, frontal, transverse) should be incorporated. **Figure 7.4** depicts the three different planes of movement.

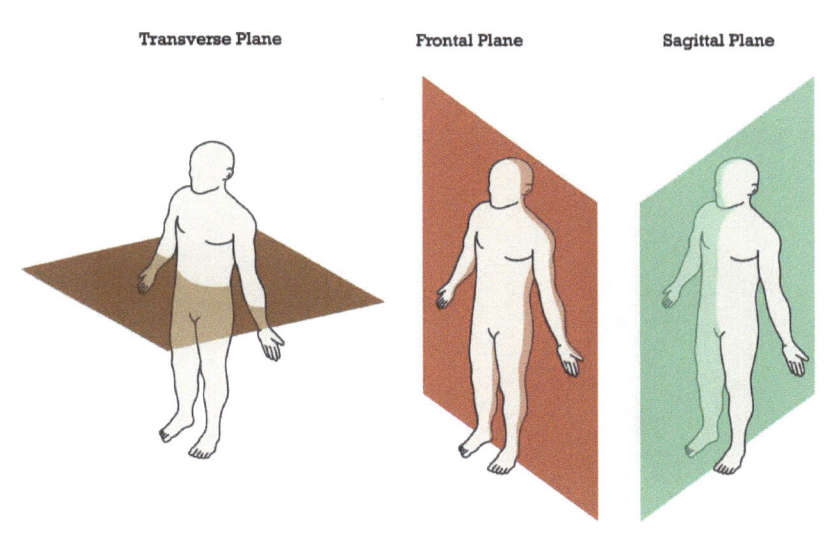

Figure 7.4. The 3 Planes of Movement

The **cool-down** should be performed immediately following physical activity and involve a gradual reduction in exercise intensity. For example, walking an additional tenth of a mile at 3.0 miles per hour or slower on the treadmill after finishing a pace / tempo workout. The purpose of a cool-down is to allow the heart rate and breathing to return to normal. Additionally, a proper cool-down helps to improve **venous return** (blood flow back to the heart) thereby aiding in the body's ability to recover. Since the muscles, tendons, and connective tissue are warmer following physical activity, and thus more elastic and pliable, the cool-down is the best time to stretch.

Stretching Types

As previously mentioned, a proper warm-up should be performed at the beginning of each training session; however, stretching should be performed at the end of each training session. The only exception to this rule is if the sport and/or exercise in which the individual is about to

Chapter 7: Training for Mobility

perform requires an extensive amount of mobility and/or flexibility in order to be successful (e.g., gymnastics, cheerleading). In total, there are four types of stretches: static, ballistic, dynamic (aka mobility drills), and proprioceptive neuromuscular facilitation (PNF).

- **Static stretching.** This type of active stretching uses a slow and constant stretch with the end position being held for at least 30 seconds. If done properly, static stretching will facilitate a central nervous system response which reduces muscle tension thereby allowing the muscle to lengthen. This reduction in muscle tension, although effective for improving flexibility and range of motion, is also associated with decreased force production, speed and reaction time. As a result, static stretching is best performed <u>after</u> a training session and not before.

- **Ballistic stretching.** This type of active stretching uses bouncing type movements to an unheld end position. Because the muscle is stretched rapidly, the **muscle spindle**, which is located in the muscle belly, is activated which causes the muscle to contract instead of relax. This autonomic reflex is called the **stretch reflex**, which is counterproductive to the purpose of stretching and increases the risk of injury. As a result, ballistic stretching is generally not recommended. **Figure 7.5** shows the location of the muscle spindle within the muscle.

Figure 7.5. Muscle Spindle vs. Golgi Tendon Organ

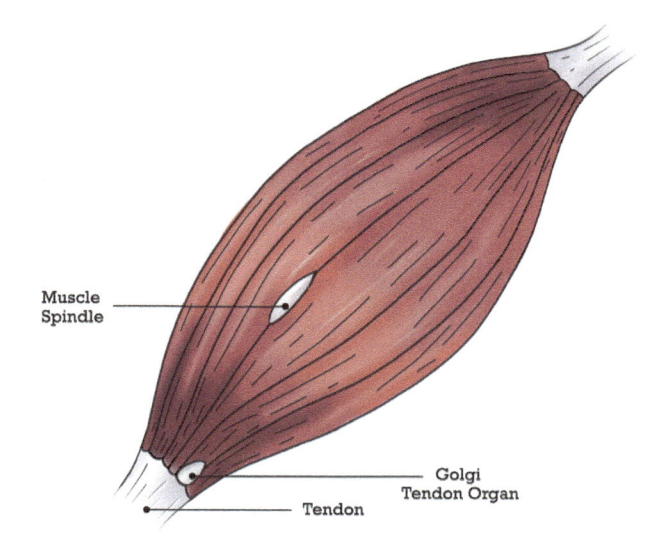

- **Dynamic stretching.** This type of active stretching uses sport-specific movements to prepare the muscles and connective tissue for the physical activity to follow. Dynamic stretching differs from ballistic stretching in that it uses slow and controlled movements instead of bouncing or jerky movements. Unlike static stretching, dynamic stretching is best performed <u>before</u> a training session as it helps to improve range of motion by raising body temperature which in turn increases the plasticity of the muscles and connective tissue. Examples of some dynamic stretches include walking toe touches, arm circles, walking knee hugs, side shuffles and backpedaling.

A CHRISTIAN GUIDE TO BODY STEWARDSHIP, DIET AND EXERCISE

- **PNF stretching.** This type of stretching uses a partner and involves both passive and active muscle actions. Similar to static stretching, PNF stretching is best performed <u>after</u> a training session. There are three basic types of PNF stretching techniques: hold-relax, contract-relax and hold-relax with agonist contraction. It is worth mentioning that this type of stretching is better suited for some muscle groups than others. For example, PNF stretching is commonly used for the chest, shoulders, hamstrings, quadriceps, groin, hip flexors and calves. [*Please note that each type of PNF stretching is hyperlinked to an instructional video on how to safely perform the stretch.*] **Figures 7.6 - 7.9** depict the proper set-up and positioning for the PNF hamstring, quadriceps, chest and shoulder stretches.

Figure 7.6. Set-Up for PNF Hamstring Stretch

Figure 7.7. Set-Up for PNF Quadriceps Stretch

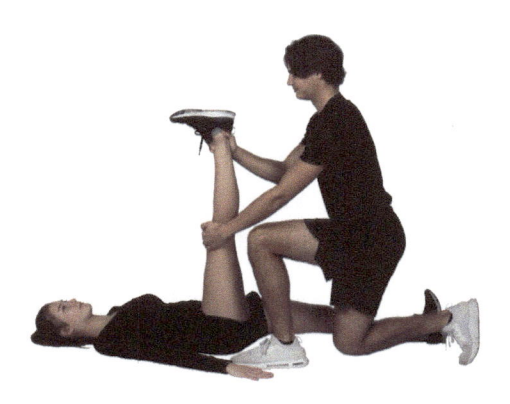

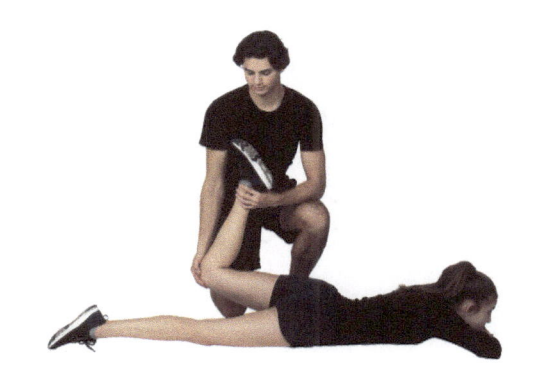

Figure 7.8. Set-Up for PNF Chest Stretch

Figure 7.9. Set-Up for PNF Shoulder Stretch

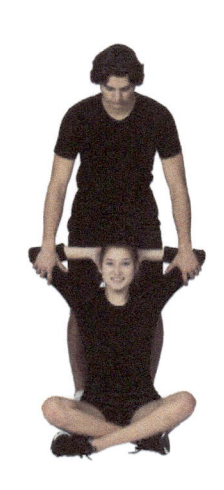

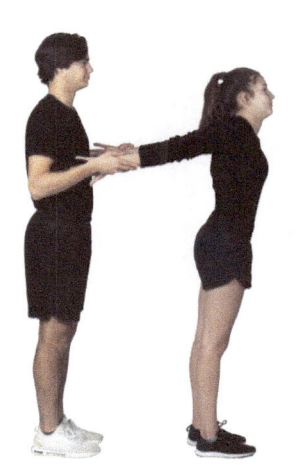

CHAPTER 7: TRAINING FOR MOBILITY

Prehab

In addition to the various types of stretches, several other techniques can be used to increase flexibility and mobility. For example, performing 10-15 minutes of **prehab** work prior to a training session can improve ROM, athletic performance, and reduce the risk of injury. The three basic phases of prehab include: soft-tissue work, dynamic stretching and movement specific activation.

Soft-tissue work. This phase of prehab involves using a massage stick, foam roller and/or lacrosse ball to help to break up scar tissue and/or adhesions within the muscle tissue. Because it is sometimes difficult to identify the exact cause of the pain or restriction, it may prove beneficial to perform soft tissue work above and below the affected area. For example, pain in the patellar tendon of the knee can sometimes be caused by tight quadriceps muscles. This phenomenon is called **referred pain**. Soft-tissue work can be performed <u>before and/or after</u> a training session.

Dynamic Stretching. As previously mentioned, this phase of prehab involves using various dynamic movements and sport-specific drills in an effort to warm-up the muscles and help improve mobility and ROM. For example, performing several sets of walking toe touches, walking knee hugs, side shuffles and backpedaling would serve as an effective warm-up prior to participation in a game of basketball or other similar activities. **Figure 7.10** provides a depiction of some of these exercises.

Figure 7.10. Walking Toe Touches (Left), Walking Knee Hugs (Center) and Side Shuffles (Right)

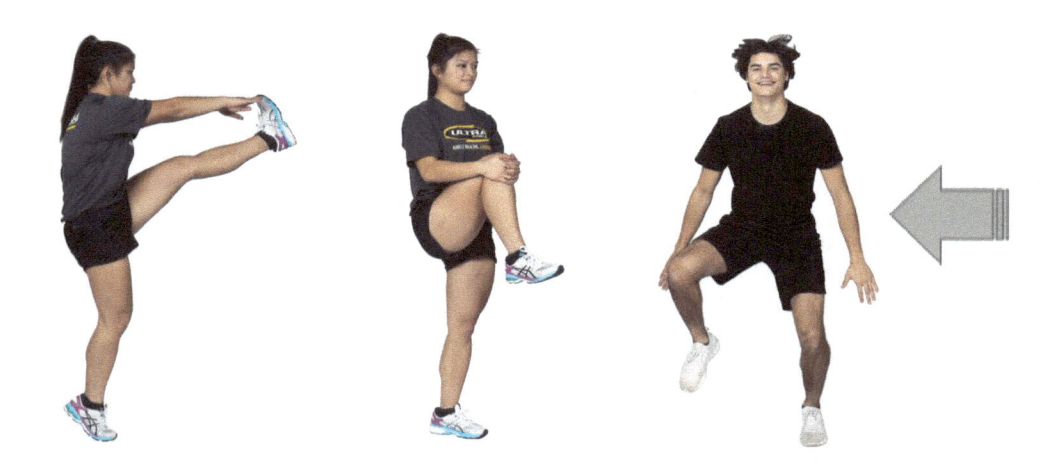

Movement Specific Activation: This phase of prehab involves using a variety of strength training exercises in order to "turn on" or activate the specific muscles that will be used in the upcoming training session. For example, performing several sets of glute bridges prior to doing the deadlift will help activate the glute muscles. **Figure 7.11** provides a depiction of the glute bridge exercise. Similar to dynamic stretching, movement-specific activation is best performed <u>before</u> a training session.

Figure 7.11. Glute Bridge

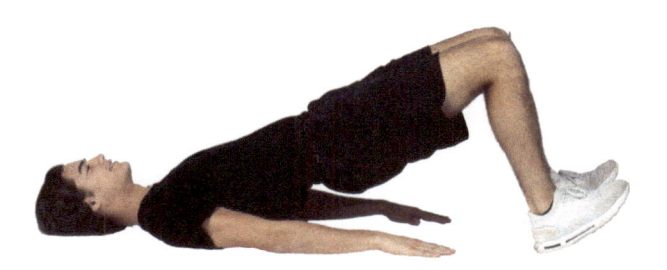

Stretching Recommendations and Precautions

As mentioned previously, individuals should work on their mobility and flexibility regularly in order to reduce the risk of certain chronic diseases as well as prevent the loss in ROM associated with prolonged sitting. In terms of flexibility training, the American College of Sports Medicine (ACSM) provides the following guidelines for static stretching (Magyari, 2018):

- **Frequency:** ≥ 3 days per week
- **Intensity:** Held to a position of mild discomfort
- **Duration:** 10-30 seconds per stretch
- **Repetitions:** 3-5 per stretch

Although a 10-30 second hold is a great place to start, most experts agree that individuals should gradually increase the hold duration over time. In fact, research shows that a hold duration of 60 seconds was more effective than either a 15 or 30 hold duration in improving hamstring flexibility (Peterson & Rittenhouse, 2019). Additionally, Starrett (2015) recommends hold durations of at least two minutes or until there is noticeable improvement. In some cases, this may mean spending up to 10 minutes in each position. A sufficient hold duration is necessary in order to stimulate the **Golgi tendon organ** (a proprioceptor located adjacent to the myotendinous junction that detects changes in muscle tension and when stimulated produces muscle contraction) (**Figure 7.5**), which in turn allows the muscle to relax and lengthen. As previously mentioned, poor flexibility is more likely a factor of CNS inhibition than it is muscle fiber length.

According to Page et al. (2010), muscle imbalances are among the top culprits for musculoskeletal pain, especially in the back, neck, shoulder, hip and knee. These imbalances can lead to patterns of tightness and weakness that can compromise joint function. Page et al. (2010) classifies muscles as either tonic or phasic. **Tonic muscles** are primarily flexor muscles and tend to tighten with age; whereas **phasic muscles** are primarily extensor muscles and tend to weaken with age. Examples of tonic muscles include the hip adductors, hamstrings, iliopsoas, and piriformis. Examples of phasic muscles include the quadriceps, glutes, and rectus abdominis. To correct imbalances, Page et al. (2010) recommends performing regular flexibility training to help lengthen the tonic muscles and regular strength training to help strengthen the phasic muscles.

Chapter 7: Training for Mobility

In terms of precautions, it is important not to bounce (e.g., ballistic stretching) or force a movement when stretching. Immediately stop stretching if you experience any sharp or shooting pains. Additionally, stretching is not recommended if you have sustained a recent injury, are within 8-12 weeks post fracture, and/or have acute inflammation in the joint or surrounding tissue.

Low Back Pain Causes

According to one online poll, it is estimated that 80% of American adults will suffer from back pain at least once in their lives (Peterson & Rittenhouse, 2019). Additionally, it is estimated that 20% of adults under the age of 60 suffer from chronic back pain (Cady, 2016). Low back pain can be caused by many factors. Some of the prominent causes of low back pain include bulging or herniated discs, **spinal stenosis** (abnormal narrowing of the spinal canal), piriformis syndrome and/or arthritis.

In addition to the aforementioned causes, low back pain can also be self-induced. For example, some of the common agitators of low back pain include prolonged sitting / standing, certain sleeping positions and poor posture. Keeping the spine in a flexed or overextended position for a prolonged period of time can lead to or exacerbate low back pain. **Figure 7.12** depicts the proper and improper body position for various daily activities.

Figure 7.12. Proper and Improper Posture for Various Daily Activities

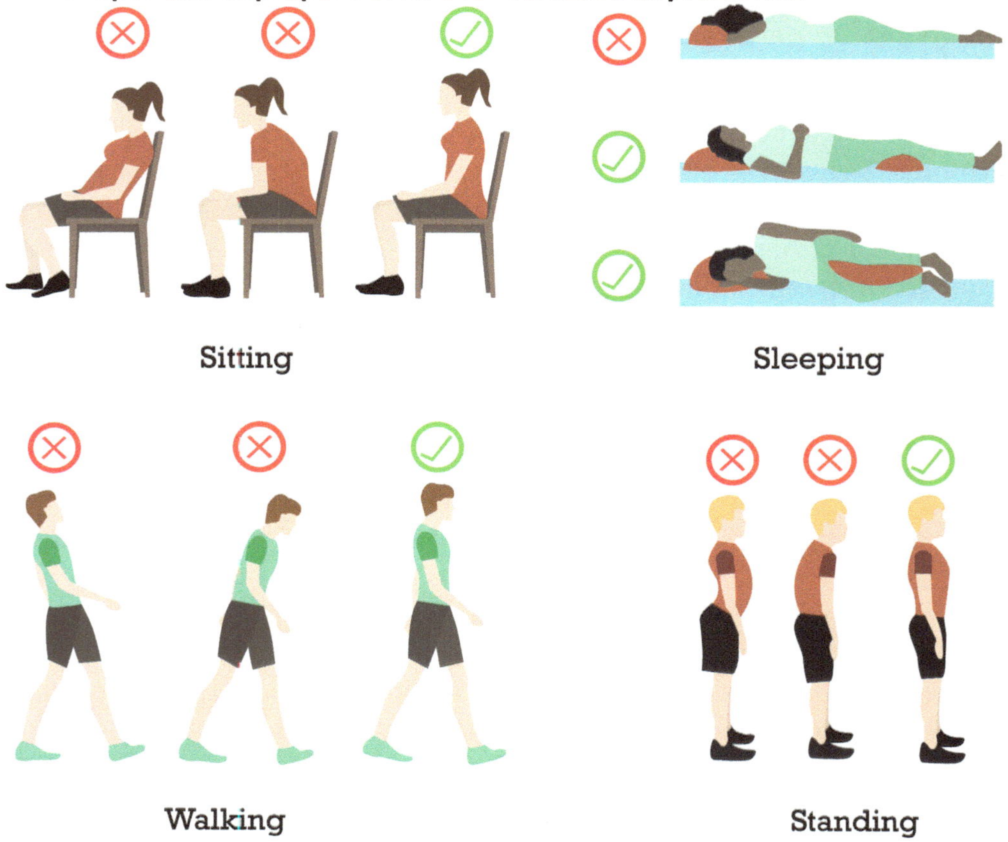

A Christian Guide to Body Stewardship, Diet and Exercise

In addition to activities susceptible to poor posture, certain strength training exercises can, in some cases, also serve as an agitator for low back pain. This is especially true with exercises that directly load the spine (e.g., squat), require a bent body position (e.g., row) or use a twisting motion (e.g., Russian twist). In fact, any exercise that involves a significant amount of **compression**, **shear** or **torsion force** on the spine can increase the risk of damaging the intervertebral discs thereby resulting in low back pain. These risks are compounded when using heavy weight and/or the exercise is performed incorrectly. **Figure 7.13** depicts the three major forces that can cause intervertebral disc damage.

Figure 7.13. 3 Forces Capable of Causing Intervertebral Disc Damage

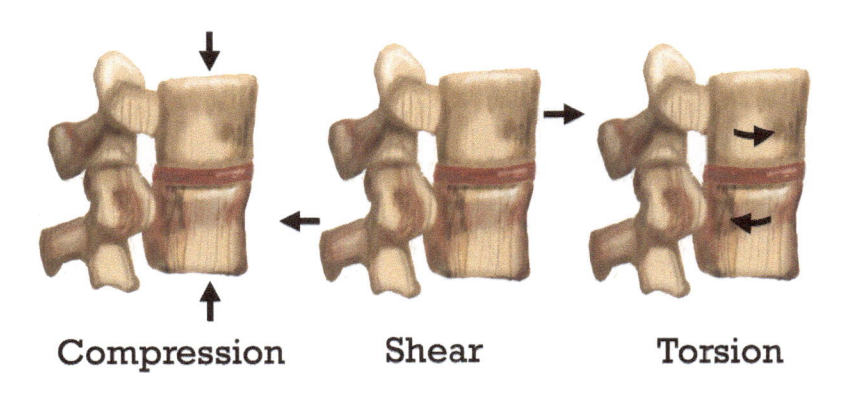

Compression   Shear   Torsion

While it may be appropriate to discontinue the use of some exercises (e.g., Russian twists), it is likely not necessary or recommended for other exercises (e.g., squat, row). Instead, use a slight modification with a similar but different strength training exercise and/or use lighter loads in order to reduce the risk of injury and prevent low back aggravation. For example, if an individual with chronic low back pain wants to incorporate the squat into their training regime, they could employ either the front squat, goblet squat or Bulgarian split squat instead of the back squat. All three of these exercises require lighter loads, which in turn reduces the magnitude of compression forces on the spine. Additionally, individuals wanting to incorporate the deadlift could elevate the bar several inches off the floor by using blocks or a trap bar. In both cases, proper execution requires a more vertical body position thereby reducing the magnitude of shear forces on the spine. Finally, individuals wanting to incorporate power exercises could employ hang cleans instead of power cleans in order to avoid the higher risk phases of movement.

Techniques for Assessing Posture

Posture plays a major role in both the prevention and cause of low back pain. Because of this role, it may be a good idea to periodically assess posture and make any necessary corrections. Two of the more common tools to assess posture include the two-hand rule and belly-whack test (Starrett, 2015). To perform the two-hand rule, place one thumb on the xiphoid process (sternum) and the other thumb on the iliac crest (top of the pelvis) with the fingers spread and palms facing down and parallel with the floor. When the spine is in a neutral position, both hands are parallel.

When the spine is flexed, the hands are closer together. When the spine is overextended, the hands are farther apart. The two-hand rule is a simple method of assessing the current position of your spine and affording feedback as to what adjustments (if any) need to be made.

The belly-whack test is another simple method of assessing posture. In essence, proper posture requires a certain amount of tension (albeit modest) from the abdominal muscles in order to maintain a neutral spine. Being able to take a quick whack to the belly ensures you have enough abdominal tension in order to support good posture. **Figure 7.14** depicts the proper set-up and execution of both the two-hand rule and belly-whack test.

Figure 7.14. Two-Hand Rule (Left) and Belly-Whack Test (Right)

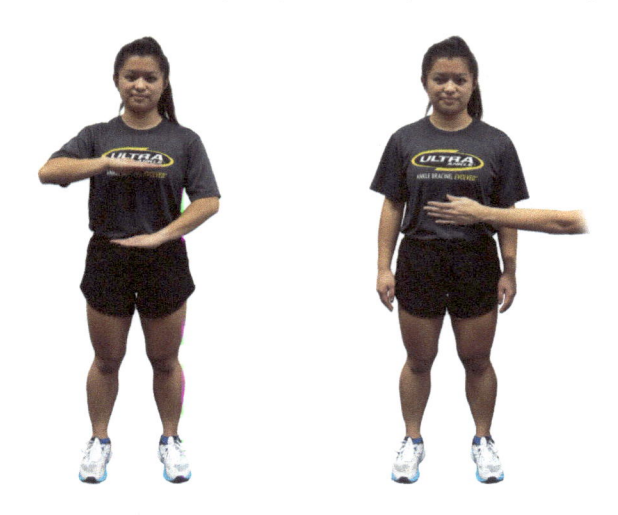

Low Back Pain Prevention and Treatment

According to Cady (2016), nearly every American adult has some form of spinal abnormality. In fact, just as with graying hair and wrinkles, changes to the spine (i.e., vertebra and intervertebral discs) are a natural part of the aging process. For example, the water content of the intervertebral discs gradually decreases with age (Zatsiorsky & Kraemer, 2006). Even so, these abnormalities of and age-related changes to the spine do not necessarily guarantee that an individual will experience low back pain. **Figure 7.15** shows the relationship between age and the percentage of individuals with a documented disc abnormality but no reported back pain (as depicted via magnetic resonance imaging (MRI)). As shown in the figure, by the age of 50 nearly 80% of adults have some degree of disc degeneration and 60% have a disc bulge.

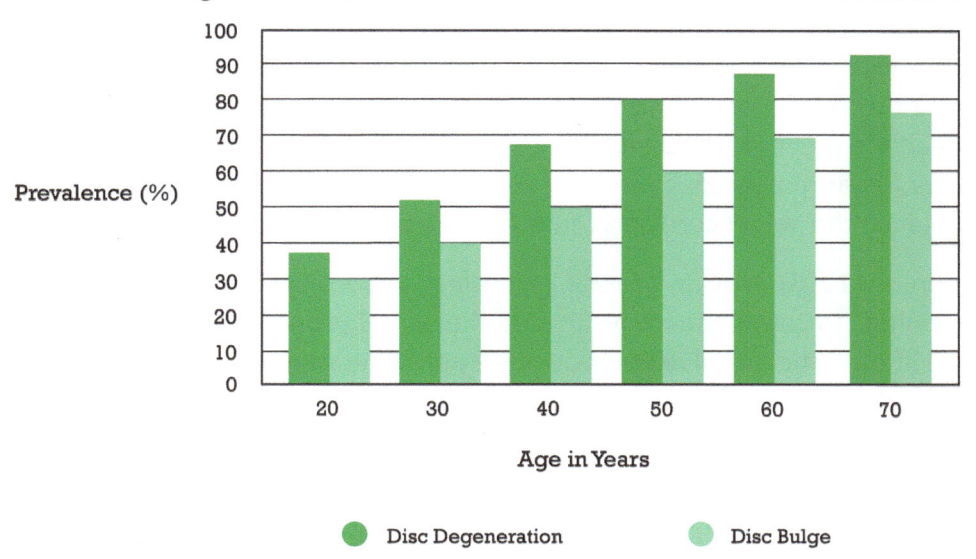

Figure 7.15. Percentage of Patients with Documented Disc Abnormalities but no Symptoms

● Disc Degeneration ● Disc Bulge

While spinal abnormalities and age-related changes of the spine do not necessarily guarantee low back pain, they can in some cases, increase the potential for low back pain. For example, heavy strength training has been shown to thicken certain portions of the lumbar vertebra (e.g., facet joints) thereby decreasing the size of the spinal canal (an opening in the lumbar vertebra that encompasses the spinal cord). These adaptations to heavy strength training are not necessarily bad, but can, when combined with other age-related disc abnormalities, increase the likelihood of the lumbar and sacral nerve roots being compressed thereby resulting in **sciatica** (a condition in which pain radiates down one or both legs). **Figure 7.16** depicts the anatomy of a lumbar vertebra.

Figure 7.16. Anatomy of a Healthy Spine (Left) and Spinal Stenosis (Right)

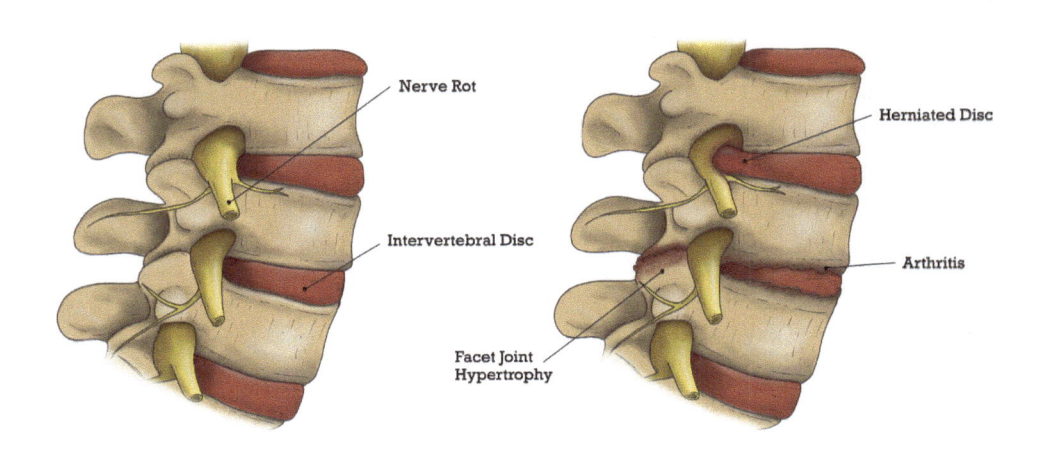

According to Zatsiorsky & Kraemer (2006), the intervertebral discs are most susceptible to damage when leaning, bending or performing rotational movements. During these movements, the nucleus pulposus (jellylike center of the intervertebral discs) is shifted to the side opposite the lean. Depending on the load used and/or condition of the intervertebral discs, the resulting pressure can exceed the mechanical strength limit of the discs and cause the nucleus pulposus to protrude from annulus fibrous (strong outward wrapping of the discs). If this happens, the disc bulge can press against the spinal cord and cause nerve pain, numbness and/or weakness.

Zatsiorsky & Kraemer (2006) provide several recommendations for protecting the lower back while strength training. Recommendations include the use of proper breathing and bracing and weight belts while lifting. The **Valsalva maneuver** is a particular method of breathing and bracing that increases intra-abdominal pressure (IAP) thereby providing additional support to the spine. If done properly, the Valsalva maneuver can reduce the compressive forces on the intervertebral discs by as much as 20-40%. Proper Valsalva performance can be achieved through the training and activation of the muscles comprising the abdominal wall (i.e., erector spinae, rectus abdominis, oblique muscles, intercostals and diaphragm). Zatsiorsky & Kraemer (2006) found that back pain occurs more frequently in individuals with weak or non-proportionally developed abdominal muscles. Similar to the Valsalva maneuver, the use of weight belts can also help increase IAP and decrease the relative spinal load on the intervertebral discs. Other methods that can be used to help restore the dimensions and properties of the intervertebral discs include massage, swimming in warm water (e.g., 30° C / 86° F) and spinal traction (Zatsiorsky & Kraemer, 2006).

In terms of treatment, most cases of low back pain resolve on their own within a couple weeks. With that in mind, seeking invasive treatment options (e.g., corticosteroid injections, surgery) immediately upon the onset of low back pain is likely unnecessary. Only when it is determined, through a formal medical evaluation, that the pain is in the same neural pathway as depicted on the MRI, should individuals consider more invasive treatment options (Cady, 2016).

Research has shown walking to be an effective treatment option for low back pain (Cole, 2019). Walking as little as 30 minutes per day can help strengthen and increase the blood flow to the muscles that support the spine. Additionally, daily walks have been shown to help improve lumbar spine mobility by increasing the flexibility and elasticity of spinal ligaments and tendons. However, individuals currently suffering from low back pain may not be able to tolerate 30 minutes of continuous walking. Instead, multiple bouts of shorter walks (e.g., 5-10 minutes) throughout the day may be a better initial strategy until a tolerance for longer walks has been established.

A Case Against Sit-Ups

For years, sit-ups have been a popular means of training the abdominal muscles. Due to their effectiveness and ease of administration, sit-ups, or some version therefore, have been used in the military and physical education programs throughout the world to assess torso muscular endurance. However, current research suggests that performing high volumes of spinal flexion (e.g., sit-ups) or rotation (e.g., Russian twists) exercises may actually cause damage to outer layers

A Christian Guide to Body Stewardship, Diet and Exercise

of the intervertebral discs thereby leading to low back pain (McGill, 2006). In fact, researchers now believe it may be more effective and safer to train the torso isometrically (Boyle, 2019). In other words, although the spine allows for movement in all three planes (i.e., frontal, sagittal, transverse), the muscles attaching to the spine primarily serve as anti-flexors, anti-extensors and anti-rotators.

Table 7.1 provides some sample exercises for training the torso. As depicted in the table, the torso is divided into three parts: midline abdominals, oblique abdominals and low back. It is important to train each part of the torso weekly in order to prevent muscle imbalances. One helpful strategy would be to incorporate torso training at the end of each strength training session and alternate between midline abdominals, oblique abdominals and low back exercises. For example, individuals participating in a 3-day per week strength training program could perform planks on Monday, side planks on Wednesday and back hypers on Friday.

Table 7.1. Sample Exercises for Midline Abdominals, Oblique Abdominals and Low Back

Midline Abdominals	Sample Exercises	Oblique Abdominals	Sample Exercises
	Plank Isometric Sit-Up Vertical Knee Raise		Side Plank Single-Arm Suitcase Hold Pallof Press
Low Back	**Sample Exercises**		
	Back Hypers Reverse Hypers Superman		

Exercises and Stretches for Low Back Pain

Prior approaches to low back pain recovery included avoiding or limiting the amount of physical activity to be performed. However, current recommendations argue against remaining sedentary and instead advocate for as much low-intensity exercise as can be tolerated (Peterson & Rittenhouse, 2019). Performing low-intensity exercise (e.g., walking, swimming) while dealing

Chapter 7: Training for Mobility

with low back pain has shown to help with pain and loosen the muscles of the lower back thereby improving ROM. The amount of physical activity that can be tolerated while dealing with low back pain will differ among individuals. Other examples of low-intensity exercises include various mobility exercises, strength training exercises and stretches.

Table 7.2 provides some basic low back mobility, strength and flexibility exercises. These simple exercises can be performed before, during and after the onset of low back pain. In an effort to help prevent low back pain, it is recommended that these exercises be performed at least 2-3 times per week. While dealing with low back pain, these exercises can be performed at least once daily (more if tolerated). Even so, it is important to not be overly aggressive when performing these exercises as doing so may lead to the worsening of pain and/or symptoms.

Often individuals start to reduce the frequency in which they are performing these exercises, or stop altogether, when their low back pain begins to subside or lessen. Obviously, this is not recommended, as the relief provided can be both temporary and reversible. If the individual stops participating in mobility training, the benefits of and results from training will slowly start to diminish and eventually dissipate altogether over time. To prevent this, at least 10 minutes of mobility training is recommended each day.

Table 7.2. Sample Mobility, Strength and Flexibility Exercises

Mobility Exercises	Strength Exercises	Flexibility Exercises
Bird Dogs	Plank	Piriformis
Cat to Cow Pose	Side Plank	Pigeon
Child's to Cobra Pose	Glute Bridge	Lizard
Rocking Hip Flexor	Back Hyperextensions	Modified Hurdler
Deep Squat	Reverse Hyperextensions	Quadriceps

Chapter 7: Training for Mobility

Summary

- Research indicates that prolonged sitting is detrimental to one's health. To combat the harmful effects of sitting, individuals should get up and stand every 10-15 minutes or perform at least four minutes of physical activity for every 30 minutes of continuous sitting.

- There are several anatomical and training-related factors that can influence an individual's range of motion, mobility and flexibility.

- Although often overlooked, a proper and thorough warm-up and cool-down are essential for performance, recovery, and injury prevention.

- Since exercise and sport are rarely one dimensional, it is important to perform regular mobility work in all three planes of movement.

- While all four types of stretches can improve flexibility and range of motion, ballistic stretching is not recommended due to its higher risk of injury. Proprioceptive neuromuscular facilitation (PNF) stretching has been shown to be the most effective but requires the use of a trained partner.

- The American College of Sports Medicine (ACSM) recommends that stretching be performed at least three days per week. However, several strength and conditioning professionals are now recommending that at least 10-15 minutes be dedicated daily to mobility work.

- Tonic muscles (flexor muscles) tend to tighten with age, whereas phasic muscles (extensor muscles) tend to weaken with age. To prevent this, it is recommended to regularly stretch tonic muscles and to perform strength training exercises for phasic muscles.

- Consistent prehab work of 10-15 minutes prior to performing physical activity can significantly improve performance and range of motion, as well as reduce the risk for injury.

- Even though there are a number of different causes of low back pain, the recommended treatment for recovery and prevention is generally the same. Performing low back specific stretches and mobility exercises daily will go a long way in helping to prevent and recover from chronic low back pain.

References

1. Boyle, M. (2019, August). *Current Concepts in Core Training*. Seminar presented at Perform Better Functional Training Summit, Providence, RI.

2. Cady, M. (2016). Paindemic: *A Practical and Holistic Look at Chronic Pain, the Medical System, and the Anti-Pain Lifestyle*. New York, NY: Morgan James Publishing.

3. Cole, A. (23 September 2019). *2 Reasons Why Walking is Good for Your Lower Back*. Retrieved from https://www.spine-health.com/blog/2-reasons-why-walking-good-your-lower-back.

4. Gordon, R., & Bloxham, S. (2016). *A Systematic Review of the Effects of Exercise and Physical Activity on Non-Specific Chronic Low Back Pain*. Healthcare, 4(2): 22.

5. Haff, G., & Triplett, N. (Eds.). (2016). Essentials of Strength Training and Conditioning. (4th ed). Champaign, IL: Human Kinetics.

6. Magyari, P. (Ed.). (2018). *ACSM's Resources for the Exercise Physiologist: A Practical Guide for the Health Fitness Professional.* Philadelphia, PA: Wolters Kluwer.

7. McGill, S. (2006). *Ultimate Back Fitness and Performance.* (3rd ed). Champagne, IL: Human Kinetics.

8. Owen, N., Sparling, P., Healy, G., Dunstan, D., & Matthews, C. (2010). *Sedentary Behavior: Emerging Evidence for a New Health Risk*. Mayo Clinic Proceedings, 85(12): 1138–1141.

9. Page, P., Frank, C., & Lardner, R. (2010). *Assessment and Treatment of Muscle Imbalance: The Janda Approach.* Champaign, IL: Human Kinetics.

10. Peterson, D., & Rittenhouse, M. (2019). *A Practical Guide to Personal Conditioning.* Burlington, MA: Jones & Bartlett Learning.

11. Starrett, K. (2015). Becoming a Supple Leopard. (2nd ed.). Las Vegas, NV: Victory Belt Publishing, Inc.

12. Vallance, J., Gardiner, P., Lynch, B., D-Silva, A., Boyle, T., Taylor, L., Johnson, S., Buman, M., & Owen, N. (2018). *Evaluating the Evidence on Sitting, Smoking, and Health: Is Sitting Really the New Smoking?* Am J Public Health, 108(11): 1478-82.

13. Zatsiorsky, V., & Kraemer, W. (2006). Science and Practice of Strength Training. (2nd ed). Champaign, IL: Human Kinetics.

Chapter 7: Training for Mobility

Chapter 8
Exercise Programming

Key Terms:

Deload
Fitness test
Frequency
Intensity
Moderate-intensity aerobic activity
Recovery
Specificity
Stimulus-recovery-adaptation (SRA) curve
Variation
Vigorous-intensity aerobic activity
Volume

Learning Objectives:

- Discuss some of the common mistakes associated with exercise programming

- Review the guidelines set forth by the American College of Sports Medicine (ACSM), American Heart Association, and Centers for Disease Control and Prevention (CDC) for endurance, strength, and mobility training

- Discuss the inverse relationship between exercise intensity, volume, and frequency and relevance to exercise program design

- List and discuss other key exercise program design variables

- Understand the importance of adequate recovery between training sessions

- Design a personalized exercise plan

Chapter 8: Exercise Programming

Introduction

In chapter 5 we learned about the five different types of endurance training (i.e., long slow distance (LSD), pace / tempo, interval, high-intensity interval, and Fartlek). In chapter 6 we learned about the four different strength training goals (i.e., endurance, hypertrophy (size), strength and power). In chapter 7 we learned about the importance of regular mobility and flexibility training. In this chapter, we will learn how to combine all of these different components of fitness into a comprehensive exercise program.

The idea of developing a personalized exercise plan can be overwhelming. As a result, some individuals opt to do nothing, only what they know or feel comfortable with, or resort to using a commercial exercise program (e.g., Insanity, P90X, LiveFit). Some of the common mistakes with exercise programming include doing too much too soon, loading bad technique (e.g., adding weight to the bar before mastering proper technique), being too vague or unrealistic with training goals or expectations, and/or being too competitive (either with someone else or a previous version of yourself). The goal of this chapter is to provide specific guidance on how to develop a personalized exercise program based on individual fitness goals, abilities, and sound exercise principles.

Components of Physical Fitness

Before we can develop a comprehensive exercise program, we must first introduce and have an understanding of the various components of physical fitness. In all, there are 12 different components of physical fitness. These components of physical fitness are categorized as either health-related or performance-related. **Table 8.1** depicts the 5 health-related and 7 performance-related components of physical fitness.

Table 8.1. Various Components of Fitness

Health-related	Performance-related
Aerobic capacity	Anaerobic capacity
Muscular strength	Power
Muscular endurance	Speed
Flexibility	Agility
Body Composition	Coordination
-	Balance
-	Reaction time

Physical Activity Guidelines

Although each component of fitness is important, some are arguably more important than others in terms of their role and impact on overall health and wellbeing. Those components of fitness deemed most important should receive priority when designing an effective exercise program.

Most fitness experts agree that the three most important components of fitness are aerobic capacity (aka cardiovascular endurance or endurance), muscular strength and flexibility (to include mobility).

In an effort to reduce disease risk and improve the quality of life, the American College of Sports Medicine (ACSM) has established and published physical activity guidelines for these three components of physical fitness. In essence, these guidelines provide the minimum frequency recommendations for endurance, strength and flexibility/mobility training. Specifically, the ACSM recommends a minimum of 30 minutes on 5 days per week of **moderate-intensity aerobic activity** or 20 minutes on 3 days per week of **vigorous-intensity aerobic activity** or an equivalent mix of moderate- and vigorous-intensity on 2 or more days per week (ACSM, 2021). Similarly, the American Heart Association (AHA) and Centers for Disease Control and Prevention (CDC) recommend at least 150 minutes per week of moderate-intensity aerobic activity or 75 minutes of vigorous-intensity aerobic activity per week or a combination of both (AHA, 2021; CDC, 2020). **Table 8.2** provides examples of moderate-intensity and vigorous-intensity aerobic activities (U.S. Department of Health and Human Services, 2020). Additionally, the ACSM, AHA, and CDC recommend a minimum of 2 days per week of strength training and 2-3 days per week of flexibility/mobility training (ACSM, 2021; AHA, 2021; CDC, 2020).

Table 8.2. Examples of Moderate- and Vigorous-Intensity Physical Activity

MODERATE-INTENSITY AEROBIC ACTIVITIES	VIGOROUS-INTENSITY AEROBIC ACTIVITIES
Brisk walking (e.g., ≥ 2.5 mph)	Running
Biking (e.g., < 10 mph)	Biking (e.g., > 10 mph)
Water aerobics	Swimming laps
Dancing (e.g., ballroom or social)	Dancing (e.g., aerobic or swing)
Tennis (e.g., doubles)	Tennis (e.g., singles)
-	Hiking uphill or with a heavy backpack
-	Jumping rope

Remember, these recommendations represent the minimum amount of physical activity that should be performed per week. In some cases, more may be required. For example, an individual who only walks, jogs, or runs for exercise will likely have good endurance but may have poor strength or mobility. In this case, their ideal program would incorporate more than 2 days per week of strength and more than 2-3 days per week of mobility training while maintaining the minimum of 5 days per week for moderate-intensity or 3 days per week for vigorous-intensity aerobic activity.

To better illustrate this point, imagine an individual's current level of fitness as a three-legged stool with each leg representing one of the three key components of physical fitness. In order for the stool to be balanced, each leg of the stool must be the same length. However, if even one leg is a different length than the others, then the stool becomes unbalanced. This is the case for most

Chapter 8: Exercise Programming

individuals. When our level of fitness is unbalanced, the result is decreased athletic potential and increased risk of injury. To prevent this unbalance, individuals should strive to identify and aggressively train the component(s) of fitness that needs work, while maintaining the component(s) in which they are already proficient. This can be done by meeting, but not exceeding, the minimum weekly requirements for the component(s) in which they are proficient and exceeding the minimum weekly requirements for the component(s) in which they are lacking.

Often, individuals prefer to only train the component(s) of fitness that they enjoy and/or are good at instead of the component(s) of fitness that need the most work. These individuals will likely always have an unbalanced level of fitness as the legs of their fitness stool are never able to achieve the same length. **Figure 8.1** depicts both a balanced and an unbalanced plan level of fitness.

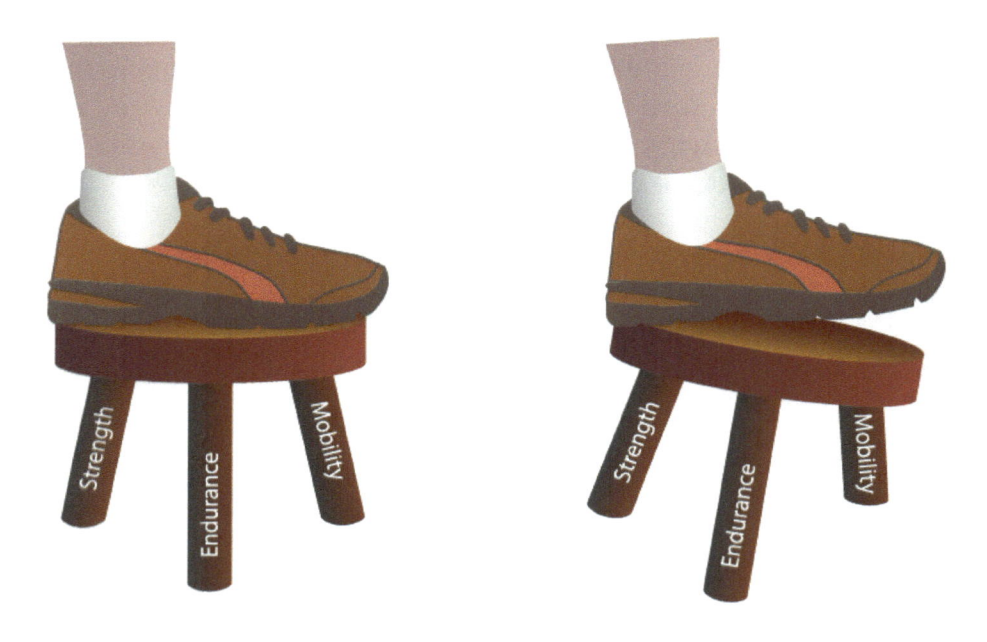

Figure 8.1. Well-Balanced (Left) vs. Unbalanced (Right) Foundation of Fitness

Fitness Testing

So how do you know which component(s) of fitness you are proficient in and which one(s) you are lacking? One of the most effective ways of assessing your level of fitness is to perform periodic fitness testing. A **fitness test** is a series of exercises designed to assess specific components of fitness (e.g., aerobic capacity, muscular strength, flexibility). In addition to identifying physiological strengths and weaknesses, periodic fitness testing can be used to track performance over time, assign training parameters (e.g., % of 1RM, MHR) and evaluate the effectiveness of an exercise program (Haff & Triplett, 2016). A sample fitness test that can be used to assess endurance, strength and mobility is provided in **Table 8.3**. Grading criteria for the deep squat is provided in **Table 8.4**.

Table 8.3. Proposed Fitness Test for Assessing Aerobic Capacity, Muscular Strength and Endurance, and Mobility

PERFORMANCE RATING	AEROBIC CAPACITY		MUSCULAR STRENGTH				MUSCULAR ENDURANCE	MOBILITY
	1-MILE RUN		1RM BENCH *		1RM HBDL *		PLANK	DEEP SQUAT
	MALE	FEMALE	MALE	FEMALE	MALE	FEMALE		
Excellent	≤ 5:45	≤ 6:25	≥ 1.6	≥ 1.1	≥ 2.5	≥ 2.3	≥ 4:20	≥ 5
Above Average	7:04-5:46	8:01-6:26	1.3-1.5	0.8-1.0	2.1-2.4	1.6-2.2	3:05-4:19	4
Average	7:05	8:02	1.2	0.7	2.0	1.5	3:04	3
Below Average	9:21-7:06	10:41-8:03	0.8-1.1	0.4-0.6	1.2-1.9	0.8-1.4	1:46-3:03	2
Poor	≥ 9:22	≥ 10:42	≤ 0.7	≤ 0.3	≤ 1.1	≤ 0.7	≤ 1:45	1

HBDL = Hexbar Deadlift
1RM Bench and HBDL are calculated by dividing weight lifted (lbs.) by bodyweight (lbs.)

Table 8.4. Deep Squat Pose Grading Criteria

	1 Point	Ability to get into the deep squat position unassisted
	1 Point	Ability to get the hips well below the knees and close to the ankles
	1 Point	Ability to position and maintain the elbows inside the knees
	1 Point	Ability to keep the entire foot flat and in contact with the floor
	1 Point	Ability to hold the deep squat position for at least 2 minutes
	1 Point	Ability to return to the upright position unassisted

Let's use our 165 lb. female from Chapter 5 as an example. After completing the proposed fitness test outlined in **Table 8.3**, she received the following scores:

- 1-mile: 7:45, which equates to a performance rating of **Above Average**

- Bench press: 80 lbs. (80 ÷ 165 = .48), which equates to a performance rating of **Poor**

- Hexbar deadlift: 150 lbs. (150 ÷ 165 = .91), which equates to a performance rating of **Below Average**

- Deep squat: 3, which equates to a performance rating of **Average**

Based on these scores and the minimum frequency recommendations provided by the ACSM, AHA, and CDC, it would be recommended that she perform strength training more than 2 times per week, mobility training at least 3 times per week, and endurance training no more than 3 times per week. It is worth mentioning that this approach works well for individuals using exercise to improve overall health and wellbeing. This approach, however, may not be recommended for individuals using exercise to improve sport performance. For example, both competitive runners and powerlifters likely have an unbalanced level of fitness. However, this is likely necessary

CHAPTER 8: EXERCISE PROGRAMMING

in order for them to be successful in their respective sport. The takeaway message is that the average individual should strive to have a balanced level of fitness, whereas, an unbalanced level of fitness may be required for competitive athletes. Even so, all individuals would benefit from identifying and training their physiological weaknesses.

Scheduling the Physical Activity Guidelines

The recommended number of days to perform endurance, strength, and mobility training will likely differ from individual to individual based on their fitness testing results and overall fitness goal (e.g., overall health versus training for a race). Provided below are some training options for an individual striving to meet the ACSM, AHA, and CDC minimum recommendations for endurance, strength, and mobility training (i.e., 3 days per week for vigorous-intensity (or 5 days per week for moderate-intensity) aerobic activity, 2 days per week for strength training, 3 days per week for mobility training). Notice that while the number of training sessions remains the same, the number of training days per week can vary (e.g., 3, 4, 5, 6 or 7).

For example, if an individual's schedule only allows for workouts 3 days per week but with no time constraints, then their best option would likely be to perform endurance, strength, and mobility training on the same day (Option 1). However, if an individual's schedule allows them to work out every day but for only 30-45 minutes, then their best option would likely be to perform endurance, strength, and mobility training on separate days (Option 7). As long as the intensity, volume, and frequency of training remains the same, the number of days per week does not appear to matter.

Option 1. Sample 3-Day per Week Training Plan

	SUN	MON	TUES	WED	THURS	FRI	SAT
Endurance		X		X		X	
Strength		X				X	
Mobility		X		X		X	

Option 2. Sample 4-Day per Week Training Plan

	SUN	MON	TUES	WED	THURS	FRI	SAT
Endurance		X		X		X	
Strength			X			X	
Mobility		X		X		X	

Option 3. Sample 5-Day per Week Training Plan

	SUN	MON	TUES	WED	THURS	FRI	SAT
Endurance		X		X		X	
Strength			X		X		
Mobility		X		X		X	

Option 4. Sample 6-Day per Week Training Plan

	SUN	MON	TUES	WED	THURS	FRI	SAT
Endurance		X		X		X	
Strength			X				X
Mobility			X		X		X

Option 5. Sample 7-Day per week Training Plan

	SUN	MON	TUES	WED	THURS	FRI	SAT
Endurance		X		X		X	
Strength	X				X		
Mobility			X		X		X

Intensity, Volume and Frequency

As mentioned previously, intensity, volume and frequency are important exercise programming variables to consider. **Intensity** refers to "how hard", **volume** refers to "how much," and **frequency** refers to "how often".

In endurance training, intensity is generally based on percentage of maximal heart rate (MHR) (e.g., pace / tempo = 80-90% MHR). In strength training, intensity is generally based on percentage of an individual's one repetition max (1RM) score (e.g., size = 67-85% 1RM). In mobility / flexibility training, intensity is generally determined by the level of discomfort while holding an exercise and/or stretch (e.g., to a position of mild discomfort).

In endurance training, volume is generally based on duration (e.g., LSD = 30-120 minutes). In strength training, volume is generally based on the number of sets and reps to be performed (e.g., strength = 3-6 sets for 6-12 reps). In mobility / flexibility training, volume is generally based

Chapter 8: Exercise Programming

on the total number of stretches and reps to be performed (e.g., 3-5 stretches for 3-5 reps per stretch).

In endurance training, strength training, and mobility / flexibility training, frequency refers to the total number of days per week. For endurance training, it is recommended that LSD, pace / tempo, and speed (which comprises interval and high-intensity interval) training each be performed at least once per week. For strength training, it is recommended that each compound lift be trained at least once per week. For mobility / flexibility training, it is recommended that some type of mobility work be performed at least three times per week.

As shown in **Figure 8.2**, there is an inverse relationship between intensity, volume and frequency (Antonio, 2015). This means that if the extent of training for one variable is increased, then there must be a subsequent decrease in one or both of the other training variables in order to prevent overtraining and/or injury. Conversely, if the extent of training for one variable is decreased, then there must be a subsequent increase in one or both of the other training variables in order to prevent training plateaus or detraining. The extent of training for each variable will be different for each individual and is based on multiple factors to include overall training goal, current fitness and injury status, and time availability.

For example, if an individual did not want to exercise every day (↓ frequency), then they would have to work out harder (↑ intensity) and/or increase either the amount of time (↑ volume) they exercised in order to achieve the same training stimulus. Similarly, if an individual wanted to work out more often (↑ frequency), they would have to decrease their intensity and/or volume in order to prevent overtraining and reduce the risk of injury. This phenomenon is illustrated in **Figure 8.3**. Generally speaking, as long as the extent of training for each variable is the same, the results should be the same regardless of how many days per week an individual trains.

Figure 8.2. Inverse Relationship Between Intensity, Volume and Frequency

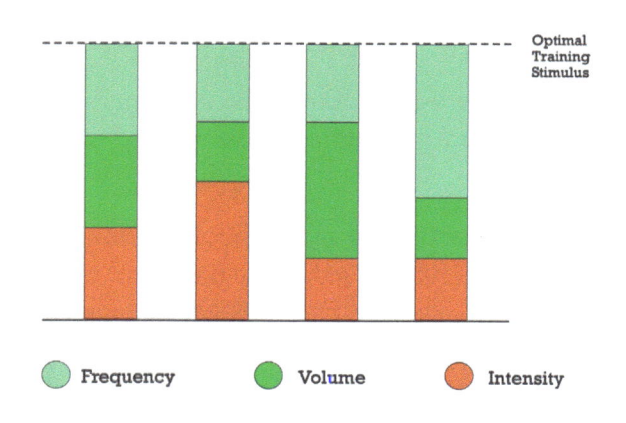

Figure 8.3. Relationship Between Intensity Volume and Frequency and Performance

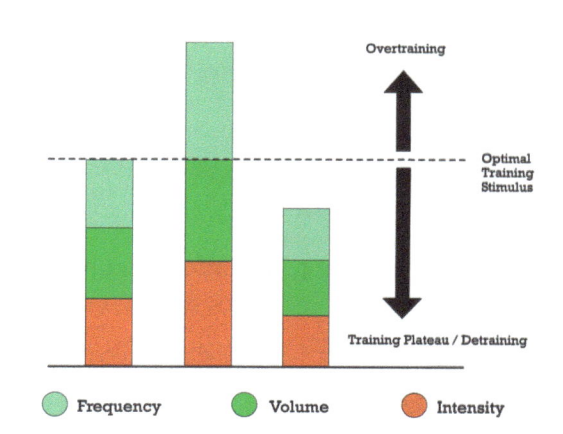

Other Exercise Programming Variables

In addition to intensity, volume and frequency, there are several other important exercise programming variables to consider. Some of these variables include specificity, recovery, and variation. Israetel et al. (2015) proposes there is a hierarchy in terms of exercise programming variables (**Figure 8.4**). In essence, some variables are more important than others in terms of their role and influence and therefore should receive priority.

Figure 8.4. Hierarchy of Training Variables

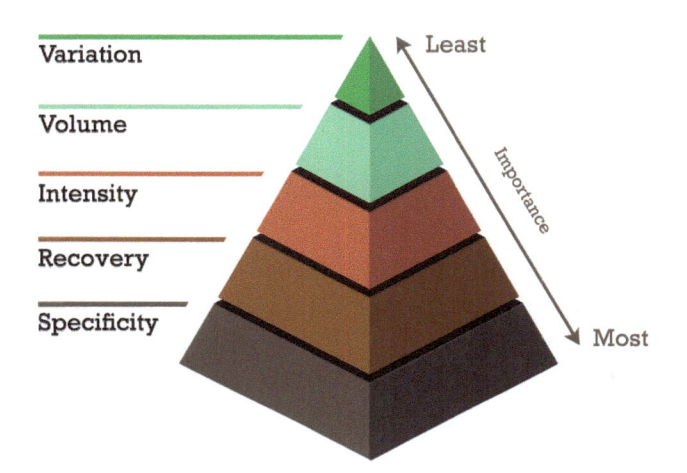

- **Specificity.** The principle of **specificity** implies that in order to become better at a particular task or skill, you must regularly perform that task or skill. According to the principle of specificity, running on a regular basis will be much more effective for improving your run performance than regular participation in biking and swimming. Additionally, regularly performing the back squat will be much more effective at improving squat performance than regular participation in cycling or lifts such as leg press or leg extensions.

- **Recovery.** Research shows that the physiological adaptations associated with hard training occur during **recovery** (Haff & Triplett, 2016; Israetel et al., 2015). Additionally, the effects of hard training are cumulative thereby affecting the body's ability to fully recover. As a result, it is recommended to introduce periods of reduced training intensity and/or volume in order to facilitate full recovery. One effective strategy to combat cumulative fatigue is to incorporate a **deload** (aka active rest) week every 3-6 weeks. Some of the different deload options include taking a week off from training or performing the same exercises but at a reduced load and volume (e.g., reduce the weight used and number of sets performed by 50%).

- **Intensity.** According to Zatsiorsky & Kraemer (2006), exercise intensity and volume are the two most important variables for producing maximal gains in muscle size and strength. Again, intensity is based on percentage of maximal heart rate (MHR) for endurance training, one repetition max (1RM) for strength training, and the level of discomfort while holding a stretch for mobility training.

Chapter 8: Exercise Programming

- **Volume.** Volume refers to the total number of exercises, sets and reps completed in a particular training session. Volume is based on the duration or distance for training, the number of sets and reps performed in strength training, and the number of stretches and reps performed in mobility training.

- **Variation.** If you recall from Chapter 6, the principle of accommodation states that the body's response to a constant stimulus decreases over time. With that in mind, it is recommended to periodically change the stimulus used in order to prevent accommodation and training plateaus. However, we also learned, according to the principle of directed adaptation, that we need to use the same stimulus long enough (up to several weeks in most cases) in order to fully develop and retain the physiological adaptations associated with that stimulus. Therefore, similar to combating cumulative fatigue, an effective strategy for implementing **variation** is to change up the exercises (stimulus) used every 3-6 weeks.

Stimulus-Recovery Adaptation Curve

It is important to remember that the physiological adaptations associated with chronic exercise occur during recovery, not training. With this in mind, it is essential that adequate rest be afforded between training sessions. The amount of time required to fully recover depends on the type and intensity of training performed. The body's response to training and its need for adequate recovery is represented in the **stimulus-recovery-adaptation (SRA) curve** depicted in **Figure 8.5**.

Figure 8.5. Stimulus-Recovery-Adaptation Curve

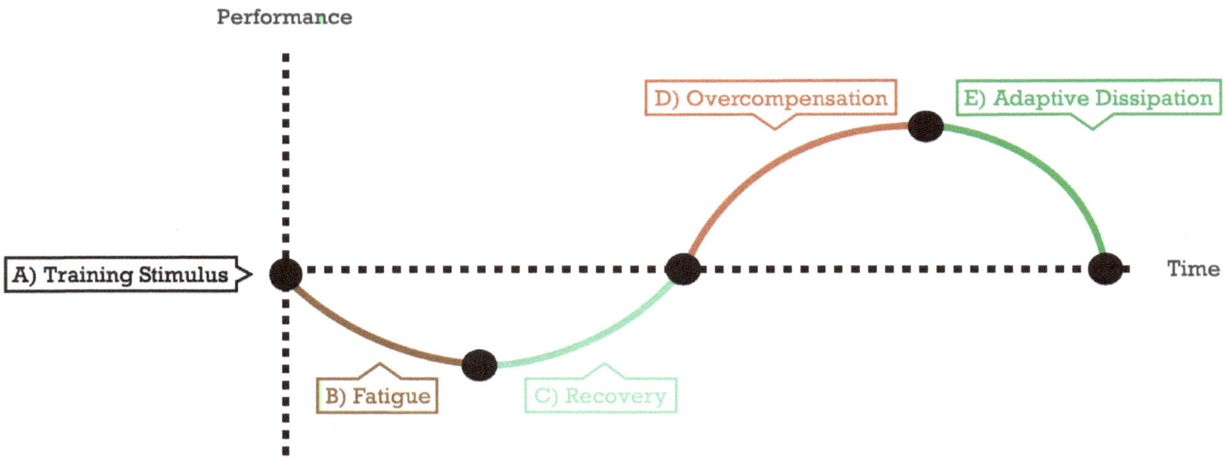

The SRA curve can be a helpful tool in determining when to conduct subsequent training sessions. Performing a training session too soon may result in the body not being fully recovered, thereby limiting the physiological adaptations, and increasing the risk of overtraining and/or injury. Similarly, waiting too long between training sessions can result in training plateaus and/or detraining. As depicted in **Figure 8.5**, Point A represents the training stimulus (e.g., 3-mile run or a deadlift workout). Point B represents the fatigue that occurs as a result of the training session. The amount of fatigue that accumulates is dependent on the type and magnitude of the training stimulus (e.g., 6 sets of 400-m sprints accumulate more fatigue than a 1-mile jog). Point C represents the initial stage of recovery where fitness levels return (go up) to where they were before the training stimulus. Point D represents the second stage of recovery, also called overcompensation, where fitness levels increase above where they were before the training stimulus. Point E represents detraining, also called adaptive dissipation, where fitness levels return (go down) to where they were before the training stimulus. In essence, the SRA curve provides guidance as to when to perform subsequent training sessions for the same or similar workout. The best time to perform a subsequent training session is at the peak of the overcompensation portion of the curve. Training before the peak can lead to overtraining or injury whereas training after the peak can lead to training plateaus or detraining.

Figure 8.6. Training Frequency and SRA Curve

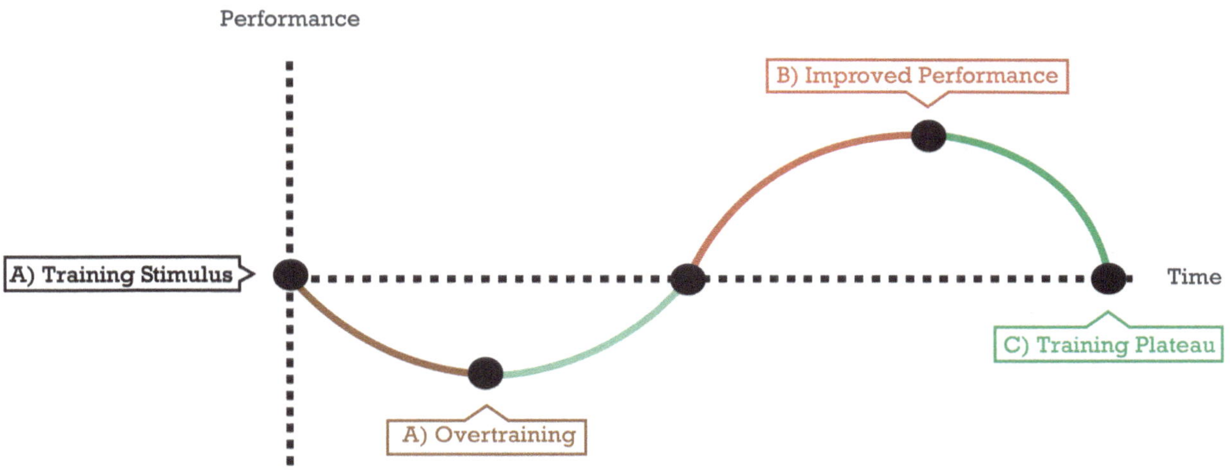

Designing a Comprehensive Exercise Program

Figure 8.6 depicts the relationship between the timing of training sessions and the physiological response to training. As previously mentioned, performing subsequent training sessions during the fatigue / recovery portion of the curve will likely result in overtraining (Point A). Performing subsequent training sessions during the adaptation portion of the curve will likely result in improved performance (Point B); while performing training sessions at the end of the adaptive dissipation portion of the curve will likely result in a training plateau and/or detraining (Point C). **Table 8.5** provides specific recommendations as to when the best time is to perform subsequent training sessions for various types of endurance and strength training.

Chapter 8: Exercise Programming

Table 8.5. SRA Recommendations for Various Types of Training

Training Type	SRA Recommendations
Moderate-intensity endurance training (e.g., long slow distance (LSD))	24 hours between training sessions
Vigorous-intensity endurance training (e.g., pace / tempo, interval, and high-intensity interval training (HIIT))	48 hours between training sessions
Moderate-intensity strength training (e.g., low to moderate intensity and/or volume strength training)	48 hours between training sessions
Vigorous-intensity strength training (e.g., high intensity and/or volume strength training)	72-96 hours between training sessions

The above recommendations are intended for individuals who are young, healthy, and have been exercising regularly. Individuals who are older, currently recovering from injury and/or have been previously sedentary, will likely require additional time to recover between training sessions. As previously mentioned, these recommendations are meant to provide guidance for when to perform subsequent sessions of similar training.

For example, at least 48 hours is required between two interval or high-intensity interval training sessions. However, long slow distance training can be performed daily. Similarly, at least 72 hours is required between two vigorous lower body strength training sessions. However, there are no restrictions as to when to perform upper body strength training following lower body strength training as the two sessions target and train different muscle groups.

While the SRA curve provides specific recommendations as to when to perform subsequent sessions of endurance training or strength training, combining the two into a single exercise plan can be challenging. For example, if both endurance training and strength training are performed on the same day, which type of training should be performed first? Likewise, should lower body strength training and speed training be performed on the same or subsequent days?

If both endurance and strength training are performed in a single training session, then the order in which they are performed does appear to matter. For example, performing endurance training first will negatively affect strength training performance to follow. Similarly, performing strength training first will negatively affect endurance training performance to follow. As a result, it is recommended to perform the type of training receiving priority first. For example, if an individual's primary goal is to improve strength, then strength training should be performed before endurance training. That said, if strength training and endurance training are performed at different times on the same day (e.g., separate morning and evening training sessions), then the order has no consequence as the body has had enough time to recover between training sessions.

Generally speaking, it would be inadvisable to perform lower body strength training within 24 hours of performing speed training as both target the fast twitch (type II) muscle fibers of the lower extremities. Instead, it would be better to conduct both on the same day (e.g., within the same training session or separate morning and evening training sessions) then wait at least 72 hours before repeating or wait at least 48 hours between the two training sessions.

3 Steps of Program Design

So far, we have discussed the different components of fitness, ACSM, AHA, CDC recommendations for endurance, strength and mobility training, the relationship between intensity, volume and frequency and the stimulus-recovery-adaptation (SRA) curve. The next step is to combine and use this information to design a weekly training template based on the individual's overall training goal (e.g., improve health, lose weight, run faster/farther, lift heavier, get bigger).

Step 1: Determine the number of days per week you plan on allotting for exercise. In doing so, be sure to meet the minimum frequency requirements set forth by the ASCM. Specifically:

- Endurance training: 5 days per week of moderate-intensity aerobic activity OR 3 days per week of vigorous-intensity aerobic activity OR an equivalent combination of moderate and vigorous intensity aerobic activity
- Strength training: 2 days per week
- Mobility training: 3 days per week

Remember, these are the minimum recommendations. Additional sessions per week will likely be required for those components of fitness considered weak or lacking. Additionally, be sure to adhere to the stimulus recovery adaptation (SRA) recommendations in regard to the timing of subsequent training sessions. Specifically:

- Moderate-intensity endurance training: 24 hours of recovery
- Vigorous-intensity endurance / moderate strength training: 48 hours of recovery
- Vigorous-intensity strength training: 72-96 hours of recovery

Provided below is a sample training template for an individual who has average endurance and mobility but below average strength (as determined through fitness testing). Although this individual's schedule permits them only one hour to workout, their schedule does allow them to work out every day. As a result, they opt for a 7-day per week training schedule. Based on ACSM, AHA, and CDC recommendations, they opt to perform both endurance and mobility training 3 days per week (for maintenance) and strength training 4 days per week (for improvement).

Mon	**Tues**	**Wed**	**Thurs**	**Fri**	**Sat**	**Sun**
Endurance	Strength	Endurance	Strength	Off	Endurance	Off
Mobility		Mobility			Mobility	

Chapter 8: Exercise Programming

Step 2: After determining the number of training days per week as well as when each type of training will be performed, the next step is to decide the type of training you plan on doing for each fitness component. In terms of endurance training, determine whether you will be performing long slow distance (LSD), pace/tempo (P/T), and/or speed work. In terms of strength training, determine which compound lifts and/or split option you plan on performing. In terms of mobility training, determine which mobility exercises and/or stretches you will be performing. Some different split options for strength training include:

- Push / Pull
    - Push: Bench, Press, Squat
    - Pull: Row, Deadlift
- Upper Body / Lower Body
    - *Upper Body (UB): Bench, Row, Press*
    - *Lower Body (LB): Squat, Deadlift*
- Total Body
    - Bench, Row, Press, Squat, Deadlift

Mon	Tues	Wed	Thurs	Fri	Sat	Sun
Endurance	Strength	Endurance	Strength	Off	Endurance	Off
Mobility		Mobility			Mobility	
Speed	Upper Body	Long Slow Distance	Lower Body	Off	Pace / Tempo	Off
Stretching		Yoga			Stretching	

Step 3: After determining the number and type of training days per week, the final step is to list the exact training parameters for each training session (e.g., run time/distance; load, reps, and sets). Because our example individual had less than 6 months of lifting experience, they were classified as a beginner and therefore only assigned 3 sets for each of the compound lifts and no assistance exercises. Additionally, since their primary training goal was strength, 6 reps were assigned per set for each of the compound lifts as outlined in **Table 6.8** (Chapter 6).

Mon	Tues	Wed	Thurs	Fri	Sat	Sun
Endurance	Strength	Endurance	Strength	Off	Endurance	Off
Mobility		Mobility			Mobility	
Speed	Upper Body	Long Slow Distance	Lower Body	Off	Pace / Tempo	Off
Stretching		Yoga			Stretching	
6 x 200-m Sprints	Bench 3 x 6	3-mi. Run	Squat 3 x 6	Off	Treadmill Tempo Run	Off
Modified Hurdler Stretch 3 x 30 sec.	Row 3 x 6	45-min. Yoga Video for Low-Back Mobility	Deadlift 3 x 6		Modified Hurdler Stretch 3 x 30 sec.	
Quad Stretch 3 x 30 sec.	Press 3 x 6		Back Hypers 3 x 6		Quad Stretch 3 x 30 sec.	
Piriformis Stretch 3 x 30 sec.	Plank 3 x 30 sec.				Piriformis Stretch 3 x 30 sec.	

CHAPTER 8: EXERCISE PROGRAMMING

Top 10 Takeaway Points

In this textbook we have covered a lot of information on a wide variety of topics to include basic nutrition, weight management, stress management and sleep, training for endurance, strength, and mobility and exercise programming. With all of the information covered, it can be overwhelming and/or difficult to know where to begin. With that in mind, provided below are the top 10 recommendations for how to live healthy lives and be good stewards of the bodies God has given us.

1. **Identify and correct for nutritional deficiencies.** Eating a variety of nutrient-dense foods like whole grains, high-fiber carbohydrates, lean meats and a variety of fresh fruits and vegetables every day can help to ensure daily macronutrient and micronutrient requirements are met. Some individuals may benefit from periodically tracking their daily food intake (e.g., MyFitnessPal) to determine if their current diet is either too high or low in a particular nutrient(s).

2. **Eat 3 or more servings of fresh fruits and vegetables every day.** Multiple servings of fruits and vegetables should be consumed daily as they are a good source of vitamins, minerals, and fiber. Additionally, fruits and vegetables are a good food option for those striving to lose weight, as they are low in fat and calories.

3. **Drink more water.** Since up to 60% of the human body is comprised of water, even a slight decrease in hydration can result in decreased physical and mental performance. Regardless of your fitness or weight management goal, drinking plenty of water is a good option.

4. **Keep track of your weight.** The average adult's weight can fluctuate up to 5-6 pounds per day. As a result, weighing yourself daily can provide misleading information. Instead, it is better to weigh yourself at the same time, and under similar circumstances, once per week. For those wanting to lose or gain weight, strive for no more than 0.5-2 lbs. per week. This information can then be used to adjust daily caloric consumption (diet) and/or expenditure (exercise) as required. [NOTE: Although this can be an effective strategy for some, weekly weigh-ins may not be appropriate for individuals who have anxiety about their weight and/or appearance.]

5. **Identify and deal with life stressors.** Similar to dehydration, stress can have a major impact on both physical and mental performance. As a result, it is important to address major life stressors early before they turn into an even bigger problem (e.g., sleep deprivation, depression).

6. **Strive for at least 8 hours of sleep every night.** In addition to decreased physical and mental performance, research has shown a link between sleep deprivation and certain chronic diseases to include diabetes, cardiovascular disease, obesity, and depression (Centers for Disease Control and Prevention, 2018).

7. **Walk at least 30 minutes every day.** There are numerous health benefits associated with daily walking. These benefits include increased cardiovascular and pulmonary fitness, decreased risk of heart disease, stroke and diabetes, improved balance, management of hypertension

and cholesterol and reduced joint / muscular pain and stiffness (Harvard Health Publishing, 2020). Additionally, walking immediately after a meal can help with digestion and improve satiety (feeling of being full).

8. **Perform all 5 compound lifts at least once per week.** Regular participation in the five compound lifts (i.e., bench, row, press, squat, and deadlift) can help to strengthen all of the major muscles groups as well as become more proficient in performing certain tasks of everyday life (e.g., lifting, pushing, carrying). In order to maximize the physiological adaptations associated with chronic strength training and prevent detraining, each compound lift should be performed at least once per week.

9. **Perform at least 10 minutes of mobility work every day.** In order to counteract the effects of prolonged sitting, it is recommended to perform at least 3-5 mobility exercises and/or stretches daily. Ideally, individuals should strive to perform at least four minutes of mobility work for every 30 minutes of continuous sitting (Starrett, 2015).

10. **Aggressively train your weaknesses while maintaining your strengths.** The tendency for most individuals is to train what they enjoy and/or are good at. However, doing so can lead to physiological imbalances that can negatively affect performance and/or increase injury risk. Instead, it would be better to identify (through periodic fitness testing) and tailor training to known weaknesses.

Summary

- Although there are 12 different components of fitness, some are more important than others and thus have training priority. The top three fundamental components of fitness include cardiovascular endurance, muscular strength, and mobility.

- According to recommendations from the American College of Sports Medicine (ACSM), American Heart Association (AHA), and Centers for Disease Control and Prevention (CDC), vigorous-intensity endurance training should be performed at least three days per week (or moderate-intensity endurance training at least five days per week); strength training should be performed at least two days per week; and mobility training should be performed at least two to three days per week. It is important to note, however, that these are the recommended minimums and if you are deficit in a particular area, you should do more than the minimums.

- There is an inverse relationship between exercise intensity, volume, and frequency. As one variable increases, reductions will need to be made in the other two in order to prevent overtraining and/or injury.

- It is important to remember that the physiological and beneficial adaptations associated with chronic exercise occur during recovery, not training. The amount of time required to fully recover depends on the type and intensity of training performed.

- The order in which exercises are performed does appear to matter when combining strength and endurance training into a single training session. Therefore, whichever component of fitness (i.e., strength or endurance) needs the most work should be performed first. However, if strength training and endurance training are performed at different times on the same day (e.g., morning and evening workouts), then the order has no consequence.

- There are essentially three steps to design a comprehensive exercise training plan based on an individual's overall training goals: 1) Determine the number of days per week to allot for exercise, 2) decide the type of exercise training plan for each fitness component, and 3) list the exact training parameters for each training session.

References

1. American College of Sports Medicine. (2021). Physical Activity Guidelines. Retrieved from https://www.acsm.org/read-research/trending-topics-resource-pages/physical-activity-guidelines.

2. American Heart Association. (2021). *American Heart Association Recommendations for Physical Activity in Adults and Kids*. Retrieved from https://www.heart.org/en/healthy-living/fitness/fitness-basics/aha-recs-for-physical-activity-in-adults.

3. Antonio, R. (2015). Deciphering the Ideal Training Frequency for Muscle Growth. Retrieved from http://www.thinkeatlift.com/deciphering-the-ideal-training-frequency-for-muscle-growth/.

4. Centers for Disease Control and Prevention. (2020). *How Much Physical Activity Do Adults Need?* Retrieved from https://www.cdc.gov/physicalactivity/basics/adults/index.htm.

5. Centers for Disease Control and Prevention. (2018). Sleep and Chronic Disease. Retrieved from https://www.cdc.gov/sleep/about_sleep/chronic_disease.html#:~:text=Notably%2C%20insufficient%20sleep%20has%20been,disease%2C%20obesity%2C%20and%20depression.

6. Haff, G., & Triplett, N. (Eds.). (2016). Essentials of Strength Training and Conditioning. (4th ed.). Champaign, IL: Human Kinetics.

7. Harvard Health Publishing: Harvard Medical School. (2020). Walking: Your Steps to Health. Retrieved from https://www.health.harvard.edu/staying-healthy/walking-your-steps-to-health.

8. Israetel, M., Hoffmann, J, & Smith, C. (2015). *Scientific Principles of Strength Training*. Renaissance Periodization.

9. Starrett, K. (2015). Becoming a Supple Leopard. (2nd ed.). Las Vegas, NV: Victory Belt Publishing, Inc.

10. U.S. Department of Health and Human Services. (2020, May 21). Physical Activity. Retrieved from https://health.gov/our-work/physical-activity.

11. Zatsiorsky, V., & Kraemer, W. (2006). Science and Practice of Strength Training (2nd ed). Champaign, IL: Human Kinetics.

Appendix A
Glycemic Index and Glycemic Load for Common Foods

Appendix A: Glycemic Index and Glycemic Load for Common Foods

Category	Food	Glycemic Index	Glycemic Load
Breads	Baguette	95	15
	Waffle	76	10
	White bread	73	10
	Bagel	72	25
	100% whole grain bread	71	9
	Pita bread	68	10
	Hamburger bun	61	9
	Pumpernickel bread	56	7
Grains	White rice	89	43
	Couscous	65	9
	Quinoa	53	13
	Brown rice	50	16
Breakfast Cereals	Cornflakes	93	23
	Coco Pops	77	20
	Special K	69	14
	Raisin Bran	61	12
	Oatmeal	55	13
	All-Bran	55	12
Pasta and Noodles	Macaroni and cheese	64	32
	Macaroni	47	23
	Spaghetti	46	22
	Fettuccini	32	15
Fruits	Watermelon	72	4
	Raisins	64	28
	Banana	62	16
	Grapes	59	11
	Peach	42	5
	Orange	40	4
	Apple	39	6
	Pear	38	4
	Grapefruit	25	3

Vegetables	Mashed potatoes	87	17
	White potato	82	21
	Green peas	51	4
	Sweet potato	70	22
	Yam	54	20
	Carrots	35	2
Beans and Nuts	Baked Beans	40	6
	Blackeye peas	33	10
	Navy beans	31	9
	Black beans	30	7
	Lentils	29	5
	Cashews	27	3
	Soy beans	15	1
	Chickpeas	10	3
	Peanuts	7	0
	Hummus	6	0
Dairy Products	Ice cream	57	6
	Full-fat milk	41	5
	Reduced-fat yogurt	33	11
	Skim milk	32	4
Snack Foods	Pretzels	83	16
	Rice cakes	82	17
	Vanilla wafers	77	14
	Graham crackers	74	14
	Microwave popcorn	55	6
	Potato chips	51	12
Beverages	Gatorade	78	12
	Cranberry juice cocktail	68	24
	Coca cola	63	16
	Orange juice	50	12
	Apple juice	44	30
	Tomato juice	38	4

Appendix A: Glycemic Index and Glycemic Load for Common Foods

Appendix B
Estimated Percent Body Fat Based on Waist Circumference

Appendix B: Estimated Percent Body Fat Based on Waist Circumference

Estimated Percent Body Fat Based on Waist Circumference for Males

WC (in.)	60	60.5	61	61.5	62	62.5	63	63.5	64	64.5	65	65.5	66	66.5	67	67.5	68	68.5	69	69.5
23	<5	<5	<5	<5	<5	<5	<5	<5	<5	<5	<5	<5	<5	<5	<5	<5	<5	<5	<5	<5
23.5	<5	<5	<5	<5	<5	<5	<5	<5	<5	<5	<5	<5	<5	<5	<5	<5	<5	<5	<5	<5
24	<5	<5	<5	<5	<5	<5	<5	<5	<5	<5	<5	<5	<5	<5	<5	<5	<5	<5	<5	<5
24.5	<5	<5	<5	<5	<5	<5	<5	<5	<5	<5	<5	<5	<5	<5	<5	<5	<5	<5	<5	<5
25	<5	<5	<5	<5	<5	<5	<5	<5	<5	<5	<5	<5	<5	<5	<5	<5	<5	<5	<5	<5
25.5	5.1	<5	<5	<5	<5	<5	<5	<5	<5	<5	<5	<5	<5	<5	<5	<5	<5	<5	<5	<5
26	6.4	5.9	5.5	5.0	<5	<5	<5	<5	<5	<5	<5	<5	<5	<5	<5	<5	<5	<5	<5	<5
26.5	7.6	7.2	6.7	6.2	5.8	5.3	<5	<5	<5	<5	<5	<5	<5	<5	<5	<5	<5	<5	<5	<5
27	8.8	8.4	7.9	7.4	7.0	6.5	6.1	5.6	5.2	<5	<5	<5	<5	<5	<5	<5	<5	<5	<5	<5
27.5	10.0	9.6	9.1	8.6	8.2	7.7	7.3	6.8	6.4	6.0	5.5	5.1	<5	<5	<5	<5	<5	<5	<5	<5
28	11.2	10.7	10.3	9.8	9.3	8.9	8.4	8.0	7.6	7.1	6.7	6.3	5.8	5.4	5.0	<5	<5	<5	<5	<5
28.5	12.3	11.9	11.4	10.9	10.5	10.0	9.6	9.1	8.7	8.3	7.8	7.4	7.0	6.5	6.1	5.7	5.3	<5	<5	<5
29	13.5	13.0	12.5	12.1	11.6	11.2	10.7	10.3	9.8	9.4	9.0	8.5	8.1	7.7	7.3	6.8	6.4	6.0	5.6	5.2
29.5	14.6	14.1	13.6	13.2	12.7	12.3	11.8	11.4	10.9	10.5	10.1	9.6	9.2	8.8	8.4	7.9	7.5	7.1	6.7	6.3
30	15.7	15.2	14.7	14.3	13.8	13.4	12.9	12.5	12.0	11.6	11.1	10.7	10.3	9.9	9.4	9.0	8.6	8.2	7.8	7.4
30.5	16.7	16.3	15.8	15.3	14.9	14.4	14.0	13.5	13.1	12.7	12.2	11.8	11.4	10.9	10.5	10.1	9.7	9.3	8.9	8.5
31	17.8	17.3	16.8	16.4	15.9	15.5	15.0	14.6	14.1	13.7	13.3	12.8	12.4	12.0	11.6	11.1	10.7	10.3	9.9	9.5
31.5	18.8	18.3	17.9	17.4	17.0	16.5	16.1	15.6	15.2	14.7	14.3	13.9	13.4	13.0	12.6	12.2	11.8	11.4	10.9	10.5
32	19.8	19.4	18.9	18.4	18.0	17.5	17.1	16.6	16.2	15.8	15.3	14.9	14.5	14.0	13.6	13.2	12.8	12.4	12.0	11.6
32.5	20.8	20.4	19.9	19.4	19.0	18.5	18.1	17.6	17.2	16.8	16.3	15.9	15.5	15.0	14.6	14.2	13.8	13.4	13.0	12.6
33	21.8	21.3	20.9	20.4	19.9	19.5	19.1	18.6	18.2	17.7	17.3	16.9	16.5	16.0	15.6	15.2	14.8	14.4	14.0	13.5
33.5	22.8	22.3	21.9	21.4	20.9	20.5	20.0	19.6	19.2	18.7	18.3	17.9	17.4	17.0	16.6	16.2	15.7	15.3	14.9	14.5
34	23.7	23.3	22.8	22.4	21.9	21.4	21.0	20.6	20.1	19.7	19.2	18.8	18.4	18.0	17.5	17.1	16.7	16.3	15.9	15.5
34.5	24.7	24.2	23.8	23.3	22.8	22.4	21.9	21.5	21.1	20.6	20.2	19.8	19.3	18.9	18.5	18.1	17.6	17.2	16.8	16.4
35	25.6	25.2	24.7	24.2	23.8	23.3	22.9	22.4	22.0	21.6	21.1	20.7	20.3	19.8	19.4	19.0	18.6	18.2	17.8	17.4
35.5	26.5	26.1	25.6	25.1	24.7	24.2	23.8	23.3	22.9	22.5	22.0	21.6	21.2	20.8	20.3	19.9	19.5	19.1	18.7	18.3
36	27.4	27.0	26.5	26.1	25.6	25.1	24.7	24.3	23.8	23.4	22.9	22.5	22.1	21.7	21.2	20.8	20.4	20.0	19.6	19.2
36.5	28.3	27.9	27.4	26.9	26.5	26.0	25.6	25.1	24.7	24.3	23.8	23.4	23.0	22.5	22.1	21.7	21.3	20.9	20.5	20.1
37	29.2	28.7	28.3	27.8	27.4	26.9	26.5	26.0	25.6	25.1	24.7	24.3	23.9	23.4	23.0	22.6	22.2	21.8	21.4	20.9
37.5	30.1	29.6	29.2	28.7	28.2	27.8	27.3	26.9	26.5	26.0	25.6	25.1	24.7	24.3	23.9	23.5	23.0	22.6	22.2	21.8
38	30.9	30.5	30.0	29.5	29.1	28.6	28.2	27.7	27.3	26.9	26.4	26.0	25.6	25.2	24.7	24.3	23.9	23.5	23.1	22.7
38.5	31.8	31.3	30.9	30.4	29.9	29.5	29.0	28.6	28.2	27.7	27.3	26.9	26.4	26.0	25.6	25.2	24.7	24.3	23.9	23.5

Height (in.)

Estimated Percent Body Fat Based on Waist Circumference for Males – Cont.

WC (in.)	Height (in.)																				
	60	60.5	61	61.5	62	62.5	63	63.5	64	64.5	65	65.5	66	66.5	67	67.5	68	68.5	69	69.5
39	32.6	32.2	31.7	31.2	30.8	30.3	29.9	29.4	29.0	28.5	28.1	27.7	27.3	26.8	26.4	26.0	25.6	25.2	24.8	24.4
39.5	33.4	33.0	32.5	32.1	31.6	31.1	30.7	30.3	29.8	29.4	28.9	28.5	28.1	27.7	27.2	26.8	26.4	26.0	25.6	25.2
40	34.3	33.8	33.3	32.9	32.4	32.0	31.5	31.1	30.6	30.2	29.8	29.3	28.9	28.5	28.0	27.6	27.2	26.8	26.4	26.0
40.5	35.1	34.6	34.1	33.7	33.2	32.8	32.3	31.9	31.4	31.0	30.6	30.1	29.7	29.3	28.9	28.4	28.0	27.6	27.2	26.8
41	35.9	35.4	34.9	34.5	34.0	33.6	33.1	32.7	32.2	31.8	31.3	30.9	30.5	30.1	29.6	29.2	28.8	28.4	28.0	27.6
41.5	36.6	36.2	35.7	35.2	34.8	34.3	33.9	33.4	33.0	32.6	32.1	31.7	31.3	30.9	30.4	30.0	29.6	29.2	28.8	28.4
42	37.4	36.9	36.5	36.0	35.6	35.1	34.7	34.2	33.8	33.3	32.9	32.5	32.0	31.6	31.2	30.8	30.4	30.0	29.5	29.1
42.5	38.2	37.7	37.2	36.8	36.3	35.9	35.4	35.0	34.5	34.1	33.7	33.2	32.8	32.4	32.0	31.6	31.1	30.7	30.3	29.9
43	>38.2	>37.7	>37.2	>36.8	>36.3	>35.9	>35.4	>35.0	>34.5	>34.1	>33.7	>33.2	>32.8	>32.4	>32.0	>31.6	>31.1	>30.7	>30.3	>29.9
43.5	>38.2	>37.7	>37.2	>36.8	>36.3	>35.9	>35.4	>35.0	>34.5	>34.1	>33.7	>33.2	>32.8	>32.4	>32.0	>31.6	>31.1	>30.7	>30.3	>29.9
44	>38.2	>37.7	>37.2	>36.8	>36.3	>35.9	>35.4	>35.0	>34.5	>34.1	>33.7	>33.2	>32.8	>32.4	>32.0	>31.6	>31.1	>30.7	>30.3	>29.9
44.5	>38.2	>37.7	>37.2	>36.8	>36.3	>35.9	>35.4	>35.0	>34.5	>34.1	>33.7	>33.2	>32.8	>32.4	>32.0	>31.6	>31.1	>30.7	>30.3	>29.9
45	>38.2	>37.7	>37.2	>36.8	>36.3	>35.9	>35.4	>35.0	>34.5	>34.1	>33.7	>33.2	>32.8	>32.4	>32.0	>31.6	>31.1	>30.7	>30.3	>29.9

Estimated Percent Body Fat Based on Waist Circumference for Males – Cont.

WC (in.)	Height (in.)																			
	70	70.5	71	71.5	72	72.5	73	73.5	74	74.5	75	75.5	76	76.5	77	77.5	78	78.5	79	79.5
23	< 5	< 5	< 5	< 5	< 5	< 5	< 5	< 5	< 5	< 5	< 5	< 5	< 5	< 5	< 5	< 5	< 5	< 5	< 5	< 5
23.5	< 5	< 5	< 5	< 5	< 5	< 5	< 5	< 5	< 5	< 5	< 5	< 5	< 5	< 5	< 5	< 5	< 5	< 5	< 5	< 5
24	< 5	< 5	< 5	< 5	< 5	< 5	< 5	< 5	< 5	< 5	< 5	< 5	< 5	< 5	< 5	< 5	< 5	< 5	< 5	< 5
24.5	< 5	< 5	< 5	< 5	< 5	< 5	< 5	< 5	< 5	< 5	< 5	< 5	< 5	< 5	< 5	< 5	< 5	< 5	< 5	< 5
25	< 5	< 5	< 5	< 5	< 5	< 5	< 5	< 5	< 5	< 5	< 5	< 5	< 5	< 5	< 5	< 5	< 5	< 5	< 5	< 5
25.5	< 5	< 5	< 5	< 5	< 5	< 5	< 5	< 5	< 5	< 5	< 5	< 5	< 5	< 5	< 5	< 5	< 5	< 5	< 5	< 5
26	< 5	< 5	< 5	< 5	< 5	< 5	< 5	< 5	< 5	< 5	< 5	< 5	< 5	< 5	< 5	< 5	< 5	< 5	< 5	< 5
26.5	< 5	< 5	< 5	< 5	< 5	< 5	< 5	< 5	< 5	< 5	< 5	< 5	< 5	< 5	< 5	< 5	< 5	< 5	< 5	< 5
27	< 5	< 5	< 5	< 5	< 5	< 5	< 5	< 5	< 5	< 5	< 5	< 5	< 5	< 5	< 5	< 5	< 5	< 5	< 5	< 5
27.5	< 5	< 5	< 5	< 5	< 5	< 5	< 5	< 5	< 5	< 5	< 5	< 5	< 5	< 5	< 5	< 5	< 5	< 5	< 5	< 5
28	< 5	< 5	< 5	< 5	< 5	< 5	< 5	< 5	< 5	< 5	< 5	< 5	< 5	< 5	< 5	< 5	< 5	< 5	< 5	< 5
28.5	< 5	< 5	< 5	< 5	< 5	< 5	< 5	< 5	< 5	< 5	< 5	< 5	< 5	< 5	< 5	< 5	< 5	< 5	< 5	< 5
29	< 5	< 5	< 5	< 5	< 5	< 5	< 5	< 5	< 5	< 5	< 5	< 5	< 5	< 5	< 5	< 5	< 5	< 5	< 5	< 5
29.5	5.9	5.5	5.1	< 5	< 5	< 5	< 5	< 5	< 5	< 5	< 5	< 5	< 5	< 5	< 5	< 5	< 5	< 5	< 5	< 5
30	7.0	6.6	6.2	5.8	5.4	5.0	< 5	< 5	< 5	< 5	< 5	< 5	< 5	< 5	< 5	< 5	< 5	< 5	< 5	< 5
30.5	8.1	7.7	7.3	6.9	6.5	6.1	5.7	5.3	< 5	< 5	< 5	< 5	< 5	< 5	< 5	< 5	< 5	< 5	< 5	< 5
31	9.1	8.7	8.3	7.9	7.5	7.1	6.7	6.4	6.0	5.6	5.2	< 5	< 5	< 5	< 5	< 5	< 5	< 5	< 5	< 5
31.5	10.1	9.7	9.3	8.9	8.6	8.2	7.8	7.4	7.0	6.6	6.3	5.9	5.5	5.1	< 5	< 5	< 5	< 5	< 5	< 5
32	11.2	10.8	10.4	10.0	9.6	9.2	8.8	8.4	8.0	7.7	7.3	6.9	6.5	6.2	5.8	5.4	5.1	< 5	< 5	< 5
32.5	12.2	11.8	11.4	11.0	10.6	10.2	9.8	9.4	9.0	8.7	8.3	7.9	7.5	7.2	6.8	6.4	6.1	5.7	5.4	5.0
33	13.1	12.7	12.3	12.0	11.6	11.2	10.8	10.4	10.0	9.6	9.3	8.9	8.5	8.2	7.8	7.4	7.1	6.7	6.3	6.0
33.5	14.1	13.7	13.3	12.9	12.5	12.1	11.8	11.4	11.0	10.6	10.2	9.9	9.5	9.1	8.8	8.4	8.0	7.7	7.3	7.0
34	15.1	14.7	14.3	13.9	13.5	13.1	12.7	12.3	12.0	11.6	11.2	10.8	10.5	10.1	9.7	9.4	9.0	8.6	8.3	7.9
34.5	16.0	15.6	15.2	14.8	14.4	14.0	13.7	13.3	12.9	12.5	12.1	11.8	11.4	11.0	10.7	10.3	9.9	9.6	9.2	8.9
35	17.0	16.5	16.2	15.8	15.4	15.0	14.6	14.2	13.8	13.4	13.1	12.7	12.3	12.0	11.6	11.2	10.9	10.5	10.1	9.8
35.5	17.9	17.5	17.1	16.7	16.3	15.9	15.5	15.1	14.7	14.4	14.0	13.6	13.2	12.9	12.5	12.1	11.8	11.4	11.1	10.7
36	18.8	18.4	18.0	17.6	17.2	16.8	16.4	16.0	15.6	15.3	14.9	14.5	14.1	13.8	13.4	13.0	12.7	12.3	12.0	11.6
36.5	19.7	19.3	18.9	18.5	18.1	17.7	17.3	16.9	16.5	16.2	15.8	15.4	15.0	14.7	14.3	13.9	13.6	13.2	12.9	12.5
37	20.5	20.1	19.7	19.4	19.0	18.6	18.2	17.8	17.4	17.0	16.7	16.3	15.9	15.6	15.2	14.8	14.5	14.1	13.7	13.4
37.5	21.4	21.0	20.6	20.2	19.8	19.4	19.1	18.7	18.3	17.9	17.5	17.2	16.8	16.4	16.1	15.7	15.3	15.0	14.6	14.3
38	22.3	21.9	21.5	21.1	20.7	20.3	19.9	19.5	19.1	18.8	18.4	18.0	17.6	17.3	16.9	16.5	16.2	15.8	15.5	15.1
38.5	23.1	22.7	22.3	21.9	21.5	21.1	20.8	20.4	20.0	19.6	19.2	18.9	18.5	18.1	17.8	17.4	17.0	16.7	16.3	16.0

A Christian Guide to Body Stewardship, Diet and Exercise

Estimated Percent Body Fat Based on Waist Circumference for Males – Cont.

WC (in.)	70	70.5	71	71.5	72	72.5	73	73.5	74	74.5	75	75.5	76	76.5	77	77.5	78	78.5	79	79.5
39	23.9	23.5	23.2	22.8	22.4	22.0	21.6	21.2	20.8	20.4	20.1	19.7	19.3	19.0	18.6	18.2	17.9	17.5	17.1	16.8
39.5	24.8	24.4	24.0	23.6	23.2	22.8	22.4	22.0	21.6	21.3	20.9	20.5	20.1	19.8	19.4	19.0	18.7	18.3	18.0	17.6
40	25.6	25.2	24.8	24.4	24.0	23.6	23.2	22.8	22.5	22.1	21.7	21.3	21.0	20.6	20.2	19.9	19.5	19.1	18.8	18.4
40.5	26.4	26.0	25.6	25.2	24.8	24.4	24.0	23.6	23.3	22.9	22.5	22.1	21.8	21.4	21.0	20.7	20.3	19.9	19.6	19.2
41	27.2	26.8	26.4	26.0	25.6	25.2	24.8	24.4	24.1	23.7	23.3	22.9	22.6	22.2	21.8	21.5	21.1	20.7	20.4	20.0
41.5	28.0	27.6	27.2	26.8	26.4	26.0	25.6	25.2	24.8	24.5	24.1	23.7	23.3	23.0	22.6	22.2	21.9	21.5	21.2	20.8
42	28.7	28.3	27.9	27.5	27.2	26.8	26.4	26.0	25.6	25.2	24.9	24.5	24.1	23.7	23.4	23.0	22.7	22.3	21.9	21.6
42.5	29.5	29.1	28.7	28.3	27.9	27.5	27.1	26.8	26.4	26.0	25.6	25.3	24.9	24.5	24.1	23.8	23.4	23.1	22.7	22.3
43	>29.5	>29.1	>28.7	>28.3	>27.9	>27.5	>27.1	>26.8	>26.4	>26.0	>25.6	>25.3	>24.9	>24.5	>24.1	>23.8	>23.4	>23.1	>22.7	>22.3
43.5	>29.5	>29.1	>28.7	>28.3	>27.9	>27.5	>27.1	>26.8	>26.4	>26.0	>25.6	>25.3	>24.9	>24.5	>24.1	>23.8	>23.4	>23.1	>22.7	>22.3
44	>29.5	>29.1	>28.7	>28.3	>27.9	>27.5	>27.1	>26.8	>26.4	>26.0	>25.6	>25.3	>24.9	>24.5	>24.1	>23.8	>23.4	>23.1	>22.7	>22.3
44.5	>29.5	>29.1	>28.7	>28.3	>27.9	>27.5	>27.1	>26.8	>26.4	>26.0	>25.6	>25.3	>24.9	>24.5	>24.1	>23.8	>23.4	>23.1	>22.7	>22.3
45	>29.5	>29.1	>28.7	>28.3	>27.9	>27.5	>27.1	>26.8	>26.4	>26.0	>25.6	>25.3	>24.9	>24.5	>24.1	>23.8	>23.4	>23.1	>22.7	>22.3

Height (in.)

Appendix B: Estimated Percent Body Fat Based on Waist Circumference

Estimated Percent Body Fat Based on Waist Circumference for Females

WC (in.)	58	58.5	59	59.5	60	60.5	61	61.5	62	62.5	63	63.5	64	64.5	65	65.5	66	66.5	67	67.5
23	9.7	9.4	9.0	8.7	8.4	8.1	7.8	7.5	7.2	6.9	6.6	6.4	6.1	5.8	5.5	5.2	5.0	<5	<5	<5
23.5	10.9	10.6	10.3	10.0	9.7	9.3	9.0	8.7	8.5	8.2	7.9	7.6	7.3	7.0	6.7	6.4	6.2	5.9	5.6	5.4
24	12.1	11.8	11.5	11.2	10.8	10.5	10.2	9.9	9.6	9.4	9.1	8.8	8.5	8.2	7.9	7.6	7.4	7.1	6.8	6.5
24.5	13.3	12.9	12.6	12.3	12.0	11.7	11.4	11.1	10.8	10.5	10.2	9.9	9.7	9.4	9.1	8.8	8.5	8.3	8.0	7.7
25	14.4	14.1	13.8	13.5	13.2	12.9	12.6	12.3	12.0	11.7	11.4	11.1	10.8	10.5	10.2	10.0	9.7	9.4	9.1	8.9
25.5	15.5	15.2	14.9	14.6	14.3	14.0	13.7	13.4	13.1	12.8	12.5	12.2	11.9	11.6	11.4	11.1	10.8	10.5	10.3	10.0
26	16.6	16.3	16.0	15.7	15.4	15.1	14.8	14.5	14.2	13.9	13.6	13.3	13.0	12.8	12.5	12.2	11.9	11.6	11.4	11.1
26.5	17.7	17.4	17.1	16.8	16.5	16.2	15.9	15.6	15.3	15.0	14.7	14.4	14.1	13.8	13.6	13.3	13.0	12.7	12.4	12.2
27	18.8	18.5	18.1	17.8	17.5	17.2	16.9	16.6	16.3	16.0	15.8	15.5	15.2	14.9	14.6	14.3	14.1	13.8	13.5	13.2
27.5	19.8	19.5	19.2	18.9	18.6	18.3	18.0	17.7	17.4	17.1	16.8	16.5	16.2	15.9	15.7	15.4	15.1	14.8	14.5	14.3
28	20.8	20.5	20.2	19.9	19.6	19.3	19.0	18.7	18.4	18.1	17.8	17.5	17.2	17.0	16.7	16.4	16.1	15.8	15.6	15.3
28.5	21.8	21.5	21.2	20.9	20.6	20.3	20.0	19.7	19.4	19.1	18.8	18.5	18.2	18.0	17.7	17.4	17.1	16.8	16.6	16.3
29	22.8	22.5	22.2	21.9	21.6	21.3	21.0	20.7	20.4	20.1	19.8	19.5	19.2	19.0	18.7	18.4	18.1	17.8	17.6	17.3
29.5	23.8	23.5	23.2	22.9	22.6	22.3	22.0	21.7	21.4	21.1	20.8	20.5	20.2	19.9	19.6	19.4	19.1	18.8	18.5	18.3
30	24.8	24.4	24.1	23.8	23.5	23.2	22.9	22.6	22.3	22.0	21.7	21.4	21.2	20.9	20.6	20.3	20.0	19.8	19.5	19.2
30.5	25.7	25.4	25.1	24.8	24.5	24.2	23.9	23.6	23.3	23.0	22.7	22.4	22.1	21.8	21.5	21.3	21.0	20.7	20.4	20.2
31	26.6	26.3	26.0	25.7	25.4	25.1	24.8	24.5	24.2	23.9	23.6	23.3	23.0	22.7	22.5	22.2	21.9	21.6	21.4	21.1
31.5	27.5	27.2	26.9	26.6	26.3	26.0	25.7	25.4	25.1	24.8	24.5	24.2	23.9	23.6	23.4	23.1	22.8	22.5	22.3	22.0
32	28.4	28.1	27.8	27.5	27.2	26.9	26.6	26.3	26.0	25.7	25.4	25.1	24.8	24.5	24.3	24.0	23.7	23.4	23.2	22.9
32.5	29.3	29.0	28.7	28.4	28.1	27.8	27.5	27.2	26.9	26.6	26.3	26.0	25.7	25.4	25.1	24.9	24.6	24.3	24.0	23.8
33	30.2	29.9	29.5	29.2	28.9	28.6	28.3	28.0	27.7	27.4	27.1	26.9	26.6	26.3	26.0	25.7	25.5	25.2	24.9	24.6
33.5	31.0	30.7	30.4	30.1	29.8	29.5	29.2	28.9	28.6	28.3	28.0	27.7	27.4	27.1	26.9	26.6	26.3	26.0	25.8	25.5
34	31.9	31.5	31.2	30.9	30.6	30.3	30.0	29.7	29.4	29.1	28.8	28.6	28.3	28.0	27.7	27.4	27.1	26.9	26.6	26.3
34.5	32.7	32.4	32.1	31.8	31.5	31.2	30.8	30.6	30.3	30.0	29.7	29.4	29.1	28.8	28.5	28.3	28.0	27.7	27.4	27.2
35	33.5	33.2	32.9	32.6	32.3	32.0	31.7	31.4	31.1	30.8	30.5	30.2	29.9	29.6	29.3	29.1	28.8	28.5	28.2	28.0
35.5	34.3	34.0	33.7	33.4	33.1	32.8	32.5	32.2	31.9	31.6	31.3	31.0	30.7	30.4	30.2	29.9	29.6	29.3	29.0	28.8
36	35.1	34.8	34.5	34.2	33.9	33.6	33.3	33.0	32.7	32.4	32.1	31.8	31.5	31.2	30.9	30.7	30.4	30.1	29.8	29.6
36.5	35.9	35.6	35.3	35.0	34.7	34.4	34.0	33.8	33.5	33.2	32.9	32.6	32.3	32.0	31.7	31.5	31.2	30.9	30.6	30.4
37	36.7	36.3	36.0	35.7	35.4	35.1	34.8	34.5	34.2	33.9	33.6	33.4	33.1	32.8	32.5	32.2	31.9	31.7	31.4	31.1
37.5	37.4	37.1	36.8	36.5	36.2	35.9	35.6	35.3	35.0	34.7	34.4	34.1	33.8	33.5	33.3	33.0	32.7	32.4	32.2	31.9
38	38.2	37.9	37.6	37.2	36.9	36.6	36.3	36.0	35.7	35.4	35.2	34.9	34.6	34.3	34.0	33.7	33.5	33.2	32.9	32.6
38.5	38.9	38.6	38.3	38.0	37.7	37.4	37.1	36.8	36.5	36.2	35.9	35.6	35.3	35.0	34.8	34.5	34.2	33.9	33.7	33.4

A CHRISTIAN GUIDE TO BODY STEWARDSHIP, DIET AND EXERCISE

Appendix B: Estimated Percent Body Fat Based on Waist Circumference for Females – Cont.

WC (in.)	58	58.5	59	59.5	60	60.5	61	61.5	62	62.5	63	63.5	64	64.5	65	65.5	66	66.5	67	67.5
39	39.7	39.3	39.0	38.7	38.4	38.1	37.8	37.5	37.2	36.9	36.6	36.3	36.1	35.8	35.5	35.2	34.9	34.7	34.4	34.1
39.5	40.4	40.1	39.8	39.4	39.1	38.8	38.5	38.2	37.9	37.6	37.4	37.1	36.8	36.5	36.2	35.9	35.7	35.4	35.1	34.8
40	41.1	40.8	40.5	40.2	39.9	39.5	39.2	39.0	38.7	38.4	38.1	37.8	37.5	37.2	36.9	36.7	36.4	36.1	35.8	35.6
40.5	41.8	41.5	41.2	40.9	40.6	40.3	40.0	39.7	39.4	39.1	38.8	38.5	38.2	37.9	37.6	37.4	37.1	36.8	36.5	36.3
41	42.5	42.2	41.9	41.6	41.3	41.0	40.7	40.4	40.1	39.8	39.5	39.2	38.9	38.6	38.3	38.1	37.8	37.5	37.2	37.0
41.5	43.2	42.9	42.6	42.2	41.9	41.6	41.3	41.0	40.7	40.5	40.2	39.9	39.6	39.3	39.0	38.7	38.5	38.2	37.9	37.6
42	43.9	43.5	43.2	42.9	42.6	42.3	42.0	41.7	41.4	41.1	40.8	40.6	40.3	40.0	39.7	39.4	39.1	38.9	38.6	38.3
42.5	44.5	44.2	43.9	43.6	43.3	43.0	42.7	42.4	42.1	41.8	41.5	41.2	40.9	40.7	40.4	40.1	39.8	39.5	39.3	39.0
43	45.2	44.9	44.6	44.3	44.0	43.7	43.4	43.1	42.8	42.5	42.2	41.9	41.6	41.3	41.0	40.8	40.5	40.2	39.9	39.7
43.5	45.9	45.5	45.2	44.9	44.6	44.3	44.0	43.7	43.4	43.1	42.8	42.5	42.3	42.0	41.7	41.4	41.1	40.9	40.6	40.3
44	46.5	46.2	45.9	45.6	45.3	45.0	44.7	44.4	44.1	43.8	43.5	43.2	42.9	42.6	42.3	42.1	41.8	41.5	41.2	41.0
44.5	47.1	46.8	46.5	46.2	45.9	45.6	45.3	45.0	44.7	44.4	44.1	43.8	43.6	43.3	43.0	42.7	42.4	42.2	41.9	41.6
45	47.8	47.5	47.2	46.8	46.5	46.2	45.9	45.6	45.3	45.1	44.8	44.5	44.2	43.9	43.6	43.3	43.1	42.8	42.5	42.2

Height (in.)

Appendix B: Estimated Percent Body Fat Based on Waist Circumference for Females – Cont.

WC (in.)	68	68.5	69	69.5	70	70.5	71	71.5	72	72.5	73	73.5	74	74.5	75	75.5	76	76.5	77	77.5
23	<5	<5	<5	<5	<5	<5	<5	<5	<5	<5	<5	<5	<5	<5	<5	<5	<5	<5	<5	<5
23.5	5.1	<5	<5	<5	<5	<5	<5	<5	<5	<5	<5	<5	<5	<5	<5	<5	<5	<5	<5	<5
24	6.3	6.0	5.7	5.5	5.2	5.0	<5	<5	<5	<5	<5	<5	<5	<5	<5	<5	<5	<5	<5	<5
24.5	7.4	7.2	6.9	6.7	6.4	6.1	5.9	5.6	5.4	5.1	<5	<5	<5	5.3	5.0	<5	<5	<5	<5	<5
25	8.6	8.3	8.1	7.8	7.5	7.3	7.0	6.8	6.5	6.3	6.0	5.8	5.5	5.3	5.0	<5	<5	<5	<5	<5
25.5	9.7	9.5	9.2	8.9	8.7	8.4	8.1	7.9	7.6	7.4	7.1	6.9	6.6	6.4	6.1	5.9	5.7	5.4	5.2	<5
26	10.8	10.6	10.3	10.0	9.8	9.5	9.2	9.0	8.7	8.5	8.2	8.0	7.7	7.5	7.2	7.0	6.8	6.5	6.3	6.0
26.5	11.9	11.6	11.4	11.1	10.8	10.6	10.3	10.1	9.8	9.6	9.3	9.1	8.8	8.6	8.3	8.1	7.8	7.6	7.4	7.1
27	13.0	12.7	12.4	12.2	11.9	11.6	11.4	11.1	10.9	10.6	10.4	10.1	9.9	9.6	9.4	9.1	8.9	8.7	8.4	8.2
27.5	14.0	13.7	13.5	13.2	12.9	12.7	12.4	12.2	11.9	11.7	11.4	11.2	10.9	10.7	10.4	10.2	9.9	9.7	9.5	9.2
28	15.0	14.8	14.5	14.2	14.0	13.7	13.5	13.2	12.9	12.7	12.4	12.2	11.9	11.7	11.5	11.2	11.0	10.7	10.5	10.3
28.5	16.0	15.8	15.5	15.2	15.0	14.7	14.5	14.2	13.9	13.7	13.4	13.2	12.9	12.7	12.5	12.2	12.0	11.7	11.5	11.3
29	17.0	16.8	16.5	16.2	16.0	15.7	15.4	15.2	14.9	14.7	14.4	14.2	13.9	13.7	13.4	13.2	13.0	12.7	12.5	12.3
29.5	18.0	17.7	17.5	17.2	16.9	16.7	16.4	16.2	15.9	15.7	15.4	15.2	14.9	14.7	14.4	14.2	13.9	13.7	13.5	13.2
30	18.9	18.7	18.4	18.2	17.9	17.6	17.4	17.1	16.9	16.6	16.4	16.1	15.9	15.6	15.4	15.1	14.9	14.6	14.4	14.2
30.5	19.9	19.6	19.4	19.1	18.8	18.6	18.3	18.1	17.8	17.5	17.3	17.0	16.8	16.6	16.3	16.1	15.8	15.6	15.4	15.1
31	20.8	20.5	20.3	20.0	19.8	19.5	19.2	19.0	18.7	18.5	18.2	18.0	17.7	17.5	17.2	17.0	16.8	16.5	16.3	16.0
31.5	21.7	21.5	21.2	20.9	20.7	20.4	20.1	19.9	19.6	19.4	19.1	18.9	18.6	18.4	18.1	17.9	17.7	17.4	17.2	16.9
32	22.6	22.3	22.1	21.8	21.6	21.3	21.0	20.8	20.5	20.3	20.0	19.8	19.5	19.3	19.0	18.8	18.6	18.3	18.1	17.8
32.5	23.5	23.2	23.0	22.7	22.4	22.2	21.9	21.7	21.4	21.2	20.9	20.7	20.4	20.2	19.9	19.7	19.4	19.2	19.0	18.7
33	24.4	24.1	23.8	23.6	23.3	23.0	22.8	22.5	22.3	22.0	21.8	21.5	21.3	21.0	20.8	20.5	20.3	20.1	19.8	19.6
33.5	25.2	24.9	24.7	24.4	24.2	23.9	23.6	23.4	23.1	22.9	22.6	22.4	22.1	21.9	21.6	21.4	21.2	20.9	20.7	20.4
34	26.1	25.8	25.5	25.3	25.0	24.7	24.5	24.2	24.0	23.7	23.5	23.2	23.0	22.7	22.5	22.2	22.0	21.8	21.5	21.3
34.5	26.9	26.6	26.4	26.1	25.8	25.6	25.3	25.1	24.8	24.5	24.3	24.0	23.8	23.6	23.3	23.1	22.8	22.6	22.3	22.1
35	27.7	27.4	27.2	26.9	26.6	26.4	26.1	25.9	25.6	25.4	25.1	24.9	24.6	24.4	24.1	23.9	23.6	23.4	23.2	22.9
35.5	28.5	28.2	28.0	27.7	27.4	27.2	26.9	26.7	26.4	26.2	25.9	25.7	25.4	25.2	24.9	24.7	24.4	24.2	24.0	23.7
36	29.3	29.0	28.8	28.5	28.2	28.0	27.7	27.5	27.2	27.0	26.7	26.5	26.2	26.0	25.7	25.5	25.2	25.0	24.8	24.5
36.5	30.1	29.8	29.6	29.3	29.0	28.8	28.5	28.3	28.0	27.7	27.5	27.2	27.0	26.8	26.5	26.3	26.0	25.8	25.5	25.3
37	30.9	30.6	30.3	30.1	29.8	29.5	29.3	29.0	28.8	28.5	28.3	28.0	27.8	27.5	27.3	27.0	26.8	26.6	26.3	26.1
37.5	31.6	31.4	31.1	30.8	30.6	30.3	30.0	29.8	29.5	29.3	29.0	28.8	28.5	28.3	28.0	27.8	27.6	27.3	27.1	26.8
38	32.4	32.1	31.8	31.6	31.3	31.1	30.8	30.5	30.3	30.0	29.8	29.5	29.3	29.0	28.8	28.6	28.3	28.1	27.8	27.6
38.5	33.1	32.8	32.6	32.3	32.1	31.8	31.5	31.3	31.0	30.8	30.5	30.3	30.0	29.8	29.5	29.3	29.1	28.8	28.6	28.3

Appendix B: Estimated Percent Body Fat Based on Waist Circumference for Females – Cont.

WC (in.)	68	68.5	69	69.5	70	70.5	71	71.5	72	72.5	73	73.5	74	74.5	75	75.5	76	76.5	77	77.5
39	33.8	33.6	33.3	33.1	32.8	32.5	32.3	32.0	31.8	31.5	31.3	31.0	30.8	30.5	30.3	30.0	29.8	29.5	29.3	29.1
39.5	34.6	34.3	34.0	33.8	33.5	33.3	33.0	32.7	32.5	32.2	32.0	31.7	31.5	31.2	31.0	30.8	30.5	30.3	30.0	29.8
40	35.3	35.0	34.8	34.5	34.2	34.0	33.7	33.5	33.2	32.9	32.7	32.4	32.2	32.0	31.7	31.5	31.2	31.0	30.7	30.5
40.5	36.0	35.7	35.5	35.2	34.9	34.7	34.4	34.2	33.9	33.7	33.4	33.2	32.9	32.7	32.4	32.2	31.9	31.7	31.5	31.2
41	36.7	36.4	36.2	35.9	35.6	35.4	35.1	34.9	34.6	34.3	34.1	33.8	33.6	33.4	33.1	32.9	32.6	32.4	32.1	31.9
41.5	37.4	37.1	36.8	36.6	36.3	36.1	35.8	35.5	35.3	35.0	34.8	34.5	34.3	34.0	33.8	33.6	33.3	33.1	32.8	32.6
42	38.1	37.8	37.5	37.3	37.0	36.7	36.5	36.2	36.0	35.7	35.5	35.2	35.0	34.7	34.5	34.2	34.0	33.8	33.5	33.3
42.5	38.7	38.5	38.2	37.9	37.7	37.4	37.2	36.9	36.6	36.4	36.1	35.9	35.6	35.4	35.2	34.9	34.7	34.4	34.2	34.0
43	39.4	39.1	38.9	38.6	38.3	38.1	37.8	37.6	37.3	37.1	36.8	36.6	36.3	36.1	35.8	35.6	35.3	35.1	34.9	34.6
43.5	40.0	39.8	39.5	39.3	39.0	38.7	38.5	38.2	38.0	37.7	37.5	37.2	37.0	36.7	36.5	36.2	36.0	35.7	35.5	35.3
44	40.7	40.4	40.2	39.9	39.6	39.4	39.1	38.9	38.6	38.4	38.1	37.9	37.6	37.4	37.1	36.9	36.6	36.4	36.2	35.9
44.5	41.3	41.1	40.8	40.5	40.3	40.0	39.8	39.5	39.3	39.0	38.7	38.5	38.3	38.0	37.8	37.5	37.3	37.0	36.8	36.6
45	42.0	41.7	41.4	41.2	40.9	40.7	40.4	40.1	39.9	39.6	39.4	39.1	38.9	38.6	38.4	38.2	37.9	37.7	37.4	37.2

APPENDIX B: ESTIMATED PERCENT BODY FAT BASED ON WAIST CIRCUMFERENCE

Appendix C
Meal Planning Made Easy

APPENDIX C: MEAL PLANNING MADE EASY

Recommended Timing of Specific Food Groups

MEAL	FRUIT	VEGETABLES	GRAINS	PROTEIN	DAIRY
Breakfast	X	-	X	X	X
Snack	X	-	-	-	X
Lunch	X	X	X	X	-
Snack	-	X	-	-	X
Dinner	-	X	X	X	-

Notes:

1. The above serving and timing recommendations were developed to ensure adequate intake of each food group. However, the timing of each food group (assuming the number of servings remain the same) can be adjusted based on food availability and preference. For example, vegetables can be consumed at breakfast and fruit can be consumed at dinner.

2. As long as a variety of healthy food items are selected and eaten daily (e.g., avocado, olives, salmon, walnuts, full-fat dairy, flax seeds, etc.), fat does need to be tracked as a separate food group.

Recommended Serving Size per Food Group

FOOD GROUP	HAND REFERENCE	AVG SERVING SIZE	AVG KCAL
Fruits	Fist	1 Cup	75
Vegetables	Fist	1 Cup	40
Grains	Fist	1 Cup	200
Protein	Palm	3 oz	160
Dairy	Fist	1 Cup	150

Note: The serving sizes provided in MPME for each food group may differ from those posted by other nutritional databases and sources.

The serving sizes used in MPME were designed to meet the average kcal requirements listed above for each food group (e.g., 75 kcal for fruits, 40 kcal for vegetables, 200 kcal for grains, etc.).

Fruit Group Examples (Includes Berries, Melons, and Fruit Juices)

Food Item	Serving Size	Food Item	Serving Size
Raisins	⅛ Cup	Apple Juice	6 oz
Mango	¾ Cup	Orange Juice	6 oz
Blueberries	1 Cup	Cranberry Juice	6 oz
Cherries	1 Cup	Plums	2 Plums
Pineapple	1 Cup	Kiwi	2 Kiwi (2" dia)
Blackberries	1¼ Cup	Apple	1 Apple (2¼" dia)
Cantaloupe	1¼ Cup	Orange	1 Orange (2¼" dia)
Grapes	1¼ Cup	Pear	1 Pear (2¼" dia)
Honeydew	1¼ Cup	Peaches	1 Peach (2⅔" dia)
Strawberries	1½ Cup	Banana	1 Banana (7-8")

Click here for more food choices

Vegetable Group Examples (Includes Dark-Green, Red and Orange Vegetables, Starchy Vegetables, Beans and Peas)

Food Item	Serving Size	Food Item	Serving Size
Corn	¼ Cup	Bell Peppers	¾ Cup
Edamame	¼ Cup	Asparagus	1 Cup
Lima Beans	¼ Cup	Broccoli	1¼ Cup
Sweet Potatoes	¼ Cup	Green Beans	1¼ Cup
White Potatoes	¼ Cup	Kale	1¼ Cup
Carrots	½ Cup	Bean Sprouts	4 Cups
Green Peas	½ Cup	Bok Choy	4 Cups
Spinach (Cooked)	½ Cup	Collard Greens	4 Cups
Acorn Squash	¾ Cup	Avocado	¼ Avocado
Beets	¾ Cup	Tomatoes	1 Tomato (2¼" dia)

Click here for more food choices

APPENDIX C: MEAL PLANNING MADE EASY

Grain Group Examples (Includes Whole and Refined Grains)

Food Item	Serving Size	Food Item	Serving Size
Brown Rice (Cooked)	1 Cup	Pretzels	2 oz
Couscous	1 Cup	Wheat Bread	2 Slices
Oatmeal	1 Cup	White Bread	2 Slices
Quinoa	1 Cup	Wheat Crackers	6 crackers (1 oz)
White Rice (Cooked)	1 Cup	Cornbread	1 Piece (60 g)
Whole Wheat Pasta	1 Cup	Bagel	1 Bagel (3½ in. dia)
Cereal (Cheerios)	1½ Cup	Biscuit	4 Biscuits (1½" dia)
Grits	1½ Cup	Pancakes	1 Pancake (7" dia)
Hominy	1¾ Cup	Pita Bread	1 Large Pita (6½ in. dia)
Popcorn	2 Cups	Naan Bread	1 Piece (6" dia)

Click here for more food choices

Protein Group Examples (Includes Meats, Beans and Peas, Soy Products, Eggs, Nuts and Seeds, and Seafood)

Food Item	Serving Size	Food Item	Serving Size
Almonds	¼ Cup	Salmon	3 oz
Cashews	¼ Cup	Turkey	3 oz
Chia Seeds	¼ Cup	Tilapia	4 oz
Walnuts	¼ Cup	Tuna	5 oz
Lentils	½ Cup	Halibut	5 oz
Black-Eyed Peas	¾ Cup	Scallops	6 oz
Pinto Beans	¾ Cup	Shrimp	6 oz
Beef	3 oz	Tofu	8 oz
Chicken	3 oz	Peanut Butter	2 Tablespoons
Pork	3 oz	Eggs	2 Large Eggs

Click here for more food choices

Dairy Group Examples (Includes Milk, Non-Dairy Alternatives, Cheeses, and Yogurt)

Food Item	Serving Size	Food Item	Serving Size
Ricotta Cheese	⅓ Cup	Brie Cheese	1.5 oz (3 dice)
Cottage Cheese (Whole Milk)	½ Cup	Cheddar Cheese	1.5 oz (3 dice)
Soy Milk Yogurt	½ Cup	Swiss Cheese	1.5 oz (3 dice)
Frozen Yogurt	¾ Cup	Mozzarella	2 oz (4 dice)
Fruit Yogurt	¾ Cup	Flavored Milks	6 oz
Feta Cheese	¾ Cup	Whole Milk	8 oz
Ice Milk	1 Cup	Soy Milk	8 oz
Plain Yogurt (Low Fat)	1 Cup	2% Milk	10 oz
Greek Yogurt	1½ Cup	1% Milk	12 oz
American Cheese	1.5 oz (2 slices)	Skim Milk	16 oz

Click here for more food choices

Appendix C: Meal Planning Made Easy

Sample Meal Plan (180 lb. / Moderately Active / Meal Plan = J)

	BREAKFAST	SNACK	LUNCH	SNACK	DINNER
Fruit	1 Med Banana + 1½ Cup Strawberries	1 Cup Blueberries	1 Med Apple + 2 Kiwi	-	-
Vegetable	-	-	1¼ Cup Broccoli + 1 Cup Asparagus	-	½ Cup Carrots + 1¼ Cup Green Beans
Grain	1 Cup Oatmeal	-	1 Cup White Rice	1 oz Wheat Crackers	1 Cup Quinoa
Protein	2 Large Eggs	-	6 oz Chicken Breast	-	6 oz Salmon
Dairy	8 oz Whole Milk	1½ Cup Greek Yogurt	-	1.5 oz Cheddar Cheese	-

Meal Planning Made Easy Template

	BREAKFAST		SNACK		LUNCH		SNACK		DINNER	
	# SVG	FOOD ITEM(S)	# SVG	FOOD ITEM(S)	# SVG	FOOD ITEM(S)	# SVG	FOOD ITEM(S)	# SVG	FOOD ITEM(S)
Fruit										
Vegetable										
Grain										
Protein										
Dairy										

Fruits: 75 kcal per serving	Vegetables: 40 kcal per serving	Grains: 200 kcal per serving	Protein: 160 kcal per serving	Dairy: 150 kcal per serving

Appendix C: Meal Planning Made Easy

Appendix D
Stress Assessment

Appendix D: Stress Assessment

Assign each question a number according to the following scale. When you are finished, add up your numbers and look at the key that follows.

0: I seldom or never feel this way.

1: I sometimes (once a month or so) feel this way.

2: I often (more than once a month) feel this way.

3: I almost always feel this way.

1. Do you feel moody in the morning and have difficulty getting up? ____
2. Do you experience slight fevers, signs of the flu, a sore throat, or tender lymph nodes? ____
3. Are mornings the worst time of your day, with evenings being better? ____
4. Do you fall asleep easily but wake early without being able to fall asleep again? ____
5. Have you ever found yourself staring at a computer monitor, keyboard, or book, barely able to keep your head from dropping? ____
6. Do you feel mentally sluggish, confused, and unresponsive? ____
7. Has your short-term memory worsened, and do you have trouble concentrating? ____
8. Has your daily activity dropped to below half of what it was before? ____
9. Are your emotions relatively blunted, and do you often feel apathetic? ____
10. Does your body ache all over, as if it is weaker than it used to be? ____
11. When you exercise, do you feel debilitated for more than 12 hours afterward? ____
12. Does your work stress you out to the point that you want to escape from it? ____
13. Do you get headaches? ____
14. Do you find yourself desperately wanting to avoid being with other people? ____
15. Are you more impatient, irritable, nervous, angry, or anxious than you used to be? ____

Total score: ____

If your score is . . .

Below 12: Your fatigue is within normal limits. Cut back on unnecessary stress wherever you can and improve your sleeping habits.

12 to 22: You have type 1 fatigue, which is temporary and not serious. You can reverse it by lowering your stress level, taking a vacation or sabbatical, or increasing your rest and sleep time. If these things don't help, consult a professional.

23 to 32: You have type 2 fatigue, which is longstanding and serious. A simple short break will not relieve it. You are suffering from chronic stress, depletion of adrenaline, and most likely a compromised immune system. You probably need to make a major lifestyle change and get professional help.

Above 33: You have type 3 fatigue, which is a "disease state." You are at risk for serious depression, hormonal imbalances, and physical illnesses such as chronic fatigue syndrome. You must get professional help.

From Walters & Byl. (2013). *Christian Paths to Health and Wellness* (2nd ed.). Champaign, IL: Human Kinetics. Adapted, by permission, from Hart. (1998). *Adrenaline and Stress*. Waco, TX: Word.

Appendix D: Stress Assessment

Appendix E
1 Repetition Max (RM) Testing Protocol

Appendix E: 1 Repetition Max (RM) Testing Protocol

1RM Testing Protocol

1. Warm-up with a light resistance that easily allows 5 - 10 repetitions
2. Afford a 1-minute rest period
3. Estimate warm-up load that can be completed for 3 - 5 repetitions
4. Afford a 2-minute rest period
5. Estimate a conservative, near-maximal load that can be completed for 2 - 3 repetitions
6. Afford a 2 - 4-minute rest period
7. Make a load increase and attempt 1RM
8. If successful, afford a 2 - 4-minute rest period, make a load increase, and attempt a new (higher) 1RM
9. If unsuccessful, afford a 2 - 4-minute rest period, make a load decrease, and attempt a new lighter) 1RM
10. Continue increasing or decreasing the load until a 1RM is determined. Ideally, the 1RM will be determined within 3 - 5 testing sets.

****

1RM Prediction Equation

If an individual is uncomfortable performing 1RM testing and/or does not have access to a spotter, 1RM can be estimated by using submaximal weight for reps to failure and a prediction equation. For example, the Epley (1985) equation calculates 1RM as follows:

- 1RM = (0.033 × number of reps × weight) + weight

Let's perform a sample equation; say an individual was able to perform 10 reps at 225 lbs. Their estimated 1RM would be ~ 300 lbs.

- 1RM = (0.033 x 10 x 225) + 225
- 1RM = (74.25) + 225
- 1RM = 299.25

Appendix F
Predicted 1RM Based on Reps to Fatigue

Appendix F: Predicted 1RM Based on Reps to Fatigue

Weight	\multicolumn{6}{c}{Repetitions Performed}						Weight	\multicolumn{6}{c}{Repetitions Performed}					
	5	6	7	8	9	10		5	6	7	8	9	10
30	34	35	36	37	38	39	140	157	163	168	174	180	187
35	40	41	42	43	44	45	145	163	168	174	180	186	193
40	46	47	49	50	51	53	150	169	174	180	186	193	200
45	51	53	55	56	58	60	155	174	180	186	192	199	207
50	56	58	60	62	64	67	160	180	186	192	199	206	213
55	62	64	66	68	71	73	165	186	192	198	205	212	220
60	67	70	72	74	77	80	170	191	197	204	211	219	227
65	73	75	78	81	84	87	175	197	203	210	217	225	233
70	79	81	84	87	90	93	180	202	209	216	223	231	240
75	84	87	90	93	96	100	185	208	215	222	230	238	247
80	90	93	96	99	103	107	190	214	221	228	236	244	253
85	96	99	102	106	109	113	195	219	226	234	242	251	260
90	101	105	108	112	116	120	200	225	232	240	248	257	267
95	107	110	114	118	122	127	205	231	238	246	254	264	273
100	112	116	120	124	129	133	210	236	244	252	261	270	280
105	118	122	126	130	135	140	215	242	250	258	267	276	287
110	124	128	132	137	141	147	220	247	255	264	273	283	293
115	129	134	138	143	148	153	225	253	261	270	279	289	300
120	135	139	144	149	154	160	230	259	267	276	286	296	307
125	141	145	150	155	161	167	235	264	273	282	292	302	313
130	146	151	158	161	167	173	240	270	279	288	298	309	320
135	152	157	162	168	174	180	245	276	285	294	304	315	327

Brzycki, M. (1993). *Predicted 1RM Based on Reps to Fatigue*. Journal of Physical Education, Recreation and Dance, 64: 88-90.

Appendix G
Strength Standards

Appendix G: Strength Standards

Bench Press Standards (lb.)

Body Weight	Beginner Male	Beginner Female	Novice Male	Novice Female	Intermediate Male	Intermediate Female	Advanced Male	Advanced Female	Elite Male	Elite Female
90	-	19	-	40	-	70	-	109	-	154
100	-	23	-	46	-	78	-	119	-	165
110	51	28	82	52	122	86	170	128	223	176
120	61	32	94	58	137	93	188	137	243	187
130	71	36	107	63	151	100	204	145	262	196
140	81	40	118	68	166	106	221	153	281	205
150	90	44	130	73	179	113	236	161	298	214
160	100	47	141	78	192	119	251	168	315	222
170	109	51	152	83	205	125	266	175	332	230
180	118	55	163	87	218	130	280	181	347	238
190	127	58	174	92	230	136	294	188	363	245
200	136	62	184	96	242	141	307	194	378	252
210	145	65	194	101	253	146	320	200	392	259
220	153	68	204	105	265	151	333	206	406	266
230	162	72	213	109	275	156	345	211	420	272
240	170	75	223	113	286	160	357	217	433	278
250	178	78	232	116	297	165	369	222	446	284
260	186	81	241	120	307	169	381	227	458	290
270	194	-	250	-	317	-	392	-	470	-
280	201	-	259	-	327	-	403	-	482	-
290	209	-	267	-	336	-	413	-	494	-
300	216	-	276	-	346	-	424	-	505	-
310	224	-	284	-	355	-	434	-	516	-

Notes: 1) Standards taken from https://strengthlevel.com/strength-standards/bench-press

2) Bench press standards include the weight of a 20 kg / 44 lb. bar

What do the strength standards mean?

Beginner	Stronger than 5% of lifters. A beginner lifter can perform the movement correctly and has practiced it for at least a month.
Novice	Stronger than 20% of lifters. A novice lifter has trained regularly in the technique for at least six months.
Intermediate	Stronger than 50% of lifters. An intermediate lifter has trained regularly in the technique for at least two years.
Advanced	Stronger than 80% of lifters. An advanced lifter has progressed for over five years.
Elite	Stronger than 95% of lifters. An elite lifter has dedicated over five years to become competitive at strength sports.

A Christian Guide to Body Stewardship, Diet and Exercise

Bent-Over Row Standards (lb.)

Body Weight	Beginner Male	Beginner Female	Novice Male	Novice Female	Intermediate Male	Intermediate Female	Advanced Male	Advanced Female	Elite Male	Elite Female
90	-	24	-	44	-	71	-	104	-	143
100	-	26	-	47	-	75	-	110	-	149
110	46	29	74	50	111	79	156	114	205	154
120	54	31	84	53	124	83	171	119	222	160
130	62	33	95	56	136	86	185	123	239	165
140	70	35	105	59	148	90	199	127	254	169
150	78	37	114	61	159	93	212	131	269	174
160	86	39	124	64	171	96	225	135	284	178
170	94	41	133	66	181	99	237	138	298	182
180	101	43	142	69	192	102	249	141	311	185
190	109	45	151	71	202	104	261	145	324	189
200	116	46	159	73	212	107	272	148	337	192
210	123	48	168	75	222	109	283	150	349	196
220	130	50	176	77	231	112	294	153	360	199
230	137	51	184	79	240	114	304	156	372	202
240	144	53	192	81	249	116	314	158	383	205
250	150	54	199	82	258	118	324	161	394	208
260	157	55	207	84	266	120	333	163	404	210
270	163	-	214	-	275	-	343	-	414	-
280	170	-	221	-	283	-	352	-	424	-
290	176	-	228	-	291	-	361	-	434	-
300	182	-	235	-	299	-	369	-	444	-
310	188	-	242	-	306	-	378	-	453	-

Notes: 1) Standards taken from https://strengthlevel.com/strength-standards/bent-over-row

2) Bent-over row standards include the weight of a 20 kg / 44 lb. bar

What do the strength standards mean?

Beginner	Stronger than 5% of lifters. A beginner lifter can perform the movement correctly and has practiced it for at least a month.
Novice	Stronger than 20% of lifters. A novice lifter has trained regularly in the technique for at least six months.
Intermediate	Stronger than 50% of lifters. An intermediate lifter has trained regularly in the technique for at least two years.
Advanced	Stronger than 80% of lifters. An advanced lifter has progressed for over five years.
Elite	Stronger than 95% of lifters. An elite lifter has dedicated over five years to become competitive at strength sports.

Appendix G: Strength Standards

Pendlay Row Standards (lb.)

Body Weight	Beginner Male	Beginner Female	Novice Male	Novice Female	Intermediate Male	Intermediate Female	Advanced Male	Advanced Female	Elite Male	Elite Female
90	-	36	-	56	-	82	-	114	-	148
100	-	40	-	61	-	89	-	121	-	157
110	53	44	81	66	115	94	156	128	201	164
120	63	48	92	71	129	100	172	134	219	172
130	72	51	103	75	142	105	187	140	235	179
140	81	55	114	79	154	110	201	146	252	185
150	90	58	124	84	167	115	215	152	267	191
160	98	61	134	87	178	120	228	157	282	197
170	107	64	144	91	190	124	241	162	296	203
180	115	67	154	95	201	128	254	167	310	208
190	124	70	164	98	212	132	266	171	324	213
200	132	73	173	101	222	136	278	176	337	218
210	140	76	182	105	233	140	289	180	349	223
220	147	79	191	108	243	143	301	184	362	227
230	155	81	200	111	252	147	311	188	374	232
240	163	84	208	114	262	150	322	192	385	236
250	170	86	216	117	271	153	332	195	396	240
260	177	89	225	119	280	157	342	199	407	244
270	184	-	233	-	289	-	352	-	418	-
280	191	-	240	-	298	-	362	-	428	-
290	198	-	248	-	306	-	371	-	439	-
300	205	-	255	-	315	-	380	-	449	-
310	211	-	263	-	323	-	389	-	458	-

Notes: 1) Standards taken from https://strengthlevel.com/strength-standards/pendlay-row

2) Pendlay row standards include the weight of a 20 kg / 44 lb. bar

What do the strength standards mean?

Beginner	Stronger than 5% of lifters. A beginner lifter can perform the movement correctly and has practiced it for at least a month.
Novice	Stronger than 20% of lifters. A novice lifter has trained regularly in the technique for at least six months.
Intermediate	Stronger than 50% of lifters. An intermediate lifter has trained regularly in the technique for at least two years.
Advanced	Stronger than 80% of lifters. An advanced lifter has progressed for over five years.
Elite	Stronger than 95% of lifters. An elite lifter has dedicated over five years to become competitive at strength sports.

Shoulder Press Standards (lb.)

Body Weight	Beginner Male	Beginner Female	Novice Male	Novice Female	Intermediate Male	Intermediate Female	Advanced Male	Advanced Female	Elite Male	Elite Female
90	-	17	-	31	-	51	-	76	-	104
100	-	20	-	35	-	56	-	82	-	111
110	32	22	53	39	80	60	113	87	150	117
120	38	25	60	42	90	65	125	92	163	123
130	44	27	68	45	99	68	136	97	176	128
140	50	30	76	48	108	72	146	101	188	133
150	56	32	83	51	117	76	156	105	199	138
160	62	34	90	54	125	79	166	109	211	143
170	68	36	97	56	134	82	176	113	221	147
180	74	38	104	59	142	86	185	117	232	151
190	79	40	111	62	149	89	194	120	241	155
200	85	42	117	64	157	92	202	124	251	159
210	91	44	124	66	165	94	211	127	260	163
220	96	46	130	69	172	97	219	130	270	167
230	101	48	136	71	179	100	227	133	278	170
240	106	50	142	73	186	102	235	136	287	173
250	111	52	148	75	192	105	242	139	295	177
260	116	53	154	77	199	107	250	142	303	180
270	121	-	160	-	205	-	257	-	311	-
280	126	-	165	-	212	-	264	-	319	-
290	131	-	171	-	218	-	271	-	327	-
300	136	-	176	-	224	-	277	-	334	-
310	140	-	181	-	230	-	284	-	341	-

Notes: 1) Standards taken from https://strengthlevel.com/strength-standards/shoulder-press

2) Shoulder press standards include the weight of a 20 kg / 44 lb. bar

What do the strength standards mean?

Beginner	Stronger than 5% of lifters. A beginner lifter can perform the movement correctly and has practiced it for at least a month.
Novice	Stronger than 20% of lifters. A novice lifter has trained regularly in the technique for at least six months.
Intermediate	Stronger than 50% of lifters. An intermediate lifter has trained regularly in the technique for at least two years.
Advanced	Stronger than 80% of lifters. An advanced lifter has progressed for over five years.
Elite	Stronger than 95% of lifters. An elite lifter has dedicated over five years to become competitive at strength sports.

Appendix G: Strength Standards

Squat Standards (lb.)

Body Weight	Beginner Male	Beginner Female	Novice Male	Novice Female	Intermediate Male	Intermediate Female	Advanced Male	Advanced Female	Elite Male	Elite Female
90	-	40	-	71	-	114	-	167	-	226
100	-	46	-	80	-	124	-	179	-	240
110	72	52	112	87	164	134	226	190	295	254
120	85	58	128	95	184	143	249	201	321	266
130	98	63	144	102	203	152	271	211	346	278
140	111	69	160	108	221	160	292	221	370	289
150	123	74	175	115	239	168	313	230	393	299
160	136	79	190	121	256	175	333	239	415	309
170	148	84	204	127	273	182	352	247	436	319
180	160	88	219	133	289	189	370	256	456	328
190	172	93	232	138	305	196	388	263	476	337
200	184	97	246	144	321	202	405	271	496	345
210	195	102	259	149	336	208	422	278	514	353
220	206	106	272	154	350	214	439	285	532	361
230	217	110	285	159	365	220	455	291	550	369
240	228	114	297	164	379	226	470	298	567	376
250	239	118	309	169	392	231	486	304	584	383
260	249	122	321	173	406	237	500	310	600	390
270	259	-	332	-	419	-	515	-	616	-
280	270	-	344	-	431	-	529	-	631	-
290	279	-	355	-	444	-	543	-	646	-
300	289	-	366	-	456	-	556	-	661	-
310	299	-	377	-	468	-	570	-	676	-

Notes: 1) Standards taken from https://strengthlevel.com/strength-standards/squat

2) Squat standards include the weight of a 20 kg / 44 lb. bar

What do the strength standards mean?

Beginner	Stronger than 5% of lifters. A beginner lifter can perform the movement correctly and has practiced it for at least a month.
Novice	Stronger than 20% of lifters. A novice lifter has trained regularly in the technique for at least six months.
Intermediate	Stronger than 50% of lifters. An intermediate lifter has trained regularly in the technique for at least two years.
Advanced	Stronger than 80% of lifters. An advanced lifter has progressed for over five years.
Elite	Stronger than 95% of lifters. An elite lifter has dedicated over five years to become competitive at strength sports.

Conventional Deadlift Standards (lb.)

Body Weight	Beginner Male	Beginner Female	Novice Male	Novice Female	Intermediate Male	Intermediate Female	Advanced Male	Advanced Female	Elite Male	Elite Female
90	-	54	-	91	-	140	-	199	-	265
100	-	61	-	100	-	151	-	212	-	280
110	94	68	141	109	201	161	272	225	349	294
120	109	75	159	117	223	171	297	236	377	308
130	123	81	177	125	244	181	321	247	404	320
140	138	87	194	132	264	190	344	258	430	332
150	152	93	211	139	283	198	366	268	455	344
160	166	98	228	146	302	207	388	277	479	354
170	180	104	243	153	321	214	408	286	502	365
180	193	109	259	159	338	222	428	295	524	374
190	206	114	274	165	356	229	448	303	545	384
200	219	119	289	171	372	236	466	311	566	393
210	231	124	303	177	389	243	485	319	586	401
220	244	128	317	183	404	249	502	326	605	410
230	256	133	331	188	420	256	519	334	624	418
240	267	137	344	193	435	262	536	341	643	426
250	279	142	357	198	449	268	552	347	660	433
260	290	146	370	203	464	273	568	354	678	440
270	301	-	383	-	478	-	584	-	695	-
280	312	-	395	-	492	-	599	-	711	-
290	323	-	407	-	505	-	614	-	727	-
300	334	-	419	-	518	-	628	-	743	-
310	344	-	430	-	531	-	642	-	758	-

Notes: 1) Standards taken from https://strengthlevel.com/strength-standards/deadlift

2) Conventional deadlift standards include the weight of a 20 kg / 44 lb. bar

What do the strength standards mean?

Beginner	Stronger than 5% of lifters. A beginner lifter can perform the movement correctly and has practiced it for at least a month.
Novice	Stronger than 20% of lifters. A novice lifter has trained regularly in the technique for at least six months.
Intermediate	Stronger than 50% of lifters. An intermediate lifter has trained regularly in the technique for at least two years.
Advanced	Stronger than 80% of lifters. An advanced lifter has progressed for over five years.
Elite	Stronger than 95% of lifters. An elite lifter has dedicated over five years to become competitive at strength sports.

APPENDIX G: STRENGTH STANDARDS

Sumo Deadlift Standards (lb.)

Body Weight	Beginner Male	Beginner Female	Novice Male	Novice Female	Intermediate Male	Intermediate Female	Advanced Male	Advanced Female	Elite Male	Elite Female
90	-	79	-	117	-	164	-	220	-	281
100	-	85	-	124	-	173	-	230	-	292
110	109	91	162	131	228	181	305	239	389	302
120	125	96	181	137	251	188	332	248	419	312
130	141	101	200	143	273	195	357	256	448	321
140	157	106	218	149	294	202	381	263	475	329
150	172	110	236	154	315	208	404	270	501	337
160	186	114	253	159	334	214	427	277	526	345
170	201	118	270	164	354	220	449	283	550	352
180	215	122	286	169	372	225	469	289	573	358
190	229	126	302	173	390	230	490	295	595	365
200	242	130	318	177	408	235	509	301	616	371
210	255	133	333	181	425	240	528	306	637	377
220	268	137	347	185	441	244	546	311	657	383
230	280	140	361	189	457	249	564	316	677	388
240	293	143	375	193	473	253	582	321	696	393
250	305	146	389	196	488	257	599	325	715	398
260	317	149	402	200	503	261	615	330	733	403
270	328	-	415	-	518	-	631	-	750	-
280	339	-	428	-	532	-	647	-	767	-
290	351	-	440	-	546	-	662	-	784	-
300	361	-	453	-	559	-	677	-	800	-
310	372	-	465	-	573	-	692	-	816	-

Notes: 1) Standards taken from https://strengthlevel.com/strength-standards/sumo-deadlift

2) Sumo deadlift standards include the weight of a 20 kg / 44 lb. bar

What do the strength standards mean?

Beginner	Stronger than 5% of lifters. A beginner lifter can perform the movement correctly and has practiced it for at least a month.
Novice	Stronger than 20% of lifters. A novice lifter has trained regularly in the technique for at least six months.
Intermediate	Stronger than 50% of lifters. An intermediate lifter has trained regularly in the technique for at least two years.
Advanced	Stronger than 80% of lifters. An advanced lifter has progressed for over five years.
Elite	Stronger than 95% of lifters. An elite lifter has dedicated over five years to become competitive at strength sports.

Hex Bar Deadlift Standards (lb.)

Body Weight	Beginner Male	Beginner Female	Novice Male	Novice Female	Intermediate Male	Intermediate Female	Advanced Male	Advanced Female	Elite Male	Elite Female
90	-	67	-	106	-	156	-	215	-	281
100	-	75	-	115	-	167	-	229	-	297
110	118	82	170	125	234	178	309	242	390	311
120	133	89	188	133	256	189	334	254	418	325
130	148	96	206	141	276	198	357	265	444	338
140	163	102	223	149	296	208	379	276	469	350
150	177	108	239	157	315	216	401	286	493	361
160	191	114	255	164	333	225	421	295	515	372
170	204	120	271	170	351	233	441	304	537	382
180	217	126	286	177	368	240	460	313	558	392
190	230	131	300	183	384	248	479	322	579	401
200	242	136	315	189	400	255	497	330	598	410
210	254	141	328	195	416	262	514	337	617	419
220	266	146	342	201	431	268	531	345	635	427
230	278	151	355	207	446	275	547	352	653	435
240	289	155	368	212	460	281	563	359	670	443
250	300	160	380	217	474	287	578	366	687	451
260	311	164	392	222	487	293	593	373	703	458
270	321	-	404	-	501	-	607	-	719	-
280	332	-	416	-	513	-	622	-	735	-
290	342	-	427	-	526	-	635	-	750	-
300	352	-	438	-	538	-	649	-	764	-
310	362	-	449	-	550	-	662	-	779	-

Notes: 1) Standards taken from https://strengthlevel.com/strength-standards/hex-bar-deadlift

2) Hex bar standards include the weight of a 30 kg / 66 lb. bar

What do the strength standards mean?

Beginner	Stronger than 5% of lifters. A beginner lifter can perform the movement correctly and has practiced it for at least a month.
Novice	Stronger than 20% of lifters. A novice lifter has trained regularly in the technique for at least six months.
Intermediate	Stronger than 50% of lifters. An intermediate lifter has trained regularly in the technique for at least two years.
Advanced	Stronger than 80% of lifters. An advanced lifter has progressed for over five years.
Elite	Stronger than 95% of lifters. An elite lifter has dedicated over five years to become competitive at strength sports.

Appendix G: Strength Standards

Appendix H
Adjustment Procedure for Nautilus Equipment

Appendix H: Adjustment Procedure for Nautilus Equipment

Adjustment Procedures for Nautilus Equipment

Machine	Priority	Adjustment Procedures
Leg Press	1	• Adjust seat height so hips are below knees and knees do not extend over toes
Leg Extension	2	• Adjust backrest so knees align with red axis of rotation (AOR) • Adjust lower foam pad so that it is positioned directly on top of the ankle
Leg Curl	2	• Adjust backrest so knees align with red axis of rotation (AOR) • Adjust upper foam pad to keep upper leg flat against the seat • Adjust lower foam pad so that it is positioned directly underneath the ankle
Glute Press	2	• Adjust foot pedal so that the ankle joint is directly under the hip joint
Abduction / Adduction	3	• Position pads on the inside of the knees for Adduction • Position pads on the outside of the knees for Abduction
Ab Crunch	1	• Adjust seat height so that mid torso (xiphoid process) aligns with red AOR
Back Extension	2	• Adjust back pad so that it is positioned on upper back (across shoulder blades)
Chest Press	1	• Adjust seat height so handles align with lower chest (across nipple line) • Position hands at or slightly wider than shoulder width
Row	1	• Adjust seat height so chest pad is positioned at mid chest
Lat Pulldown	1	• Adjust seat height to allow for full arm extension • Position hands at or slightly wider than shoulder width
Shoulder Press	1	• Adjust seat height so handles are at shoulder level • Position hands at or slightly wider than shoulder width
Pec Fly / Rear Deltoid	3	• Position back against pad for Pec Fly • Position chest against pad for Rear Deltoid • Adjust seat height so arms are parallel with the floor
Deltoid Raise	3	• Adjust seat height so shoulders align with red AOR
Biceps Curl	2	• Adjust seat height so elbows align with red AOR
Triceps Press	2	• Adjust seat height so elbows are higher than 90 degrees (same height as shoulders)

General Strength Training Recommendations:

1. Priority 1 exercises represent one of the five compound lifts and are a must. Priority 2 exercises represent one of the various assistance exercises are good to include if you have time. Priority 3 exercises target the same muscles groups already used in Priority 1 and/or 2 exercises and thus are not required/optional.

2. Breath out during exertion and breath in while returning to the start position

3. The exertion (aka concentric) phase should last for 2 seconds while the return (aka eccentric) phase should last for 3 seconds

4. Perform 3 sets of 12-15 reps for all exercises

5. Exercises can be performed back to back (e.g., 3 consecutive sets of Leg Press followed by 3 consecutive sets of Chest Press...) or via a circuit (e.g., 1 set of Leg Press followed by 1 set of Chest Press... and repeat 3 times).

Appendix I
Sample Strength Training Exercises for Weekly Exercise Log

APPENDIX I: SAMPLE STRENGTH TRAINING EXERCISES FOR WEEKLY EXERCISE LOG

	FREE WEIGHTS	**MACHINES (NAUTILUS)**	**RESISTANCE BANDS**	**BODYWEIGHT**
Bench / Chest	Bench Press Cable Cross-Overs	Chest Press Pec Fly	Push-Up Pec Fly	Push-Ups Dips
Press / Shoulders	Standing Military Press Seated Military Press	Shoulder Press Deltoid Raise	Shoulder Press Lateral Raise	Pike Push-Ups Atlas Press
Row / Back	Bent-Over Row Lat Pull-Downs	Row Lat Pull-Down	Row Seated Row	Pull-Ups Australian Row
Squat / Quadriceps	Back Squat Goblet Squat	Leg Press Leg Extension	Squat Lunge	Wall Squat Split Squats
Deadlift / Hamstrings	Conventional Deadlift Hex-Bar Deadlift	Glute Press Leg Curl	Romanian Deadlift Stiff-Leg Deadlift	Roman Chair Good Mornings
Torso / Abdominals	Back Hyperextensions Ab Roller	Ab Crunch Back Extension	Bicycles Kneeling Crunch	Plank Side Plank

Appendix J
QR Codes for Instructional Content

Appendix J : QR Codes for Instructional Content

Chapter Lectures

Fitness Pre- and Post-Test Events

Nautilus Equipment

Compound Lifts

Abdominal Exercises

McGill Big 3

5N1 Lower Body Trainer

Body Composition Assessment

Glossary of Terms

Glossary of Terms

1-Repetition maximum (1RM): Greatest amount of weight that can be lifted for one repetition.

Accommodation: The principle of accommodation states the body's response to a constant stimulus decreases over time.

Actin: A cellular protein found in microfilaments that is active in muscular contraction, cellular movement, and maintenance of cell shape.

Adenosine: A nucleoside involved in the energy metabolism of cells.

Adenosine diphosphate (ADP): A nucleotide composed of adenosine and two phosphate groups that is formed as an intermediate between ATP and AMP and that is reversibly converted to ATP by the addition of a high-energy phosphate group.

Adenosine triphosphate (ATP): Principal molecule for storing and transferring energy in cells.

Aerobic activity: Any form of sustained exercise (e.g., jogging, rowing, swimming, or cycling) that stimulates and strengthens the heart and lungs thereby improving the body's utilization of oxygen.

Aerobic metabolism: Means of producing energy through the combustion of carbohydrates, amino acids, and fats in the presence of oxygen.

Age-predicted maximum heart rate equation: A simple equation (i.e., 220- Age) used to estimate maximum heart rate.

Agonist muscle: Most skeletal muscle is arranged in opposing pairs. The contracting muscle is the agonist muscle during an exercise.

Air displacement plethysmography (aka BodPod): A method that uses air displacement to determine body volume in order to calculate percent body fat.

Alarm stage: First stage of stress, also known as the fight-or-flight stage, that results in the heart beating faster, thereby sending more blood to your arms and legs, in the event you need to fight or flee.

Alkaloid: Any class of nitrogenous organic compounds of plant origin that have pronounced physiological actions in humans.

Alveoli: The tiny air sacs within the lungs that allow for rapid gaseous exchange.

Amino acids: Amino acids are the building blocks of proteins. The body absorbs amino acids through the small intestine into the blood.

Amortization phase: One of the three plyometric phases of movement that occurs between the concentric and eccentric phases and is considered to be the most crucial phase in the body's ability to produce power.

Anabolism: Synthesis of complex molecules from simpler ones.

Anaerobic metabolism: Means of producing energy through the combustion of carbohydrates in the absence of oxygen.

Android: Apple-shaped fat distribution mainly around the trunk and upper body, such as the abdomen, chest, shoulder and neck.

Antagonist muscle: Most skeletal muscle is arranged in opposing pairs. The contracting muscle is the agonist muscle during an exercise. The antagonist muscle is the opposite (opposing) the agonist muscle.

Anthropometry: Study of the measurements and proportions of the human body.

Antioxidant: Substance that removes potentially damaging oxidizing agents in the body.

Appendicular skeleton: Bones that comprise the limbs as well as shoulder and pelvic girdles.

Artery: A large diameter blood vessel that carries blood from the heart to another part of the body.

Arteriole: A small diameter blood vessel in the microcirculation that extends and branches out from an artery and leads to capillaries.

Arthritis: Painful inflammation and/or stiffness of the joints.

Assistance exercises: Recruit smaller muscle areas, involve only one primary joint, and are considered less important to improving sport performance.

Atrium: Either of the two upper chambers of the heart that receive blood from the veins and in turn push it into the ventricles.

Axial skeleton: Bones that comprise the skull and vertebral column.

Balance: The ability to stay upright or stay in control of body movement; coordination is the ability to move two or more body parts under control, smoothly and efficiently. There are two types of balance: static and dynamic.

Bands: Are a method of strength training for advanced lifters in which bands are added to the bar to add elastic pressure thereby making the lockout portion of the lift more difficult.

Basal metabolic rate: The rate at which the body uses energy at rest. Used for breathing and to keep vital organs functioning.

Beta oxidation: Catabolic process by which fatty acid molecules are broken down in the mitochondria to form acetyl-CoA and enter the Krebs cycle.

Bioavailability: Proportion of a drug or other substance that enters circulation that is able to have an active effect.

Bioelectrical impedance (BIA): A method of estimating percent body fat that uses a painless electrical current to determine the amount of fat mass and fat-free mass within the body.

Glossary of Terms

Bioenergetics: Study of the transformation of energy in living organisms.

Biological age: Subjective age based of an individual's development.

Body composition: method (e.g., circumference measurements, skinfolds) used to estimate a person's percent body fat.

Body mass index (BMI): A weight-to-height ratio, calculated by dividing weight in kilograms by the square of height in meters, which is used as an indicator of obesity and underweight.

Bone density: Refers to the amount of bone mineral in bone tissue.

Bronchi: Either of the two main branches of the trachea leading into the lungs where they divide into smaller branches (bronchioles).

Bronchioles: Tiny branch of air tubes within the lungs that connect the bronchi to the alveoli (air sacs).

Caloric balance: States the calories consumed through diet equals the calories expended through physical activity.

Caloric density: Refers to the calorie content of food. Examples of calorie dense (in contrast to nutrient dense) foods include potato chips, desserts, and candy.

Caloric expenditure: Refers to the number of calories expended during physical activity or exercise.

Capillary: Any of the minute blood vessels that form networks throughout the tissues and used to carry oxygen, nutrients, and waste products between the blood and tissues.

Carbohydrate: One of the three essential macronutrients, along with fats and protein, used as an energy source by the body. Carbohydrates come in simple forms such as sugars and in complex forms such as starches and fiber. The body breaks down most sugars and starches into glucose, which the body uses to fuel the cells. Complex carbohydrates are derived from plants.

Catabolism: Breakdown of complex molecules from simpler ones.

Catecholamines: Class of aromatic amines (organic compound derived from ammonia) that includes neurotransmitters such as epinephrine and dopamine.

Carbonic anhydrase: An enzyme that catalyzes the decomposition of carbonic acid into carbon dioxide and water, facilitating transfer of carbon dioxide from tissues to blood and from blood to alveolar air.

Cardiac Output: The amount of blood the heart pumps through the circulatory system in a minute. Stroke volume and the heart rate determine cardiac output.

Cardiovascular fitness: The ability of the heart and lungs to efficiently deliver oxygenated blood to the working muscles as well as the muscle's ability to extract and use the oxygen being provided.

Cartilaginous joints: Joint covered with cartilage to allow movement between bones.

Celiac disease: A disease in which the small intestine is hypersensitive to gluten thereby leading to issues with digestion.

Chains: Are a method of strength training for advanced lifters in which chains are added to the bar thereby making the lockout portion of the lift more difficult.

Circuit training: A form of conditioning or resistance training that incorporates both strength building and muscular endurance. A "circuit" is one completion of all prescribed exercises in the program.

Circumference measurements (aka girth measurements): A method used to assess body composition that involves taking measurements at various sites in order to predict percent body fat.

Cholesterol: Cholesterol is a waxy, fat-like substance found in all cells of the body. The body needs some cholesterol to make hormones, vitamin D, and substances that help in digestion. The body can manufacture all the cholesterol it needs; however, cholesterol can also be found in food (animal products). High levels of cholesterol in the blood can increase the risk of heart disease.

Chronic sleep deprivation: Refers to the condition of getting insufficient sleep or experiencing sleeplessness over an extended period of time.

Chronological age: Number of years that an individual has lived.

Circadian biological clock: Refers to the 24-hour cycle regulating the timing of certain biological processes like eating, sleeping, and temperature.

Closed kinetic chain (CKC): Exercises where the hand (for arm movement) or foot (for leg movement) are fixed, cannot move, and remains in constant contact with an immobile surface, usually the ground or base of a machine (e.g., leg press).

Cluster sets: Sets that incorporate intra-set rest periods that allow for better manipulation of volume and intensity.

Collagen: Main structural protein found in connective tissue.

Complete protein: A protein food source that contains each of the nine essential amino acids. Examples of food sources with complete proteins are red meat, poultry, fish, eggs, milk, cheese, yogurt, and quinoa.

Compound exercise (aka core exercise): A movement that recruits one or more major muscle groups (e.g., pectoralis major, latissimus dorsi, quadriceps) and involves two or more joints.

Complex carbohydrates: Excess glucose linked together for storage.

Compound set: A compound set involves sequentially performing two different exercises for the same muscle group.

Glossary of Terms

Concentric contraction: A type of muscle activation that increases tension on a muscle as it shortens.

Conditional amino acids: Are considered conditionally essential because their synthesis can be limited under special pathophysiological conditions. The six conditional amino acids are arginine, cysteine, glycine, glutamine, proline, and tyrosine.

Conjugate method: A specific type of non-linear periodization developed by powerlifter and strength coach Louie Simmons.

Cool-down: Easy exercise completed immediately after more intense activity to allow the body to gradually transition to a resting or near-resting state.

Compression force (aka compressive force): A force that presses inward on a segment of the spine that causes it to become compacted.

Cortisol: A glucocorticoid produced by the adrenal cortex that mediates various metabolic processes, had anti-inflammatory and immosuppressive properties.

Creatine kinase: An enzyme that when elevated in the blood is a marker of damaged tissue in either the brain, skeletal muscle, or heart.

Creatine phosphate (CP): A phosphate group found in muscle cells that stores phosphates to provide energy for muscular contraction.

Crepitus: Any grinding, creaking, cracking, grating, crunching, or popping sound that occurs when moving a joint.

Criterion standards: Use normative data that ranks individuals against an established standard (e.g., pass/fail cut-off score).

Cytokine: Substances secreted by immune system cells that have an effect on other cells within the body.

Deload: A short planned period of recovery. A typical deload period will last a week.

Depression: Feelings of severe despondency and dejection.

Detraining: Physiological adaptations associated with chronic exercise are not permanent. Once the stimulus is reduced or eliminated, the biological system(s) will revert back to pre-training levels.

Dietary supplements: A dietary supplement is a product taken to supplement the diet and typically contain one or more of the following ingredients: vitamins, minerals, herbs or other botanicals (of or pertaining to plants), amino acids, as well as various other substances. Supplements are not required to go through the testing of effectiveness and safety that drugs do.

Diffusion: The passive movement of molecules (e.g., oxygen, carbon dioxide) along a concentration gradient traveling from regions of higher to regions of lower concentration.

Directed adaptation: A fundamental principle to exercise programming that states that in order to get better at something, you must train it over and over.

Disaccharide: Two monosaccharides linked together.

Distal attachment: Being situated far from the point of attachment to the body.

Distress: Refers to bad or negative stress.

Drive theory: This theory states that the more arousal and anxiety an individual experiences, the higher their performance will be.

Dual energy x-ray absorptiometry (DEXA): A method of estimating percent body fat that uses two x-ray beams of different energy levels to determine fat mass, lean mass, and muscle mass.

Duration: Amount of time spent exercising within a specific training session.

Dynamic effort method: One of the three methods of strength training used by powerlifters to develop muscular contraction speed.

Dyspnea: Difficult or labored breathing.

Eccentric contraction: A type of muscle activation that increases tension on a muscle as it lengthens.

Eccentric training: A method of strength training for advanced lifters in which more weight Is added to the bar than can be lifted concentrically.

Ectomorph: A person with a lean and delicate body build.

Elasticity: Ability of connective tissue to return to its original length after a passive stretch.

Electrolytes: Electrolytes are minerals found in the body fluids. They include sodium, potassium, magnesium, and chloride. When you are dehydrated, your body does not have enough fluid and electrolytes.

Electron transport chain (ETC): A series of complexes that transfer electrons from electron donors to electron acceptors and couples with the transfer of protons across a membrane.

Endergonic reaction: A reaction that requires energy to be driven.

Endomorph: A person with a round body build and high proportion of body fat.

Epinephrine: A hormone secreted by the adrenal glands, especially in conditions of stress, increasing rates of blood circulation, breathing, and carbohydrate metabolism and preparing muscles for exertion.

Ergogenic aid: Any method or product used to enhance mental and physical performance or recovery.

Glossary of Terms

Essential amino acids (aka indispensable amino acids): Amino acids that must be consumed in the diet because the body cannot make them.

Eustress: Refers to good or positive stress.

Excess post-exercise oxygen consumption (EPOC): A measurably increased rate of oxygen intake following strenuous activity intended to erase the body's "oxygen deficit".

Exercise activity thermogenesis: Refers to the energy expended during exercise. This does not include the energy expended while performing normal daily tasks (e.g., working, studying, walking to class).

Exercise economy: Relates to the quantity of oxygen (ml/kg/min) required to move at a given speed or generate a specific amount of power and influenced by a number of factors including: neuro-muscular co-ordination, percentage of type I muscle fibers, elastic energy storage, and joint stability and flexibility.

Exercise energy expenditure: Amount of energy expended during physical activity (e.g., endurance training, strength training).

Exergonic reaction: A reaction that loses energy as a result of the reaction.

Exhaustion stage: Final stage of the stress response. After an extended period of stress, the body has depleted all of its energy resources by continually trying, but failing, to recover from the initial alarm reaction stage.

Fat cell theory: A theory that states obesity is caused by having too many fat cells.

Fad diet: A diet that promises quick weight loss through unhealthy and unbalanced dietary means.

Fartlek training: Swedish for "speed play", is a form of endurance training that combines long slow distance (LSD) with interval training.

Fast glycolysis: Method of providing energy for activities of short duration (i.e., 10-30 seconds), that replenishes very quickly and produces 2 ATP molecules per glucose molecule.

Fast-twitch muscle fiber: A type of muscle fiber that is composed of strong, rapidly contracting fibers, adapted for high-intensity, low-endurance activities.

Fiber type transition: Refers to the change in fiber sub-type classification as a result of aerobic and/or anaerobic conditioning.

Fat: Along with carbohydrates and protein, fat is one of the three major sources of energy in the diet. Fat contains 9 calories per gram, which is more than twice that provided by carbohydrates or protein (4 calories per gram). Due to its high caloric content, a high intake of fat increases the risk for obesity. Fat is used to help insulate the body as well aid in the absorption of certain vitamins.

Fat-soluble vitamins: A *vitamin* that can dissolve in *fats* and oils. The *Fat-soluble vitamins* are *vitamins* A, D, E, and K.

Fatigue management: After several weeks of hard training, recovery becomes incomplete as fatigue accumulates over time thereby requiring an intentional decrease in training volume and/or intensity.

Fatty acids: Fatty acids are a major component of fats and are used by the body for energy and tissue development.

Feasibility: Practicality of a test in terms of cost, man-power, equipment, and space.

Fiber: Fiber is a carbohydrate substance found in plants. Fiber helps you feel full faster and stay full longer – which can help in terms of weight control. Fiber also aids in digestion and helps prevent constipation.

Fiber type transition: Adaptation of specific muscle fibers (typically the intermediate muscle fibers) to become more aerobic or anaerobic in nature as a result of training.

Fibrosis: Process in which fibrous connective tissue starts to replace degenerating muscle fibers.

Fibrous joints: Form of articulation in which bones are connected by a fibrous tissue. Fibrous joints have no joint cavity and movement is minimal or nonexistent.

Field test: A test used to assess ability that is performed away from the laboratory and does not require extensive training or expensive equipment to administer.

Fight-or-flight response: The instinctive physiological response to a threatening situation, which readies one either to resist forcibly or to run away.

Fitness test: A series of exercises designed to assess fitness (e.g., endurance, strength, agility, etc.).

Fitness trident: Depicts the three most important components of fitness and foundation of any strength and conditioning program. Specifically: strength, endurance, and mobility.

Flavin adenine dinucleotide (FADH): One of two redox cofactors created during the Krebs cycle that is used during the electron transport chain to produce energy (ATP).

Flexibility: Range of motion of the joints or the ability of the joints to move freely through their entire range of motion.

Food composition: Describes what other nutrition is obtained along with the macronutrient and how the food is digested and utilized by the body.

Frequency: Number of times one exercises within a specified period of time.

General physical preparedness: Refers to any training method used to improve general conditioning such as strength, power, endurance, speed and flexibility.

Glossary of Terms

Genetic potential: Theoretical optimum performance capability which an individual could achieve in a specific activity, after an ideal upbringing, nutrition and training.

Glandular disorder theory: A theory that states obesity is caused by hypothyroidism.

Gluconeogenesis: Formation of glucose from precursors other than carbohydrates (e.g., amino acids, glycerol from fats, or lactate produced by muscle during anaerobic glycolysis).

Gluten: Gluten (derived from the Latin word glue) is a mixture of proteins found in wheat, rye, and barley which gives elasticity to dough, helping it rise, and gives the final product a chewing texture. It can also be found in products such as vitamin and nutrient supplements, lip balms, and certain medicines. It is important to note that less than 1% of the general population has Celiac disease (autoimmune disorder of the small intestines) which would require a gluten-free diet.

Glycemic index: Instead of counting the total amount of carbohydrates in foods in their unconsumed state, Glycemic Index (GI) measures the actual impact of these foods on blood sugar. Foods are ranked as being very low, low, medium, or high in their GI value. Low-GI diets have been associated with decreased risk of cardiovascular disease, type 2 diabetes, metabolic syndrome, stroke, depression, chronic kidney disease, formation of gall stones, neural tube defects, formation of uterine fibroids, and cancers of the breast, colon, prostate, and pancreas.

Glycemic load: Takes into account the number of grams of carbohydrate in a food to determine how quickly the food raises blood glucose levels. It can be calculated by multiplying the glycemic index of the food by the grams of carbohydrate in a serving of that food, divided by 100.

Glycogen: Storage form of carbohydrates in skeletal muscles and the liver.

Glycolysis: process in cell metabolism by which carbohydrates and sugars, especially glucose, are broken down to produce ATP and pyruvic acid.

Golgi tendon organ: Proprioceptive sensory receptor organ that senses changes in muscle tension.

Gynoid: Pear-shaped fat distribution pattern mainly around the lower upper body, such as the hips, thighs, and butt.

Half-life: Time taken for the radioactivity of a specified isotope to fall to half of its original value.

Heme: Non-protein part of hemoglobin found in animal products.

Hemoglobin: The oxygen-carrying pigment and predominate protein found in red blood cells.

Henneman's size principle: Under load, motor units are recruited from smallest to largest.

Herniated disk: A rupture of the annulus fibrosis (fibrocartilagenous material that surrounds the intervertebral disk) enabling the nucleus pulposus (gelatinous substance in the center portion of the intervertebral disk) to extrude through the fibers.

Hierarchy of fat loss: States the four major factors in determining fat loss are (in order of precedence): nutrition, sleep & stress, resistance training, and hormonal balance.

High-intensity interval training: A form of endurance training that uses high-intensity intervals (typically 30-90 seconds in duration) at intensities greater than VO_2max.

High-intensity resistance training: A method of strength training used for fat loss in which a number of exercises are performed in succession without rest.

High-tension exercises: Exercises in which one tenses a specific muscle then moves that muscle against tension as if simulating that a heavy weight was being lifted.

Hyperthyroidism: Condition of overactivity of the thyroid gland resulting in a rapid heartbeat and increased metabolism.

Hypertrophy: a method of strength training intended to induce muscle growth.

Hypoxia training: a type of training that uses a specially designed mask or device to reduce the amount of oxygen being taken in by the lungs and/or being delivered to the working muscles. In theory, doing so allows the body to become more efficient at consuming, delivering, and utilizing oxygen.

Incomplete protein: Is a protein food source that does not contain all nine of the essential amino acids. Examples of incomplete proteins include beans, specific nuts and tofu.

Incontinence: Lack of voluntary control over urination or defecation.

Individual zones of optimal functioning (IZOF): This theory takes into account that people have different levels of anxiety and arousal that are unique in making them perform at their best. Some people perform their best with low anxiety, some with a medium amount and others with a high amount. The amount of anxiety/arousal that an individual requires to perform their best is based on individual characteristics.

Individuality: Genetics plays a major role in how fast and to what degree one will respond to a particular training program.

Inferior attachment: Being situated closer to or towards the feet.

Injury analysis: Part of the needs analysis that evaluates common sites for joint and muscle injuries as well as causative factors.

Insomnia: Refers to habitual sleeplessness or the inability to sleep.

Intensity: Amount of effort or work that must be invested into a specific training session.

Intermediate muscle fiber (aka fast oxidative-glycolytic fibers): Are fast twitch muscle fibers that have been converted via endurance training. These fibers are slightly larger in diameter, have more mitochondria, greater blood supply, and more fatigue resistance than typical fast twitch fibers.

Glossary of Terms

Intermittent fasting: Specific dietary strategy that requires an intentional abstention from food, drink, or both, for a period of time for the primary purpose of losing weight.

Interval training: A form of endurance training that involves high-intensity intervals (typically 3-5 minutes in duration) close to VO$_2$max.

Inverted-U theory: This theory suggests there is a medium amount of arousal and anxiety that causes an individual to perform better. Too little arousal and anxiety or too much arousal and anxiety will result in decreased performance.

Ischemia: Inadequate blood supply to an organ (especially the heart) or part of the body.

Isokinetic contraction: Muscular contraction that occurs at a constant speed. A piece of equipment called an Isokinetic Dynamometer is used to measure the (constant) speed of isokinetic muscle contraction.

Isometric contraction: A type of strength training in which the joint angle and muscle length do not change during contraction (as compared to isotonic contractions).

Insoluble fiber: A type of fiber that does not dissolve in water. Insoluble fiber in found in wheat bran, vegetables and whole grains.

Isotonic contraction: Muscular contraction against resistance in which the length of the muscle changes. Isotonic movements are either concentric or eccentric.

Jet lag: Refers to the extreme tiredness and other physical effects felt by a person after a long flight across several time zones.

Joint: Point of articulation between two or more bones.

Ketoacidosis: A life-threatening condition resulting from dangerously high levels of ketones in the blood.

Ketones: Organic compound containing a carbonyl group bonded to two hydrocarbon groups formed when fats (instead of carbohydrates) are broken down for energy.

Lactate: Byproduct of glucose utilization by muscle cells during anaerobic glycolysis.

Lactate threshold: The intensity of exercise at which lactate begins to accumulate in the blood at a faster rate than it can be removed.

Linear periodization: Traditional model with gradual progressive increases in intensity over time.

Load: Amount of weight assigned to an exercise set.

Long slow distance (LSD) training: A form of continuous training performed at a constant pace of low to moderate intensity over an extended distance or duration.

Low intensity steady state (LISS): Any form cardio- and aerobic-based activity that's performed at a low intensity but for a prolonged period of time (typically 30-60 minutes).

Macronutrient: Type of food (e.g., fat, protein, carbohydrate) required in large amounts in the human diet.

Magnetic resonance imaging: A procedure that uses magnetism, radio waves, and a computer to create pictures from inside the body.

Major minerals: Minerals your body needs in relatively large (or major) quantities. Major minerals include sodium, potassium, chloride, calcium, phosphorus, magnesium and sulfur.

Maximal effort method: One of the three methods of strength training used by powerlifters to develop muscular strength.

Maximal lactate steady state (MLSS): Highest blood lactate concentration and work load that can be maintained over time without a continual blood lactate accumulation.

Maximum heart rate: The maximum number of beats made by the heart in 1-minute during physical exertion.

Meal planning made easy (MPME): A dietary strategy that implements MyPlate guidance in terms of daily caloric intake and recommended number of servings of fruits, vegetables, grains, protein and dairy.

Mesomorph: A person with a compact and muscular build.

Metabolism: Metabolism is the total processes (both anabolic and catabolic) used by the body to get or make energy from food.

Metabolic equivalent (MET): A MET also is defined as oxygen uptake in ml/kg/min with one MET equal to the oxygen cost of sitting quietly, equivalent to 3.5 ml/kg/min.

Metabolic resistance training: A method of strength training used for fat loss that incorporates super-setting certain core lifts (e.g., bench + bent-over row) and finishes with a drop sets of another core lift (e.g., deadlift).

Micronutrient: Type of food (e.g., vitamins, minerals) required in trace amounts in the human diet.

Minerals: Consist of inorganic elements found in foods that are essential to certain metabolic functions. Examples include sodium, potassium, chloride, calcium, phosphate, sulfate, magnesium, iron, copper, zinc, manganese, iodine, selenium, and molybdenum.

Mobility: Degree to which a joint is allowed to move before being restricted by surrounding tissue.

Moderate-intensity aerobic activity: Physical activity performed hard enough to raise heart rate and break a sweat, but easy enough to still be able to talk, but not sing.

Monosaccharide: Single sugar unit, such as glucose.

Glossary of Terms

Monounsaturated fat: Type of fat found in avocados, canola oil, nuts, olives and olive oil, and seeds. Monounsaturated fats (aka "healthy fats") are thought to help lower cholesterol and reduce heart disease risk. However, monounsaturated fat has the same number of calories as other types of fat and may contribute to weight gain if eaten in excess.

Motor neuron: A nerve cell (neuron) whose cell body is located in the spinal cord and whose fiber (axon) projects outward from the spinal cord to innervate and control muscle cells.

Motor unit: Physiological unit comprised of a motor neuron and the skeletal muscle fibers innervated by that motor neuron's axonal terminals.

Movement analysis: Part of the needs analysis that evaluates body and limb movement and muscular involvement of the sport.

Muscle fiber type: Skeletal muscle fibers can be categorized into two types: slow-twitch (Type I) and fast-twitch (Type II). Type I fibers are better suited for long duration, low-intensity activities such long distance running; whereas type II fibers are be suited for short duration, high-intensity activities such as resistance training and sprinting.

Muscle spindle: A sensory organ located within the muscle that is sensitive to the stretch of the muscle.

Myofibril: Long, cylindrical organelle in striated muscle cells, composed mainly of actin and myosin filaments, that run the entire length of the cell.

Myofibrillar hypertrophy: One of the two methods of muscle hypertrophy in which the number of actin and myosin contractile proteins increase in number.

Myoglobin: An iron-containing protein found in muscle fibers that combines with oxygen released by red blood cells and transfers it to the mitochondria of muscle cells to produce energy.

Myosin: Globulin that combines with actin to form actomyosin (protein complex in muscle fibers that shortens when stimulated and causes muscle contractions).

Myosin heavy chain (MHC): Portion of the myosin filament responsible for muscle contraction. There are three types of MHC (i.e., type I, IIa, IIx), each with a different contractile speed. MHC IIx has the fastest contractile speed (and is called fast-twitch), whereas MHC I has the slowest (and is called slow-twitch).

MyPlate: Is the current nutrition guide published by the U.S. Department of Agriculture that depicts a place setting consisting of a plate and glass divided into five food groups (e.g., fruits, vegetables, grains, protein, dairy). MyPlate replaced MyPyramid in 2011.

Near-infrared interactance (NIR): A method of estimating percent body fat that uses near infrared light to differentiate between fat mass and fat-free mass within the body.

Needs analysis: A two-stage process in developing a strength and conditioning program to include an evaluation of the sport and an assessment of the athlete.

Neuromuscular junction: A chemical synapse (junction) formed by the contact between the presynaptic terminal of a motor neuron and the postsynaptic membrane of a muscle fiber.

Nicotinamide adenine dinucleotide (NADH): One of two redox cofactors created during the Krebs cycle that is used during the electron transport chain to produce energy (ATP).

Nonessential amino acids: An amino acid that can be made by humans thus is not essential to the human diet. There are 11 nonessential amino acids: alanine, arginine, asparagine, aspartic acid, cysteine, glutamic acid, glutamine, glycine, proline, serine, and tyrosine.

Non-exercise activity thermogenesis (NEAT): Energy expended from anything other than sleeping, eating or exercise.

Non-linear periodization: Refers to a type of periodization that varies the different training phases by adjusting exercise selection, volume, and intensity.

Norepinephrine: A hormone that is released by the adrenal medulla and sympathetic nerves that functions as a neurotransmitter.

Nutrient density: Refers to food choices based off the nutrients they provide (e.g., vitamins, minerals, fiber). Examples of nutrient dense foods include milk, vegetables, protein foods, and grains.

Nutrient timing: Is the application of knowing what and when to eat before, during and after exercise.

Nutrition facts label: Lists nutrients supplied and is based on a daily diet of 2,000 kilocalories (kcal). The label was mandated by the 1990 Nutrition Labeling and Education Act (NEA).

Obesity: A condition of being grossly overweight or fat. Equates to a body mass index (BMI) rating of 30.0 or higher.

Objectivity: Degree to which a test is free from individual bias.

Omega-3 fatty acids: Unsaturated fatty acid, mainly found in fish oils, that have three double bonds within the hydrocarbon chain.

Omege-6 fatty acids: Family of pro-inflammatory and anti-inflammatory polyunsaturated fatty acids that have a final carbon-carbon double bond in the sixth bond (counting from the methyl end).

Olympic lifting: Type of strength (power) training in which athletes attempt to lift near maximum loads that are mounted on barbells.

Operational relevance: Refers to the degree to which a test represents a specific job task or set of skills.

Osteoporosis: A medical condition in which the bones become brittle and fragile from loss of bone tissue.

Glossary of Terms

Overload: Greater than normal stress (load) is required in order for training adaptations to occur. These adaptations lead to increased athletic performance in terms of speed, strength, power, endurance, etc.

Overtraining: The point where a person displays a decrease in performance and/or plateauing as a result of consistently performing at a level or training load that exceeds their recovery capacity.

Oxidation: Reaction that occurs when oxygen combines with molecules in food to produce energy, water, and carbon dioxide.

Oxidative system: One of the 3 basic energy systems used to produce ATP. This system converts carbohydrates and fats into ATP, requires the presence of oxygen to function and takes place in the mitochondria of the cell.

Oxygen debt: Period of time after high intensity exercise when the demand for oxygen is greater than the supply.

Oxygen deficit: Difference between the oxygen required and what is actually taken in during about of high intensity exercise.

Pace/tempo training: A form of endurance training that uses intensities at or slightly higher than race pace intensity.

Partials: A method of strength training for advanced lifters in which the range of motion of a particular exercise is limited in order to lift heavier loads.

Peak height velocity (PHV): Period of adolescent maturation where the maximum rate of growth occurs.

Peak weight velocity (PWV): Period of adolescent maturation associated with a rapid increase in body weight due to significant increases in the amount of muscle and bone mass.

Peaking: The traditional approach to periodization divides training into various periods to include preparation, competition, and transition periods. As the competition draws closer, training becomes more specific and intense. This buildup to in training intensity prior to competition is referred to as "peaking".

Percent body fat: Is a measurement of body composition telling how much of your body weight is comprised of fat.

Perimysium: Thin layer of connective tissue that surrounds each individual muscle fiber.

Periodization: A form of strength training that uses a strategic implementation of training phases (e.g., hypertrophy, strength, power). These phases periodically increase and decrease both volume and intensity in order to prevent overtraining and maximize gains.

Phase potentiation: Logical stringing together of dedicated strength training phases in order to get the best long-term gains in performance.

Phasic muscles: Extensor muscles that tend to get weaker with age.

Physical activity level factors: Refers to an individual's total energy expenditure over a 24-hour period and is categorized by the amount and intensity of daily exercise performed (e.g., sedentary, lightly active, moderately active, very active, super active).

Physiological analysis: Part of the needs analysis that evaluates the strength, power, size, and muscular endurance priorities of the sport.

Pilates: A system of exercises using a special apparatus intended to improve physical strength, flexibility, and posture, and enhance mental awareness.

Piriformis syndrome: An uncommon neuromuscular disorder caused when the piriformis muscle compresses the sciatic nerve.

Plasticity: Ability of connective tissue to assume a new or greater length after a passive stretch.

Plyometrics (aka jump training): A form of conditioning in which muscles exert maximum force in short intervals of time with the goal of increasing muscular power.

Phosphagen system: Fastest method to resynthesize ATP used for all-out exercise lasting up to about 10 seconds. However, since there is a limited amount of stored CP and ATP in the muscle, fatigue occurs rapidly.

Phytochemical: biologically active compounds found in plants.

Polysaccharide: Several monosaccharides linked together.

Polyunsaturated fat: Type of fat that is liquid at room temperature. There are two types of polyunsaturated fatty acids (PUFAs): omega-6 and omega-3. Omega-6 fatty acids are found in liquid vegetable oils, such as corn oil, safflower oil, and soybean oil. Omega-3 fatty acids come from plant sources such as canola oil, flaxseed, soybean oil, walnuts as well as from fish and shellfish.

Positive energy balance: Occurs when caloric intake exceeds caloric expenditure.

Positive nitrogen balance (PNB): Occurs when the intake of nitrogen into the body is greater than the loss of nitrogen from the body resulting in an increase in the total body pool of protein. PNB is associated with periods of growth, hypothyroidism, tissue repair, and pregnancy.

Post-activation potentiation: A theory that purports that the contractile history of a muscle influences the mechanical performance of subsequent muscle contractions.

Power exercises: Specific strength training exercises that are performed quickly or explosively (e.g., power cleans, snatch).

Prebiotics: Plant fibers that feed the healthy bacteria already in the gut to promote further healthy bacterial growth.

Glossary of Terms

Pre-exhaustion: Reverse exercise arrangement where the athlete purposely fatigues a large muscle group as a result of performance of a single-joint exercise prior to a multi-joint exercise involving the same muscle.

Prehab: Series of exercises and activities that if performed regularly will help to improve athletic performance and reduce the risk of injury.

Pre-stretch: To extend a limb or body part to its full length or range of motion.

Probiotics: Live microorganisms thought to increase the healthy bacteria in the gut, thereby reducing GI issues, and respiratory illness.

Progressive overload: Periodic increases in training variables (e.g., load, intensity, duration, frequency) in order for improvements to continue over time.

Progressive overload: Gradual increase in volume, intensity, frequency or time in order to prevent training plateaus and achieve the targeted goal.

Protein: An essential macronutrient, along with carbohydrates and fat, the body needs for good health. Proteins are made up of essential and nonessential amino acids. The body manufactures 13 nonessential amino acids, which aren't available from food.

Proteolysis: Breakdown of proteins or peptides into amino acids by enzymes.

Proximal attachment: Being situated close to the point of attachment to the body.

Pyruvate: The end product of glycolysis, which is converted into acetyl coA and enters the Krebs cycle when sufficient oxygen is available.

Qigong: A Chinese system of physical exercises and breathing control similar to tai chi.

Range of motion (ROM): Measurement of movement around a specific joint or body part.

Rate of perceived exertion (RPE): A method of measuring physical activity intensity level based off how hard you feel like your body is working.

Recovery: Time required between exercise sessions to allow the body to repair and replenish depends on the type and intensity of the exercise performed.

Referred pain: Pain that is felt in a part of the body other than its actual source.

Reliability: Degree of consistency or repeatability of a test.

Repetition (rep): A complete motion of a particular exercise or movement pattern.

Repetition method (aka submaximal or repeated method): One of the three methods used by powerlifters to develop muscular size.

Residual volume: Volume of air remaining in the lungs after maximal expiration.

Resistance stage: Refers to the second stage of the stress response in which the body has increased capacity to respond to the stressor. However, due to high energetic costs, the body cannot maintain high levels of resistance indefinitely. If the stressor persists, the body advances to exhaustion phase.

Rest-pause: A method that involves stopping during the completion of a set, resting for a short period and then continuing on with the set.

Resting metabolic rate (RMR): Energy expended to maintain life. RMR makes up 70-75% of our total daily energy expenditure

Reversibility: The principle of reversibility states that the physiological adaptations associated with training are lost when training is stopped; however, detraining effects can be reversed when training is resumed.

Sarcomere: Fundamental unit of muscle structure, comprised of actin and myosin filaments, responsible for muscle contraction.

Sarcopenia: Age related loss of skeletal muscle mass and strength.

Sarcoplasm: The colorless material comprising the living cell, excluding the nucleus.

Sarcoplasmic hypertrophy: One of the two methods of muscle hypertrophy in which there is an increase in the volume of sarcoplasmic fluid in the muscle cell, with no actual increase in muscular strength.

Satiety: Feeling of being full.

Saturated fat: Type of fat that is solid at room temperature. Saturated fat is found in full-fat dairy products (e.g., butter, cheese, cream, ice cream, and whole milk), coconut oil, lard, palm oil, ready-to-eat meats, and the skin and fat of chicken and turkey, among other foods. Saturated fats have the same number of calories as other types of fat, and may contribute to weight gain if eaten in excess.

Self-induced stressors: A type of stress resulting from uncontrolled thinking or mismanagement of things in a person's control.

Serotonin: A neurotransmitter involved in sleep, depression, memory, and other neurological processes.

Set: A group of repetitions sequentially per-formed before the athlete stops to rest.

Set point theory: A theory that states obesity is caused by internal programming that causes the body to carry a certain amount of weight. This programming is set and determined by the hypothalamus.

Shear force: A *force* acting in a direction parallel to the surface of a segment of the spine.

Skinfolds: A method of body composition that uses the thickness of skin at various sites in order to predict percent body fat.

Glossary of Terms

Sleep deprivation: Condition that occurs when an individual gets less sleep than they need to feel awake and alert.

Sleep hygiene: Habits and practices that are conducive to sleeping well on a regular basis.

Sleep-wake homeostasis: An internal biological system responsible for regulating the balance between sleep and wakefulness.

Sliding-filament theory: Actin (thin) filaments of muscle fibers slide past the myosin (thick) filaments during muscle contraction.

Slow glycolysis: Method of providing energy for activities of relatively short duration (i.e., 2-3 minutes), that replenishes quickly and produces 2 ATP molecules per glucose molecule.

Slow-twitch muscle fiber: A type of muscle fiber that develops less tension more slowly than a fast-twitch fiber but is more fatigue resistant due to its high oxygen content and enzyme activity.

Soluble fiber: A type of fiber that dissolves in water. Soluble fiber is found in oat bran, barley, nuts, seeds, beans, lentils, peas, and some fruits and vegetables.

Specific physical preparedness (aka sports-specific physical preparedness): Refers to training specific to movements in a specified activity, usually a sport.

Specificity: Training should be relevant to the activity the individual is training for in order to produce the desired training effect.

Spinal stenosis: An abnormal narrowing of the spinal canal, which may occur in any of the regions of the spine, resulting in a neurological deficit. Symptoms include pain, numbness, loss of motor control, and paraesthesia (tingling or pricking sensation caused by pressure on or damage to peripheral nerves).

Stability: Ability to maintain or control joint movement or position.

Stabilizer muscle: A muscle that contracts with no significant movement to maintain posture or fixate a joint.

Starch: Storage form of carbohydrates in plants.

Stimulus-recovery-adaptation (SRA): Physiological adaptations take place during recovery, not training. As a result, frequency recommendations for each of the different types of exercise types should be based off the amount of time required to recover.

Strength training (aka resistance training): Type of physical exercise specializing in the use of resistance in order to improve the strength, anaerobic endurance, and size of skeletal muscle.

Stretch reflex: A muscle contraction in response to stretching which provides automatic regulation of skeletal muscle length.

Stretch-shortening cycle (SSC): An active stretch (eccentric contraction) of a muscle followed by an immediate shortening (concentric contraction) of that same muscle.

Stress: Is a feeling of emotional strain and pressure.

Stress management: Is a wide spectrum of techniques aimed at controlling a person's level of *stress*, especially chronic *stress*, usually for the purpose of improving everyday functioning.

Stress response: Refers to the physiological and psychological *responses* to various situations.

Stressor: Something that causes a state of strain or tension.

Stroke volume: Amount of blood ejected from the left ventricle in one contraction.

Structural exercises: Exercises that load the spine directly or indirectly.

Subcutaneous fat: Fat stored below the dermis layer of the skin and is not necessarily hazardous to your health.

Subjectivity: Degree to which a test is influenced by individual bias.

Super set: A superset involves two sequentially performed exercises that stress two opposing muscles or muscle areas (i.e., an agonist and its antagonist).

Superior attachment: Being situated closer to or towards the head of the body.

Supplement facts label: Lists the names and quantities of dietary ingredients present in the product, **the serving size and the servings per container.**

Sympathetic nervous system: A part of the nervous system that serves to accelerate the heart rate, constrict blood vessels, and raise blood pressure.

Synergist muscle: A muscle that assists another muscle to accomplish a movement.

Synovial joints: Joint that has fibrous capsule surrounding the articulating surfaces of adjoining bones and is filled with synovial fluid.

Tai chi: An ancient Chinese form of exercise that was originally created as a fighting art. The words Tai Chi Chuan loosely translate to mean supreme ultimate exercise or skill.

Talk test: A simple way to measure exercise intensity. In general, during moderate-intensity activity you can talk, but not sing. During vigorous-intensity activity, you will not be able to say more than a few words without pausing for a breath.

Tapering: Practice of reducing exercise volume (40-50%), while maintaining exercise intensity, in the days just prior to competition to ensure adequate recovery.

Target muscle: The primary muscle intended to train or exercise.

Tempo: Refers to the pace or rhythm at which a movement is performed.

Glossary of Terms

Tend-and-befriend response: Is an instinctive behavior exhibited by some individuals, generally females, in response to threat. It refers to protection of offspring (tending) and seeking out their social group for mutual defense (befriending).

Thermic effect of food (TEF): Calories burned to digest food and accounts for roughly 10% of the total calories burned in a day.

Time under tension (TUT): Refers to how long the muscle is under strain during a set.

Tonic muscles: Flexor muscles and tend to get tighter with age.

Torsion force: A force that causes twisting of the spine as a result of one segment turning about a longitudinal axis while the other is held fast or turned in the opposite direction.

Trace minerals: Essential *minerals* that the human body must get from food, but unlike major *minerals*, they are only needed in very small amounts.

Trachea: A large membranous tube reinforced by rings of cartilage that extends from the larynx to the bronchial tubes and conveys air to and from the lungs.

Traction exercise: Refers to an exercise in which the range of motion unloads the spine by expanding the space between the intervertebral disks.

Traditional resistance training: A type of strength training that uses a prescribed number of sets and reps per exercise in order to accomplish a specific goal (e.g., endurance, hypertrophy (size), strength, power).

Training age: Number of years that an individual has spent training and participating in various sports.

Trans fat: Type of fat that is created when liquid oils are changed into solid fats, like shortening and some margarines. This is done to make food last longer without going bad. Trans fat are found in crackers, cookies, and snack foods. Trans fat are believed to raise LDL (bad) cholesterol and lower HDL (good) cholesterol.

Treadmill tempo run: New type of pace / tempo training aimed at targeting a desired run time for a specific race distance (e.g., 1-0-mile).

Triglycerides: Triglycerides are a type of fat found in the blood. High levels of triglycerides may increase the risk of coronary artery heart disease, especially in women.

Troponin: Globular protein complex involved in muscle contraction and occurs with tropomyosin in the thin filaments of muscle tissue.

Tropomyosin: Protein involved in muscle contraction that is related to myosin and occurs together with troponin in the thin filaments of muscle tissue.

Tryptophan: An essential amino acid and precursor of serotonin.

Underwater weighing (aka hydrostatic weighing): A method that uses the displacement of water in order to determine body volume and calculate percent body fat.

Undulating (non-linear) periodization: An alternative method that involves large fluctuations in load and volume assignments.

Valgus: Form deficiency caused by the oblique displacement of a limb away from the midline of the body.

Validity: Degree to which a test measures what it is supposed to measure, and is the most important characteristic of testing.

Valsalva maneuver: Particular method of breathing and bracing that increases intra-abdominal pressure (IAP) thereby providing additional support to the spine.

Variation: Periodic rotation of exercises in order to prevent training plateaus and/or overtraining.

Varus: Form deficiency caused by the oblique displacement of a limb towards the midline of the body.

Vegan: A person who does not eat or use animal products.

Vegetarian: A person who does not eat meat, and sometimes other animal products.

Vein: A large diameter blood vessel that carries blood low in oxygen content from the body back to the heart.

Venous return: Rate of blood flow back to the heart.

Ventricle: Either of the two lower chambers of the heart that receive blood from the atria and in turn push it into the arteries.

Venule: A small diameter blood vessel that connects the capillaries to the veins.

Vigorous-intensity aerobic activity: Physical activity performed at a high level of effort, resulting in a substantially higher heart rate and rapid breathing.

Visceral fat: Unseen fat stored around your organs and is linked to several metabolic disorders and diseases.

Vitamins: Various organic substances, either found in food or produced by the body, that are essential in minute quantities and act as coenzymes/precursors of coenzymes in the regulation of certain metabolic processes. Vitamins do not provide energy or serve as building units.

VO_2max: Maximum amount of oxygen that an individual can utilize during intense or maximal exercise. It is measured as milliliters of oxygen used in one minute per kilogram of body weight (ml/kg/min).

Volume: The total amount of weight lifted in a training session.

Glossary of Terms

Waist circumference: Measurement taken around the abdomen at the level of the umbilicus used as a screen for certain weight-related health risks.

Waist-to-hip ratio (WHR): An indicator of health risk that is calculated by dividing the waist measurement by the hip measurement.

Warm-up: Gradual increase in exercise intensity intended to prepare the body for the more intense and demanding activity to follow.

Water-soluble vitamins: Vitamins that can dissolve in water but are not stored in the body. Water-soluble vitamins include vitamin C and members of the vitamin B complex.

Weight management: Is the process of adopting long-term lifestyle modification in order to achieve and maintain a healthy bodyweight.

Work:rest ratio: Is the comparison between how much time spent exercising to the amount of time spent resting.

Yoga: A Hindu spiritual and ascetic discipline that includes breath control, simple meditation, and the adoption of specific bodily postures used for health and relaxation.